Phage Therapy: Current Research and Applications

Phage Therapy: Current Research and Applications

Editor: Tara Simon

hayle medical

New York

Hayle Medical,
750 Third Avenue, 9th Floor,
New York, NY 10017, USA

Visit us on the World Wide Web at:
www.haylemedical.com

ISBN 978-1-64647-574-2 (Hardback)

Cataloging-in-Publication Data

Phage therapy : current research and applications / edited by Tara Simon.
p. cm.
Includes bibliographical references and index.
ISBN 978-1-64647-574-2
1. Bacteriophages--Therapeutic use. 2. Bacteriophages. 3. Diagnostic bacteriology.
4. Medical bacteriology. 5. Antibacterial agents. 6. Drug resistance in microorganisms.
I. Simon, Tara.
QR342 .P433 2023
579.26--dc23

Contents

Preface

Over the recent decade, advancements and applications have progressed exponentially. This has led to the increased interest in this field and projects are being conducted to enhance knowledge. The main objective of this book is to present some of the critical challenges and provide insights into possible solutions. This book will answer the varied questions that arise in the field and also provide an increased scope for furthering studies.

Phage therapy refers to the therapeutic usage of bacteriophages to treat and manage pathogenic bacterial infections. Bacteriophages are a type of virus, which attaches to the bacterial cells and injects their genome in the cells. The viral genome replaces the bacterial genome and stops the bacterial infection from spreading. The bacterial cell responsible for causing the infection is not able to reproduce and new phages are generated as a result. Phages are selective towards those bacterial strains against which they are effective. They are commonly bacterium-specific, which makes it important to get a swab and culture it before initiating a treatment. Phages can also be applied topically or orally on the infected wounds, can be spread on the surface or can be utilized while surgical procedures are underway. This book provides significant information to help develop a good understanding of phage therapy. It presents researches and studies performed by experts across the globe. The extensive content of this book provides the readers with a thorough understanding of the subject.

I hope that this book, with its visionary approach, will be a valuable addition and will promote interest among readers. Each of the authors has provided their extraordinary competence in their specific fields by providing different perspectives as they come from diverse nations and regions. I thank them for their contributions.

Editor

1

Promises and Pitfalls of In Vivo Evolution to Improve Phage Therapy

James J. Bull [1,*], Bruce R. Levin [2] and Ian J. Molineux [3]

1 Department of Biological Sciences, University of Idaho, Moscow, ID 83844, USA
2 Department of Biology, Emory University, Atlanta, GA 30307, USA; blevin@emory.edu
3 Department of Molecular Biosciences, University of Texas, Austin, TX 78712, USA; molineux@austin.utexas.edu
* Correspondence: bull@utexas.edu

Abstract: Phage therapy is the use of bacterial viruses (phages) to treat bacterial infections, a medical intervention long abandoned in the West but now experiencing a revival. Currently, therapeutic phages are often chosen based on limited criteria, sometimes merely an ability to plate on the pathogenic bacterium. Better treatment might result from an informed choice of phages. Here we consider whether phages used to treat the bacterial infection in a patient may specifically evolve to improve treatment on that patient or benefit subsequent patients. With mathematical and computational models, we explore in vivo evolution for four phage properties expected to influence therapeutic success: generalized phage growth, phage decay rate, excreted enzymes to degrade protective bacterial layers, and growth on resistant bacteria. Within-host phage evolution is strongly aligned with treatment success for phage decay rate but only partially aligned for phage growth rate and growth on resistant bacteria. Excreted enzymes are mostly not selected for treatment success. Even when evolution and treatment success are aligned, evolution may not be rapid enough to keep pace with bacterial evolution for maximum benefit. An informed use of phages is invariably superior to naive reliance on within-host evolution.

Keywords: mathematical model; evolutionary prediction; dynamics; cocktail; within-host

---

1. Introduction

Driven by well-warranted concerns about the growing numbers of infections with antibiotic resistant pathogens, there has been a resurrection of interest in, research on, and even patient trials with a therapy that predates antibiotics by more than fifteen years: bacteriophages [1–4]. Fueling this enterprise, which is now becoming increasingly commercialized (see above references), are well-publicized successes of a handful of compassionate uses of phage to treat chronic, recalcitrant bacterial infections. Patients who were on their way to succumbing to or remaining infected with antibiotic resistant, *Acinetobacter baumannii*, *Mycobacterium abscessus*, or *Pseudomonas aeruginosa* survived and in some cases were cleared of the infecting bacteria following treatment with phages [5–8]. The role of phages in these successes is not always clear, as these treatments were necessarily uncontrolled and involved single patients. Also not apparent is whether other (and how many) compassionate use trials fail. Indeed, recent clinical trials of phage therapy that did involve controls have often been failures (e.g., [9–11]).

Could the difference between success and failure in these therapeutic efforts be simply a matter of phage suitability for treatment—that some phages are better that others? There are certainly properties that a priori seem to be ideal candidates for therapy and that might guide choices of phages (Table 1). Against this possibility, host range was the sole criterion for phages used in some patient successes, suggesting that treatment outcomes might be indifferent to phage choice. Yet, some experimental work indicates that phage characteristics can influence success ([12,13], and see below). Furthermore, given that therapeutic success with patients often required weeks to months and multiple administrations of phages, it is entirely plausible that a wise choice of phages could vastly improve the progress of treatment, even when the long term outcome is the same for arbitrarily-chosen phages.

If phage characteristics matter to treatment success, might there be a shortcut to identifying the best phages? Motivated by the highly visible field of directed evolution of biological molecules [14], it is tempting to consider a directed evolution parallel for phage therapy: can phages evolve themselves to improve treatment? There is even an historical precedent for a similar approach: in his earliest phage therapy experiments, D'Herelle [15] used phages isolated from patients to treat other patients. The idea also has intrinsic appeal: one of the oft-cited benefits of phages over antibiotics is that, by amplifying within the host, they can evolve and perhaps keep abreast of any bacterial resistance evolution. Within-host evolution might then obviate the need to design treatments wisely, instead letting evolution rather than engineers identify good treatment practices. However intrinsically worthy that idea might seem, it is not a simple one to evaluate from first principles: processes of phage dynamics and evolution can be highly unintuitive, and their effects on treatment adds a second layer of complexity. To avoid reliance on intuition, we approach the problem of within-host phage evolution using mathematical and computational models.

Here we evaluate the premise that, during the course of therapy, selection favors phages and phage combinations that are specifically effective at killing the bacteria causing an infection. Use of the phage 'effluent' from one patient to treat another assumes that the infections in different patients will be suitably similar, and thus possibly of limited utility. Even if not, however, the study of phage evolution from convalescent patients might at least help identify principles that apply to other infections. Given that therapeutic use of phages in humans is so limited at present (at least in the U.S. and much of Europe), initial research on within-host evolution will likely need to use non-human animals and identify principles that could be applied to humans. Indeed, widespread adoption of the One Health perspective, coupled with the problem of drug resistant infections in non-human animals and the need to limit antibiotic use in those settings [16], provides many reasons to develop phage therapy for animals—with the added benefit of helping formulate practices that would work on humans as well. Although established animal infections may prove at least as useful as human infections in discovering principles that work well for treatment, experimental infections may need to be chosen carefully to avoid artefacts.

Table 1. Phage properties ideal for therapy.

Characteristic	How Beneficial
Broad host range	can be applied rapidly, with minimal testing of pathogen sensitivity
Good in vivo growth and persistence	single dosing sufficient for treatment
Bacterial resistance difficult	single phage type sufficient for treatment
Synergistic with antibiotics *	can be used in combination with standard treatment
Disrupts bacterial extracellular protections	makes vulnerable bacterial clusters (e.g., biofilms and aggregates) that are otherwise recalcitrant to treatment

* synergy means that phages and antibiotics work better together than expected from their independent effects.

1.1. *A Precedent for the Need to Choose Phages Wisely*

One critical understanding in the development of good phage therapy practices is the extent to which different phages matter to treatment success—beyond the obvious one of whether the phages can grow on the infecting bacterium. If a phage's ability to plate on a bacterium is all that matters, phage therapy might unfold with nearly the same generality as did antibiotic use. Conversely, if phage characteristics greatly affect outcomes, success may hinge on careful choice of the best phages—unless within-host evolution is self-correcting. Even when different phages are each capable of effecting long term recovery, they might differ in speed of recovery, cost of recovery, and morbidity.

A 1982 study suggested that phage choice can have a profound effect. Using an experimental mouse infection with a K1-capsulated bacterium, Smith and Huggins [12] discovered that lytic phages isolated from the wild fell into two classes regarding treatment success. With simultaneous infection and treatment, one class of phages provided almost 100% recovery, the other closer to 30%. The underlying basis of the difference was that the 'good' phages required the bacterial capsule for infection, the 'poor' phages did not. The work set a precedent in demonstrating that phage therapy could work in vivo and in exploring the dynamic basis of success (although it is less often noted that treatment success fell off dramatically with an 8 hr delay in treatment [12], the cells rapidly becoming recalcitrant to treatment [17]). The work Smith and Huggins [12] was especially important in revealing that differences among phages could profoundly affect treatment success. It thus follows that, if we can identify or even generate good phages, better treatment should follow.

1.2. Phage Properties Subject to Selection in Patients

Smith and Huggins [12] sets the stage for our study, but the emphasis here is one step beyond: to what extent can in vivo evolution and cocktail competition be used to improve treatment or at least identify the best phages? It is obvious from the Smith and Huggins experiment that the 'poor' phages were not themselves evolving fast enough in vivo to achieve the high success rates of the good phages, or the rescue rates would not have differed between the phages. But we may instead ask about the effect of within-host phage competition: if both types of phages were injected together into the mouse, would the 'better' phage come to dominate the phage population? One can do a formal within-host competition experiment to answer the question for these phages (e.g., [18]), but we seek principles that will allow us to predict the outcome more broadly.

At a general level, predicting the outcome of phage competition requires understanding how the entire suite of characteristics for each phage affects its growth and killing of bacteria—i.e., the phage as a whole. It is also possible to consider the evolution of individual phage characteristics that we expect to influence treatment success: (a) phage decay rates [19], (b) enzymatic digestion of a protective bacterial extracellular matrix [20,21], and (c) ability to block bacterial resistance evolution [4]. Considering the phage as a whole might seem to make the most sense, but it may be a single characteristic that determines treatment success, as with the Smith and Huggins [12] example.

A technical note is that we apply the concept of within-host 'evolution' in both a narrow sense and a broad one. The narrow sense is the standard Darwinian process of natural selection: mutations arise and ascend based on their merits, eventually resulting in most of the phage population carrying the mutations, all during the interval of treatment. Our broad-sense use is a competition of different phage types within cocktails: the different phage types increase or decrease as a proportion of the total within-host phage pool, their relative fitnesses depending on their intrinsic properties. (For an overview of issues with cocktail pharmacology, see [22]). Both processes will occur in any host treated with a cocktail. The main differences between evolution in the narrow sense versus cocktail dynamics are: (i) with cocktail dynamics, the phages may differ in several characteristics that affect their competition with other phages in the mix, so the selective advantage of one trait may be overwhelmed by other differences, and (ii) because cocktails start with high levels of variation, cocktail dynamics will typically be much faster than Darwinian dynamics. However, reliance on cocktail dynamics to inform and improve treatment can only be applied when different phages are available, but this may not always be the case.

A second application for in vivo phage evolution is engineered phages—genetically modified to improve treatment [7,21,23]. Engineering may inadvertently introduce imperfections due to imbalanced gene expression or incompatibilities between wild-type proteins and the engineered protein. Within-host evolution offers a simple means to correct imperfections without even needing to diagnose the causes.

The focus here is two-fold. First, does within-host phage evolution work in favor of treatment? Second, can it work fast enough within one patient to plausibly augment that patient's outcome? Regardless of the second answer, if within-host dynamics and evolution at least work in favor of treatment, then we might collect phage from a treated patient to use in treating subsequent patients—D'Herelle's method. Any understanding of these processes is most accurately studied in vivo, but in vitro work and modeling is often all that is available or even practical. In any case, modeling is often necessary to interpret the in vivo work. New results provided here are limited to modeling, using a mix of mathematical models and computater simulations. Some processes can be analyzed as simple optimization problems, but others must be embedded in non-linear dynamics that involve interactions and feedbacks. Even the simplest evolutionary problems require quantitation to appreciate the impact on treatment success. Treatment outcomes may be qualitative (infection clearance or not), but the difference between controlling an infection versus bacterial escape may rest on minor quantitative differences, thus requiring a models framework.

2. Methods: Models

2.1. The Standard Model and Anomalies from Phage Therapy Results

For over half a century, the standard models of phage-bacterial dynamics assumed mass action—full mixing—with homogeneity of bacterial and phage states [24–26]. Mass action was depicted mathematically as the product kPB to represent all infections, with B as bacterial density, P as phage density, and k as an adsorption rate constant. With kPB as the loss to the bacterial population, an important consequence of mass action is that bacteria cannot persist in high densities of phage, hence the bacterial population crashes to miniscule (decimal) levels. This model was appropriate for bacterial growth in flasks or chemostats, which was the experimental norm and allowed for easy parameter estimation. The tight coupling between models and experiments and the ease of analysis afforded by this model resulted in most of our current understanding about phages being based on a mass action perspective. The typical outcome is that phages quickly amplify and profoundly depress high densities of sensitive bacteria. From this framework, the attraction of using phages to control bacterial populations is easily understood: a single application of even a small number of phages can virtually wipe out the bacterial population in hours, leaving only a handful of survivors for the immune system to clear.

Full mixing is a poor approximation to phage dynamics in bacterial biofilms and other structured environments. Indeed, in early laboratory experiments, sensitive bacteria were discovered to have found refuge from phage predation in the walls of chemostats. Aggregates, abscesses, and other highly structured populations are now also recognized as important features of bacterial infections [2,27,28]. Furthermore, recent successes with phages in treating individual patients has revealed that some key mass action outcomes are violated (reviewed in [2,4]). First, success in clearing or even suppressing an infection with phages is gradual and sometimes requires months—violating the principle that phages quickly outnumber and kill their sensitive prey. Second, single infusions of phages are often not sufficient: multiple infusions of high doses of phages are required. Both outcomes are difficult to reconcile with the standard model, and although there could be varied causes, spatial structure of bacterial populations (and the associated bacterial inhomogeneity in susceptibility to phages) is one obvious and empirically-justified alternative to consider.

2.2. A Dynamics Model to Accommodate Spatial Structure

The observations from successful therapies pose a dilemma: high densities of genetically sensitive bacteria persist in the presence of phage. This behavior is a clear violation of the law of mass action. Resolution of this anomaly would seem to require that much of the bacterial population is protected from attack, whether by a polysaccharide matrix, ionic gradients, low receptor expression, or even by some property of the animal host. Taking as inspiration the high-resolution imaging study of Darch et al. [29] on *Pseudomonas* in a structured environment, we model the bacterial population as consisting of a mix of individual cells (density B) and multi-cellular aggregates density (B_A). The individual cells are fully sensitive to phage attack and obey standard mass action dynamics (and for convenience will be referred to as 'planktonic'), whereas aggregates are protected from phage attack. However, aggregates convert into planktonic cells and vice versa, so the protection is not permanent; this switching of states accommodates the observation that aggregate numbers are somewhat reduced by phage attack but much less so than isolated cells [29]. Our formulation constitutes a refuge model (also true of [27] but we present a more explicit refuge).

Equations and parameters are given in Appendix A. For the model of a single bacterial strain (Appendix A.1), the main change from the standard model is to protect aggregates from phages and to allow bacteria to move between planktonic and aggregate states (some of B move to B_A and vice versa). Mass action applies to phage-bacterial interactions in the planktonic population, as they are fully sensitive. For the model that incorporates both sensitive and resistant bacteria (Appendix A.2), each bacterial strain is modeled as switching between an individual state (planktonic) and aggregates, but all states of the resistant strain are protected against phage infection.

Numerical trials of the equations were run in Mathematica 12.0.0.0, which was used to generate the figures. Mathematica files are uploaded as supplements, but the equations used in those files are given in Appendix A and can be numerically solved with other software.

3. Results

3.1. Growth on a Single Bacterium

A basic question is how phage evolution works to suppress bacterial numbers. For example, can phage evolution ever allow bacterial density to increase? From a therapeutic perspective, we suppose that decreasing bacterial numbers improves treatment success. In the simplest system—well mixed with a single, sensitive bacterial state—the answer from modeling efforts is straightforward: bacterial evolution may lead to higher bacterial densities, but phage evolution does not. At dynamical equilibrium, one phage type will prevail, the phage that most depresses bacterial density [26]. Dynamic equilibrium is not necessarily applicable to therapeutic success, but a similar theoretical result applies to phages invading a bacterial population: the phage with fastest growth will prevail while bacteria are abundant, which means that selection is for the fastest growth and killing [30]. These results apply equally to phage evolution in the narrow sense and to dynamics of different cocktail phages within the therapeutic regime.

A simple use of this principle in a cocktail setting would be 'phage sorting'—separating poorly-growing phages from those that grow well. In vitro growth—easily determined in advance of treatment—may poorly reflect in vivo growth [13], so the appropriate environment is within the patient. Adding a cocktail of phages to an infected patient and then sampling hours or days later should easily determine which phages grow (and survive) at least moderately well in the host. Sorting could be used in a highly quantitative manner, but such refinement is not advisable, as considered below. Phage sorting overlaps with D'Herelle's approach of isolating therapeutic phages from convalescing patients, the difference being that here, the phages are being administered to the patient and then collected later. D'Herelle's method recovered phages that the patient acquired naturally.

Within-host evolution is especially relevant to genetically engineered phages. On a uniform population of bacteria, selection will be for better growth. Any growth impairment caused by the engineering will be selected for improvement, which could result in loss of the engineering—if the engineering introduced a gene that is non-essential, for example [23]. This problem occurs when the engineering enhances treatment success in ways that are not aligned with phage growth (such examples are presented in subsequent sections).

The simple nature of phage selection and evolution changes when multiple bacterial states exist—bacterial heterogeneity. We assume initially that all states are sensitive to the phage and merely differ in phage-infection properties—burst size, adsorption rate, or lysis time. Different bacterial states could be driven by environmental or physiological heterogeneity, as might be represented by planktonic versus aggregate/biofilm/abscess cells, growth on different substrates, or variation in surface molecules, e.g., capsules or O antigens affecting adsorption. These kinds of heterogeneity would develop prior to phage administration and typically have a non-genetic or 'phenotypic' basis. (Genetic bacterial resistance evolution is addressed in a different section.)

Well-mixed systems with heterogeneous cell states present several unintuitive outcomes that violate a direct link between phage evolution and treatment success. Notably, selection can favor phages to avoid some types of hosts, even when the phage can productively infect those hosts [30,31]. In essence, the phage evolves to specialize on the most productive bacterial states. However, we conjecture that the types of phenotypic variation most relevant to infections will be spatially structured, such as planktonic cells dominating liquid tissues, and biofilms, aggregates or abscesses in solid tissues. With spatial structure, different phage types or mutants will differentially amplify in patches of cells where they grow best. In these settings, phage evolution and competition should often work loosely in favor of treatment, at least on a local level, but dynamical complexities allow for exceptions.

With phage cocktails or in vivo evolution of phage mutants, the composition of actively growing phages exuded from patients will typically change over time as bacterial densities are suppressed at different rates in different locations. The cumulative phage composition should mirror the phages with the biggest numerical effect on bacterial killing at the time. However, one dilemma faced in phage collection from the patient is that the relative abundance of different phages in the collection need not match phage importance to reduction of the patient's symptoms. If the bacteria responsible for morbidity or maintenance of the infection are confined to small or semi-protected bacterial populations, or slowly growing ones, the patient's phage output may be dominated by phages that kill large numbers of bacteria in other tissues that contribute only slightly to virulence. Phage evolution itself will be driven by growth on the larger, rapidly growing populations of bacteria in the host. As a consequence of these varied processes and possibilities, there is no predicted time to harvest phages from one patient that would ensure maximum benefit for use on subsequent patients.

Conclusions. Intrinsic processes of phage evolution work unambiguously in favor of bacterial killing when bacteria exist in a single, well-mixed state. When multiple bacterial phenotypic states exist and are well mixed, phage evolution and cocktail competition can give rise to unintuitive outcomes whereby phages are selected even to avoid some bacteria. Spatial structure of bacterial states, as with biofilms (aggregates or abscesses) versus planktonic cells, may align phage evolution with suppressing bacterial numbers locally, but these processes are not easy to study and are not well understood in vivo. Importantly, global phage growth rate need not be closely aligned with treatment success in a heterogeneous infection.

Although encouraging, these results do little more than suggest an expected, qualitative direction of evolution regarding treatment. They offer nothing on the speed or magnitude of infection clearance. Nor do we have any sense of how much within-host evolution to expect, given a potentially short duration of treatment. Deeper insight to the uses of in vivo evolution to improve treatment comes by addressing specific phage characteristics, next.

3.2. Phage Decay Rates

Using two well-characterized tailed phages (λ and P22), Merril et al. [19] (i) showed that the initial or 'wildtype' isolate of each phage was rapidly cleared from mice (in the absence of bacteria), and (ii) evolved mutants of each that were cleared more slowly (a clearance rate approximately 20% of the initial). The study further showed that the long-persisting phages were advantageous in prophylactic therapy—administered in advance of the infection—presumably from their ability to persist up to the

time of bacterial introduction. The interval in which phage decay was measured was short, less than a day after inoculation, too fast for adaptive immunity to develop in the naive mice. The suggestion was that phage clearance was due to the reticuloendothelial system.

These results raise two questions. (i) Is the benefit of long-persisting phages large enough to affect treatment outcomes? If phages amplify during treatment, phage differences in survival might have little benefit, except when phage amplification is weak. (ii) Will long-persisting phages evolve during treatment and evolve quickly enough that there is little to be gained by starting treatment with long-persisting phages? Phage clearance rate is not something easily predicted or measured outside of the patient, so if clearance rate is important to treatment success, it is a property that might be improved only via within-host evolution.

Of the phage characteristics analyzed in this paper, this one experiences the simplest evolutionary process: each phage type and mutant evolves independently of other phages, and the selection does not involve frequency- or density-dependence. Simple calculations can be informative as a first step. Let phage survival follow exponential decay, $\mathrm{e}^{-\mathrm{w}t}$ for the 'wildtype' and $\mathrm{e}^{-\mathrm{m}t}$ for the mutant ($m < w$, with t in minutes). If the mutant starts at frequency p_0, the ratio of the mutant to wildtype will change in time according to $R(t)$:

$$R(t) \;=\; \frac{p_0}{1-p_0}\left(\frac{\mathrm{e}^{-\mathrm{m}}}{\mathrm{e}^{-\mathrm{w}}}\right)^{t} \quad . \tag{1}$$

$R(t)$ increases without bound over time, but only as long as both phage types are abundant enough to approximate deterministic dynamics.

The time at which the mutant comprises half the phage population is approximately

$$t \;\approx\; \frac{-\ln(p_0)}{w-m} \quad . \tag{2}$$

For new mutations, the numerator will typically lie in the range of 10 to 20. Although this calculation ignores phage amplification (which should have little impact on relative phage abundances in the absence of other differences between the phages), this formula shows that the time for an initially rare mutant to dominate the phage population depends on the reciprocal of the log of its relative advantage $[(w-m)^{-1}]$. Given that both rates must be positive (and $w > m$), the magnitude of $w - m$ cannot exceed w. A wild-type phage with a very low clearance rate ($w << 1$), cannot be quickly displaced even for a mutant that is never cleared ($m = 0$). Evolution works fastest the more important the change, but of course, if w is small, there is little benefit from further reductions.

Are clearance rates of wild phages high enough to evolve during an infection? Calculations from the results in Merril et al. [19] and Westwater et al. [32] gave wildtype clearance rates on the order of $2-6\times10^{-3}$ (see calculations in [33]). A five-fold improvement (say from 5×10^{-3} to 1×10^{-3}) and $p_0 = 10^{-6}$ requires just over 2 days for the mutant to comprise half the population. This may be a long time to wait for any treatment benefit afforded by the mutant. Furthermore, if the phage population was declining (e.g., unable to maintain itself), the phages might be too rare after 2 days to observe any improvement in treatment from mutant ascendance.

When phages are used prophylactically, it is obvious that any benefit of reduced clearance must be achieved by evolving the phage before administration. The goal of prophylaxis is to maintain the phages as long as possible in a non-growing state in anticipation of a possible bacterial infection. The drawback of starting with a pure rapidly-decaying phage cannot be overcome by phage evolution when the phage are not growing. However, the situation changes if phages are administered to an infection, because now a slow-decaying phage may arise by mutation and could in principle take over the within-host population rapidly. If this process was rapid, one could rely on within-host evolution to improve treatment of that patient. To address this possibility, we rely on a numerical model (Figure 1). As described in our Methods section, this model attempts to capture more realistic dynamics than is typical of the standard 'mass action' model of phage-bacterial dynamics. This new model assumes both a sensitive bacterial population and a 'refuge' population of bacteria protected from infection, leading to reduced oscillations and (sometimes) a need to serially inoculate repeated doses of phage to keep bacterial numbers low. With this model (Figure 1), it is seen that (i) decay rate matters to rapid bacterial suppression (compare panels (B) and (D)), and (ii) early in treatment, evolution is not as effective as is dosing with the pure, slowly-decaying phage (compare (C) and (D) at time 5000).

The decay rate of engineered phages may also be improved by within-host evolution. Given the inherent problem that an engineered phage may be predisposed to evolve reversal of the engineering, one ideal aspect of in vivo evolution of decay rate is that it can be done in the absence of phage growth. Thus, if the engineering does not affect virion proteins, selection for reduced decay can be done in the absence of selecting properties affecting phage replication. In contrast, even if the phage is not growing, in vivo selection for reduced decay may directly select against engineering that does alter the virion surface, as with phage display (e.g., [34]).

Conclusions. If the wildtype phage has a suitably high in vivo decay rate, evolving the phage to a lower decay rate can offer a significant improvement in treatment. Evolution of phages in the within-host environment seems to be the only means at present of obtaining slow-decay phages, and it thus presents a compelling case for the use of within-host evolution to improve treatment. However, there is no assurance that the outcome of within-host evolution will be of significant benefit in a different host. With this caveat, evolving slow decay in advance of treatment is the only solution to improve phage prophylaxis, but evolution in advance may also offer a significant improvement over relying on evolution during treatment.

The treatment benefit of decay-rate evolution depends on the wildtype decay rate and the magnitude of improvement afforded by available mutations. Relying on within-host evolution during treatment to achieve dominance by a slow-decaying phage becomes feasible only when the treatment phages actively grow and maintain themselves in the host for days. Phages recovered from a patient, as in D'Herelle's approach, may well have evolved lower decay rates that could be used with subsequent patients.

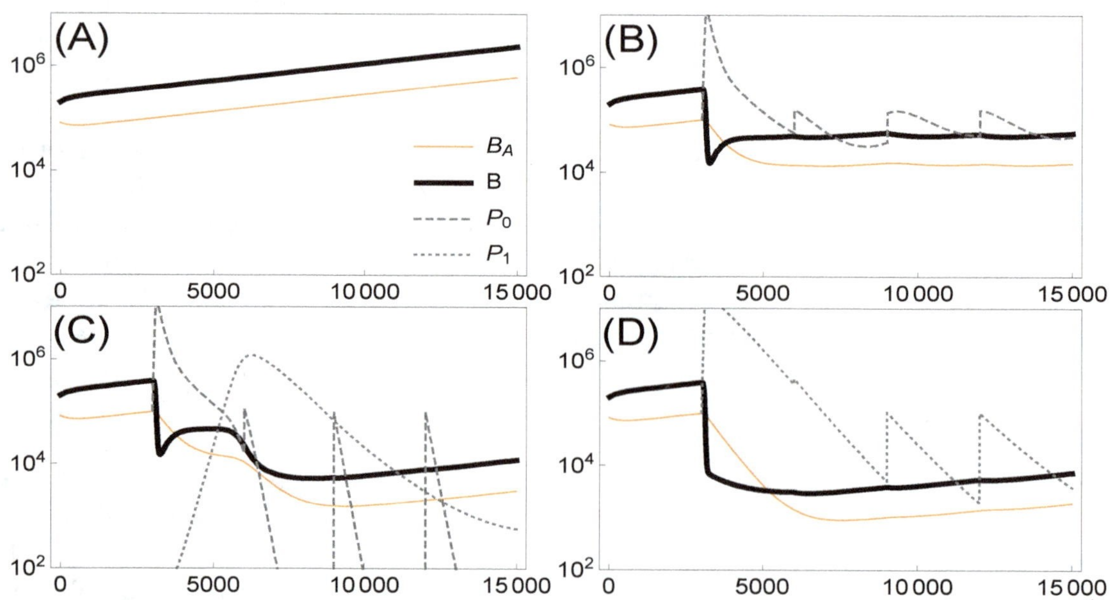

Figure 1. Phage dynamics and evolution as a property of phage decay rate. The vertical axis gives density, the horizontal axis time (minutes). Thin orange curves are protected bacteria in refuges, thick blue curves are susceptible, planktonic bacteria. Dashed grey indicates the fast-decaying phage (P_0, decay rate of 0.008 per min), dotted grey indicates the better, slow-decaying phage (P_1, decay rate of 0.002 per min). The inset key (A) applies to all panels. All trials use the same bacterial growth parameters and initial bacterial densities (given in Appendix A.1). When phage are present, they are first added at 3000 min and added every 3000 min thereafter. (**A**) Bacterial densities slowly increase in

the absence of phages. (**B**) Treatment with 10^5 rapidly-decaying phages causes a sudden decline in free bacterial densities, a somewhat slower decline in aggregate bacteria. The system is approaching equilibrium in that phage and bacterial densities are being approximately maintained between inoculations. (**C**) The phage inoculum consists of 10^5 rapidly-decaying phage and 0.1 slowly-decaying phage, the latter value to represent mutation. The slowly-decaying phage ascends profoundly but then drops when bacterial densities are too low to sustain it. (**D**) The phage inoculum consists of just 10^5 slowly-decaying phage. There is a substantial difference between the treatments with a pure fast-decaying phage or a pure slow-decaying phage. The main effect of starting with a slow-decay phage (D) instead of relying on within-host evolution (C) lies in the early dynamics, although a modest lingering benefit is apparent. Parameter values and initial conditions are given in Appendix A.1. Outcomes vary with parameter values, and the actual effect of within-host evolution or treatment with pre-evolved, slowly decaying phages would need to be evaluated for each specific application.

3.3. Matrix Degrading Activities: Depolymerases

Some phages encode enzymes (depolymerases and lysins) that may have important direct or indirect antibacterial activities. Depolymerases (the focus here) degrade bacterial secretions and may foster bacterial killing and clearance [20,21,35–39]. Thus those enzymes have the interesting property that they do not kill per se but enable killing by other agents. It is now known that the superior phage type discovered by Smith and Huggins [12] differs from the poor phage type by encoding a depolymerase that degrades the bacterial capsule [40]. The free enzyme is likely critical to treatment success—the pure depolymerase can successfully treat an infection even in the absence of phage [41–45]. Protective bacterial secretions include more than just bacterial capsules, such as the chemically complex matrices in biofilms and aggregates [21,29,38,46–48]. Phage-encoded enzymes do not necessarily exist for all bacterial matrix components, but enzyme-encoding genes from other sources (bacteria, fungi) can be engineered into and expressed from phages to achieve degradation (e.g., [21,49,50]).

In wild phages, depolymerases are assembled as tailspikes used in the initial, specific recognition of the host. The enzymes allow the virion to penetrate the protective surface layers of the bacterium and thus provide a direct benefit to the individual phage much as does any phage-encoded contribution to infection. But depolymerases also provide a dispersed benefit for treatment: considerable free enzyme, that not assembled onto virions before cell lysis, is released and can diffuse into the surrounding environment where it acts separately from the phage. The effect of the diffusing enzyme can often be observed on plates as an expanding halo beyond the plaque [46,51–53].

Interest here is primarily in the dispersed benefit of phage-encoded enzymes—a benefit beyond the phage killing itself. Free enzyme augments other forms of bacterial killing by degrading the protective layers around many bacteria. Loss of those layers exposes the bacteria to attack by complement, immune cells, drugs, and even by other types of phages that would not otherwise be able to access the bacteria. From a treatment perspective, free enzyme is ideal because it augments treatment by multiple antibacterial agents and immunity. Furthermore, genetic engineering greatly expands the capacity of phages to degrade substrates that do not directly aid infection [21]. If this property of a phage or cocktail can be evolved and maintained, it has the potential to greatly augment treatment.

Evolution of a dispersed effect from an enzyme is not straightforward. Released enzyme diffuses into the local environment and acts as a 'public good' that can benefit phages which do not produce the enzyme. By benefiting others, the producer phage is subjected to a 'tragedy of the commons' that works against its success in competition with non-producing mutants and phage types [23,53]. The 'tragedy' can be especially acute for phages engineered to encode depolymerases, as those enzymes are usually encoded entirely as free enzymes and not part of the virion [21]: evolution can quickly dispense with the engineered gene because it is not essential and even benefits mutants lacking the gene [23]. In contrast, enzymes encoded as tailspikes are genetically (evolutionarily) stable because they are essential to infection; even in this case, the excess enzyme can work against the producer phage by benefiting other phages in a cocktail. Maintenance of an enzyme-producing phage in cocktails thus has little to do with its public-good benefit in clearing the infection, and such phages can be lost even if bacterial clearance depends on their presence [53]. Evolution and dynamics can work in favor of enzyme-producing phages when the bacterial environment is spatially structured, where the free enzyme does not diffuse far to help other phages [23], but there is as yet no evidence on whether appropriate spatial structure applies to natural infections. Exogenous addition of enzyme is a possible alternative to relying on phage-carried enzymes [44,45,54] should within-host evolution prove inimical to maintaining phages encoding the enzyme.

Conclusions. Although the dispersed benefits of enzyme-producing phages can greatly enhance clearance of structured bacterial populations, within-host evolution and competition among phages are not aligned with maintaining enzymes for that reason. Within-host phage competition will not typically improve the collective enzyme-degrading activities of the input phages. Retaining the treatment benefit from engineered depolymerases requires that the engineered phages be specifically designed to avoid evolutionary loss of the enzyme. Cocktails should be administered with an a priori understanding of dynamics that may work against them.

3.4. Phage Evolution to Overcome Bacterial Resistance

The most-studied evolutionary process involving phages is their impact on and response to bacterial resistance evolution. The problem has long been considered from the perspective of genetic and molecular mechanisms, both from the perspective of bacterial defenses and phage escape [24,55–62]. The process has also been studied as phenotypic outcomes of phage-bacterial arms races in co-culture, both in conditions of natural or semi-natural dynamics [63–68] as well as highly contrived conditions in which vast numbers of phage were amplified on a permissive host and forced to grow on resistant hosts [55–58]. Our interest here is in observations from (semi-)natural dynamics.

Although many types of bacterial defenses against phages are known, many of them are irrelevant to within-host evolution during treatment. Anti-phage defenses will affect the initial choice of phages for treatment; phages that fail, for whatever reason, to grow on the pathogen at hand will not usually be further studied. Bacterial mutation in surface element genes affecting phage adsorption appears to be the most commonly-observed evolutionary response to phages, and most other bacterial defense systems will not evolve to block phage growth in the patient. For example, restriction–modification (R-M) systems—a well known mechanism blocking phage infections [69–72]—will not evolve within the patient to change specifically in response to phages. However, CRISPR loci, if present in the infecting bacterium, may evolve in vivo to block phage infection. The degree to which this process operates is under active investigation [62,73–76], but CRISPR is notably absent from at least some multidrug-resistant pathogens [73,77,78], and it is too early to tell if it will prove an important evolutionary escape in vivo.

The ascent of resistant bacteria within the patient will typically be inimical to treatment success and should be avoided. Furthermore, there remains the formal possibility that a phage-resistant bacterium will have increased virulence, perhaps by becoming mucoid and thus less sensitive to immune system components; reports of such outcomes so far seem to be lacking. Experimental work indicates that evolution of bacterial resistance is a seemingly ubiquitous and easy response to a high abundance of phages. From in vitro co-culture studies of phages grown on single bacterial strains in simple media, a common outcome of arms race evolution is ultimate dominance by resistant bacteria [64]. The arms race may involve a few steps of phages evolving to overcome bacterial resistance and new bacterial resistance evolving, but ultimately a bacterial resistance evolves that cannot be overcome by phage evolution; phage are subsequently lost or their abundance greatly suppressed. This simple story is often violated when bacteria are grown under more complex in vitro environments or in natural ones: resistant bacteria may fail to ascend, with the phage persisting and permanently suppressing the bacteria [79,80]. However, other outcomes have also been observed [65,66,68]. The hope is for in vivo outcomes that avoid bacterial resistance, but in fact, resistant bacteria have been observed to ascend within patients [61,81]). So the hope then turns to learning how to choose phages to direct the outcome toward blocking bacterial resistance evolution.

3.4.1. Intrinsic Phage Evolution to Overcome Bacterial Resistance Is Not Assured

Bacteria are selected to avoid killing by phages. Likewise, phages are selected to overcome bacterial resistance, both in vivo and in vitro. Nonetheless, reliance on de novo mutation and Darwinian evolution to overcome bacterial resistance faces two problems. First, the requisite mutations may not arise—the jump to utilize a new bacterial receptor may require an improbable combination of multiple mutations in the phage genome. (If a CRISPR-based immunity evolves within the host, there may be no way for a phage to overcome it). Second, the population dynamics work against evolution because of a mismatch between selection and phage population size (opportunity for mutation): selection is strongest when the resistant bacterial population is largest, but the phage population may already have plummeted from a declining number of sensitive hosts. These dynamics commonly lead experimentalists to evolve new phage host ranges by allowing amplification on permissive hosts between bouts of selection on resistant hosts (e.g., [55,56]).

3.4.2. Cocktails Can Be Designed to Block Stepwise Bacterial Escape, but They Can Experience Lags and Phage Loss

Natural phage evolution is not the only solution to bacterial resistance. One alternative is to isolate wild phages that grow on the resistant hosts, then use those in the therapeutic cocktail. Engineering is another possibility for generating resistance-blocking phages [50,82–85]. Advance selection of resistance-blocking phages is possible because bacterial evolution to resist a single phage often follows a common molecular pathway, enabling the investigator to replicate in vitro the within-patient arms race. One simply evolves resistant bacteria in vitro and then selects resistance-blocking phages in advance of treatment, ultimately including them in the cocktail at sufficiently high concentrations that they are not lost before substantial numbers of resistant bacteria have arisen. Indeed, our mechanistic understanding of resistance evolution is so advanced as to realize that phages infecting the same host by using different receptors will provide complementary blocks to bacterial resistance evolution—pathways of resistance evolution can thus be anticipated even before the patient experiences the resistant bacteria. Unfortunately, the approach of designing a cocktail to anticipate bacterial evolution may only be applicable to chronic infections, as the time and effort to identify phages and their specific receptors, and then formulating an appropriate cocktail, is considerable.

The dynamics of multiple, resistance-complementing phages in a cocktail works in favor of suppressing bacterial resistance, but the timing is not ideal. The main complication is that phage dynamics are not anticipatory, responding to what is present rather than what is about to occur. Given the intrinsic differences in growth likely to exist among wild phages, the initial dynamics of the cocktail will typically be dominated by one phage, with the other phages dropping to low numbers (or even disappearing) before resistant bacteria ascend (Figure 2B and [71]). Resistant bacteria will ascend and potentially exacerbate symptoms before being suppressed by other phages in the cocktail (Figure 2C), and the cycle may repeat. If the cocktail contains resistance-blocking phages, it would seem that the ascent of resistant bacteria could be avoided by periodic dosing with the cocktail, but a very high dose may be needed (see Figure 2D,E). Overall, therefore, cocktail dynamics can ultimately work in favor of overcoming bacterial resistance (provided that appropriate phages are present), but the best treatment may require an informed design and application of cocktails.

The successive collection of phages from the patient should reveal much about the dynamics before and during bacterial resistance evolution. Recovered phages may be a source of improved phages that can be used on other patients infected with the same strain, as may be likely in an epidemic. Such phages may also have been selected for lower rates of clearance by the reticuloendothelial or other systems.

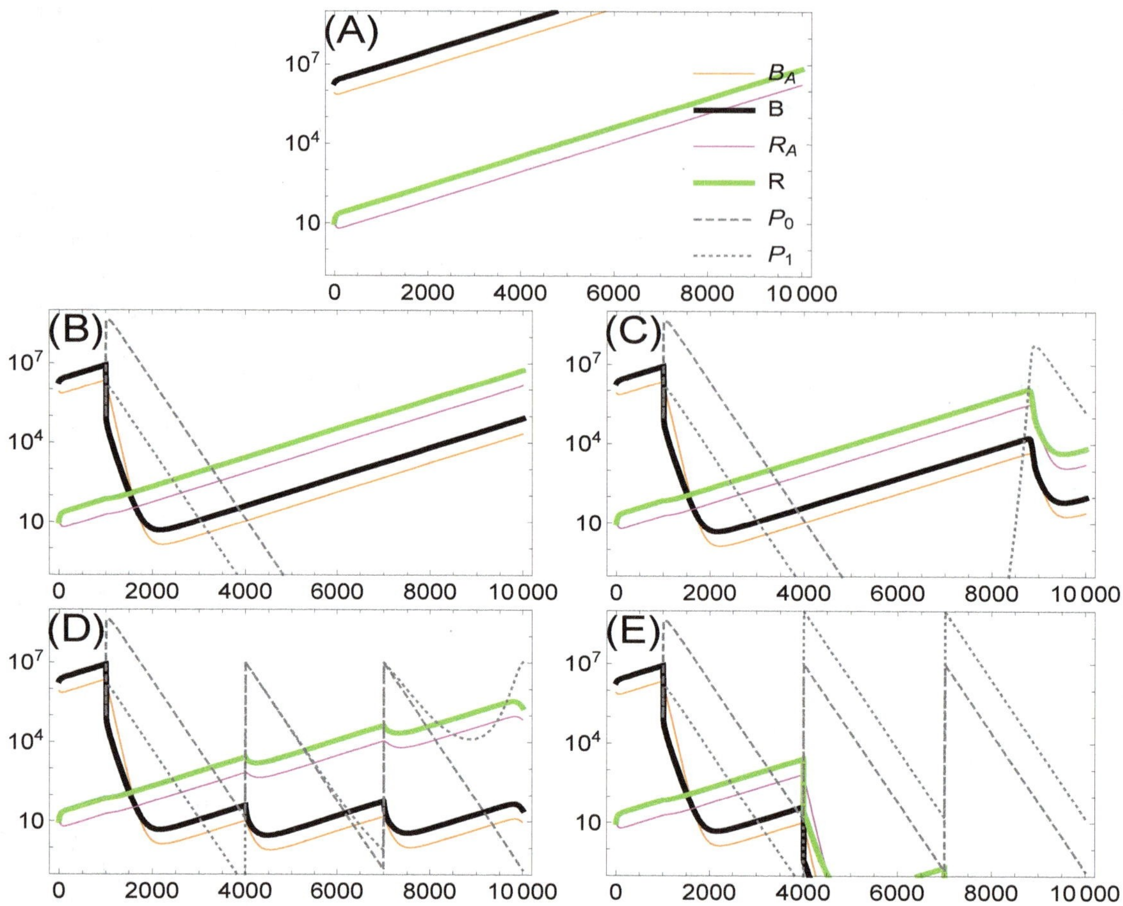

Figure 2. A 'broad' host-range phage that blocks bacterial resistance is subject to delayed ascendency. Periodic dosing may be only moderately more useful in suppressing bacterial resistance than is relying on intrinsic dynamics. The model assumes two strains of bacteria, each in two states (solid colored curves) and two strains of phage (dashed and dotted gray); the inset legend in (**A**) applies throughout, with equations and parameters given in Appendix A.2. The vertical axis gives density, the horizontal axis time (minutes). The phages differ in whether they can infect both bacteria (the 'broad' phage, given by P_1, dotted curves) or just one bacterium (the 'narrow' phage, given by P_0, dashed curves); the narrow phage has the advantage of a slightly higher adsorption rate. The bacterial strain given by blue and orange curves is sensitive to both phages, the other (green and pink curves) is resistant to the narrow phage and is initially rare. Each bacterium exists both planktonically (thick curves) and in aggregates (thin curves), with aggregates being protected from all phages. The two bacteria differ only in sensitivity to the phages. (**A**): Growth of the bacteria in the absence of phages. (**B**): Both phages are introduced at time t = 1000 at a density of 10^5 but are considered to be extinct when densities drop below 0.1. They have a rapid effect of driving the sensitive bacterial strain to low numbers, allowing the resistant bacterium to become the majority. Both phages are lost when the bacterial density is too low to sustain them, and all bacteria begin to recover, maintaining their relative abundances. (**C**): The same as in (**B**), except that phages are never considered to be extinct. The broad phage eventually rebounds in response to the high numbers of 'resistant' bacteria, and it suppresses both strains. (**D**): A cocktail of both phages is applied, each at a dose of 10^5 (time 1000) and then each at a dose of 10^7 (times 4000 and 7000). The narrow-host range phage gains early because of its superior adsorption rate. Resistant bacteria eventually ascend and allow the broad phage to maintain itself. Note that there is a substantial lag before the broad phage dominates. (**E**) The same as in (**D**), but the inocula at times 4000 and 7000 are increased to 10^9 of the broad phage. All bacteria are now pushed to near extinction.

3.4.3. Resistance-Proof Phages Can Avoid Evolutionary Arms Races, but In Vivo Dynamics Do Not Ensure Their Ascendancy in Cocktails

Resistant bacteria do not invariably ascend ([4,12] and references above). Failure to ascend occurs when bacterial resistance seriously impairs bacterial growth in the local environment. Thus, Smith and Huggins [12] observed that their 'good' phages required the bacterial capsule for growth; bacterial resistance resulted in loss of the capsule, which rendered the bacterium susceptible to the immune system and thereby prevented ascendancy. Other trade-offs between bacterial resistance to phages and bacterial growth are known; they often depend on the environmental context [4,86]. These observations suggest that single phages might be chosen wisely to prevent the ascendance of resistant bacteria. Use of such 'resistance-proof' phages has an obvious advantage, even over cocktails, as such treatments do not face the even temporary ascendance of resistant bacteria (although resistance-proof phages are subject to the same predator-prey cycles of other phages). A resistance-proof strategy has even been employed successfully with patients [4,8]. (Again, if CRISPR-based immunity evolves, there may be no possibility of a resistance-proof strategy using a single phage.)

As a possible source of resistance-proof phages, narrow host-range phages may be evolved to overcome bacterial resistance, thereby changing their host range. This selection works well in a laboratory setting where defined cultures are employed, and may lead to resistance-proofing because most host range mutations confer an expansion of host range, rather than a switch. However, the result is usually a compromise, with the rate of adsorption to both the old and new hosts being less than of specialist phages that only infect one or the other strain. Reduced adsorption may allow sensitive bacteria to persist at moderate densities or in refuges that might be suppressed by other phages; reduced adsorption will generally affect therapeutic success if rapid phage multiplication is required in vivo.

Although resistance-proof phages have sometimes been chosen a priori by design [4], a scientific basis for choosing them may not always be available in advance of treatment. Might in vivo competitions be used to dynamically evolve such phages? That is, if a cocktail of phages is used in treatment and the cocktail were to contain a resistance-proof phage, would it automatically ascend and displace the others? Not necessarily, at least not because of its resistance-proof status. At the outset, a resistance-proof phage has no advantage when the cocktail is first introduced on the sensitive strain, and whichever phage grows the fastest will predominate (e.g., [71]). When the bacterial population evolves resistance to this first phage—a potentially slow process if bacteria exist in protected states (e.g., Figure 2)—the resistance-proof phage may be one of several remaining phages capable of growing on the resistant bacteria. Again, the fastest-growing phage will predominate, not necessarily the one that is resistance-proof. Beyond this phase, there are countless possibilities as to preclude generalities—from phage competitions, bacterial competitions, bacterial protected states, and delayed, density-dependent dynamics. We thus lack assurance that a resistance-proof phage will prevail. Treatment with a single phage known to be resistance-proof appears to be the surest way to maintain a lasting block against bacterial resistance evolution, but the phage must be chosen intelligently rather than by relying on within-host evolution.

As noted above, our presentation of bacterial resistance has implicitly emphasized changes in surface receptors affecting phage adsorption. Other mechanisms of bacterial resistance to phages are known [59], but most are not prone to evolve new resistance profiles in vivo and so only affect the initial choice of treatment phages. Furthermore, changes in surface receptors may evolve in deference to other changes [76]. Nonetheless, the dynamics of phage evolution to overcome bacterial resistance by other mechanisms will face the same types of issues identified here.

Engineering phages with altered or broad host ranges is increasingly feasible [50,82–85]. To minimize the time lag problem, perhaps the goal should be to engineer a single, broad phage rather than a collection of mutants that collectively spans multiple host strains (e.g., [85]). In vivo evolution of phages engineered for host range should usually be compatible with maintaining the engineering. Such in vivo evolution may improve adsorption and tail stability, for example. But any evolution may also favor specialization that will limit phage growth on other strains.

Conclusions. Within-host evolution favors bacterial resistance to phages, but the ascendance of resistant bacteria then favors phages that grow on the resistant strains. Within-host evolution of single phages is not assured of overcoming bacterial resistance, if only because the requisite mutations may not occur. Cocktails may be designed to anticipate and block bacterial resistance evolution, but timing remains a problem: phage evolution in response to resistant bacteria necessarily lags the ascendance of resistant bacteria. Phage engineering to overcome bacterial resistance is gaining attention and may offer a shortcut from laboriously screening wild phages. Because of the time-lag problem, repeated dosing with a cocktail may be required to prevent the temporary ascent of resistant bacteria. Resistance-proof phages offer a solution to a bacteria-phage arms race, but there is no in vivo protocol that ensures automatic selection of single, resistance-proof phages, even when a resistance-proof phage is present in the initial cocktail. They must therefore be chosen from experience or an a priori understanding of the costs and benefits of bacterial resistance to phages.

4. Discussion

It is already clear that, whatever its ultimate utility, phage therapy of bacterial infections will not afford the simplicity of treatment that has been true of antibiotics. Perhaps phage treatments will need to be tailored to the infecting strain and may even need to be tailored to the nature of the infection. However, one hope for phage therapy that does not apply to antibiotics is evolution. When starting a treatment with one or more phages that infects the pathogen, either Darwinian phage evolution or cocktail dynamics within the patient might be aligned with treatment success and 'automatically' yield the best phages, obviating the need for a sophisticated understanding of best treatment practices.

Evaluating the potential utility of within-host evolution has special merit in light of the fact that current treatment protocols have been rather simplistic. This is not a criticism, one needs to know what the problems are before designing more complex protocols. In some cases, phages were selected for treatment based on no more than a demonstrated host range in vitro. In other cases, phages were chosen merely to grow on the infecting strain and also block the ascent of resistant bacteria, again based on in vitro assays. Although infections have been successfully suppressed by some of these protocols, improvements may be warranted to shorten recovery periods or to depress bacterial densities beyond that which was attained. Furthermore, in vivo phage evolution may not only augment treatment, but studying it may lead us to new insights that could improve treatment.

The thesis that in vivo phage evolution is aligned with treatment success applies to some phage properties but not others. The reason for the different effects of within-host evolution on phage improvement is that the different phage properties evolve under different dynamic processes, and only some processes are aligned with treatment. Properties improved by within-host evolution are phage growth rate and (reduced) clearance rate, as well as the ability to overcome bacterial resistance. However, phage evolution to overcome bacterial resistance has a time lag problem: phage evolution tracks bacterial resistance, so resistant bacteria ascend before being suppressed again. Resistance-proof phages avoid the emergence of resistant bacteria if they are the only phages administered, but when given as one of several phages, they do not ensure against the cyclical rise of resistant bacteria. Wise cocktail design and delivery timing is the more assured way of limiting the ascent of resistant bacteria.

Intrinsic dynamics/evolution within the patient offer no assurance for the maintenance of phage-encoded enzymes that degrade extra-bacterial substances. The release of free, phage-encoded enzymes may profoundly help clear an infection, but this benefit does not help maintain the phages producing the enzymes—unless the infection is highly structured. Again, wise choice of phages, cocktail composition, and dosing times may be required to optimize treatment.

Phages may act in synergy with antibiotics [87–89] and other therapies, although there appears to be no grand generality—some drug-phage combinations are synergistic, others antagonistic [90].

The performance of individual phages may thus well be affected by interactions with other therapies. Indeed, phage therapy with humans may invariably require co-treatment with antibiotics, so phage–drug interactions may well be critical to success. However, we do not expect the principles underlying the alignment of within-host evolution and treatment success to change because of antibiotic use.

The concept of engineering a 'super' phage for therapy has often been raised. Such a phage would likely have a broad host range and encode one or more enzymes that degrade extracellular matrices. A priori, it may be desirable to encode anti-R-M and anti-CRISPR functions, methylases, and other proteins that antagonize host defenses. However, as the maximum capacity of a phage capsid for DNA is limited, extensive engineering of a phage genome is likely to require removal of "non-essential" (within a laboratory setting) genes. The engineering may thus be self-defeating unless carefully designed. Nevertheless, within-host evolution could be used to improve such a 'super' phage in several respects, and where evolution led to undesired outcomes (e.g., loss of a phage-encoded enzyme), the evolution could at least help identify where the engineering needed improvement. Indeed, a within-host competition of different engineered phages could quickly identify which phages were the most genetically stable.

Depressing Bacterial Densities versus Improving Infection Outcomes

The perspective here has assumed that decreasing bacterial numbers invariably improves the patient's outcome. Depressing bacterial numbers will no doubt be essential to cure, but there are hints that the relationship between bacterial killing and treatment success is not always straightforward: bacterial lysis releases endotoxins. In an experimental mouse model, lethal but non-lysing phages given at very high doses were shown to improve host survival over lytic phages [91]. Although that experimental system was highly artificial, the result fits with known principles of the immune response, and it points to a wider realm of possible deviations from a simple relationship between bacterial killing by lysis and treatment improvement. For example, treatment with a phage that releases capsular depolymerases may boost immune-mediated killing, which does not entail lysis (e.g., [41,42,44,45]).

A second possible concern with 'successful' phage therapy is whether bacterial resistance to phages might increase virulence. Bacterial resistance to phages often entails a reduction in bacterial growth rates or densities, but if bacterial density is not the sole determinant of virulence, then an increase in virulence is possible despite reduced bacterial growth. Indeed, some extremely slow-growing bacteria cause serious infections. Bacterial resistance to phages may impart simultaneous protection against immunity, as with bacterial mucoidy. It is thus conceivable that some virulent bacterial mutants may have an advantage within the host only when favored by phage pressure, in which case they would not be observed in the absence of treatment. Although this possibility is speculative, there are unconfirmed reports of symptoms made worse by phage treatment. One conceivable scenario is where the use of broad host range phages and/or complex phage cocktails inadvertently targets benign commensal bacteria that themselves are antagonistic to proliferation of the pathogen.

Author Contributions: All three authors contributed to all aspects of the paper, except that J.J.B. wrote the Mathematica files to generate the figures.

Acknowledgments: We thank Steve Abedon for comments and insight to the literature. Two reviewers gave useful advice on the manuscript.

Appendix A. Model Details

The standard model of bacterial–phage interactions is one of ordinary differential equations assuming mass action, whereby the number of infections occurring per unit time is simply the product of the phage and bacterial concentrations (scaled by an adsorption rate parameter, [25,26]). This type of model typically leads to a rapid and profound depression of bacteria, followed by a bacterial resurgence and ensuing oscillations of phage and bacterial densities. These dynamics are apparently not representative of phage therapy patients [2]. We instead offer two models of ordinary differential equations that deviate from the standard model and can generate some key outcomes mirroring those of observed with phage therapy: bacteria exist in protected states, phage may slowly decay during treatment, and multiple dosing may be required [2]. Although our models explicitly include many components (minimally four variables and nine parameters), they are proposed heuristically in that they cannot be empirically parameterized. Instead, many parameters need be chosen so that the baseline behavior allows phage to have only a moderate effect on bacterial densities in the short term, and indeed for some trials, that multiple phage inoculations are needed to depress bacterial densities to low levels. Any numerical trial of this model is useful chiefly in illustrating possibilities that are incompatible with the standard model.

Appendix A.1. One Bacterial Strain with Two Bacterial States and Two Phages

In model (A1), a single strain of bacterium switches between a planktonic state and aggregates. Planktonic bacteria are susceptible to phages, aggregates are not. Two phage strains are included, differing only in decay rate. Parameters are defined in Table A1.

$$\begin{aligned} \dot{B}_A &= -\rho B_A + \beta B \\ \dot{B} &= \rho c B_A - k_0 P_0 B - k_1 P_1 B - d_B B \\ \dot{P}_0 &= b_0 k_0 \, B P_0 - d_0 P_0 \\ \dot{P}_1 &= b_1 k_1 \, B P_1 - d_1 P_1 \quad . \end{aligned} \tag{A1}$$

Parameter values used in Figure 1 are: k_0, $k_1 = 3 \times 10^{-9}$, $d_0 = 0.008$, $d_1 = 0.002$, $d_B = 0.001$, b_0, $b_1 = 50$, $c = 2.5$, $\rho = 0.0018$, $\beta = 5 \times 10^{-4}$. Initial bacterial densities are: $B(0) = 2 \times 10^5$, $B_A(0) = 8 \times 10^4$.

Table A1. Model variables and parameters.

Notation	Description	Units
Variables (Functions of Time)	**Description**	**Units**
B_A	density of bacteria in aggregates (protected)	/mL
B	density of susceptible, planktonic bacteria	/mL
P_0	density of strain 0 phage	/mL
P_1	density of strain 1 phage	/mL
Parameters	**Description**	**Units**
k_i	adsorption rate of phage strain i to planktonic bacteria	mL/min
d_i	death rate of phage strain i	/min
d_B	loss rate of bacteria from death or conversion to aggregates ($d_B \geq \beta$)	/min
b_i	burst size of phage strain i	individuals
c	conversion rate of aggregates to planktonic bacteria	
ρ	loss rate of aggregates to become planktonic bacteria	/min
β	aggregate formation rate by planktonic bacteria	/min

Appendix A.2. Two Bacterial States with Two Bacterial States and Two Phages

This model is similar to that in (A1), except that it adds a second strain of bacteria, one whose planktonic state is resistant to one of the phages, necessarily also resistant as aggregates. To keep the emphasis on the effect of resistance, many of the same parameter values are used for the two types of bacteria and for phage infection of the bacteria.

$$\begin{aligned}\dot{B}_A &= -\rho B_A + \beta B \\ \dot{B} &= \rho c B_A - k_0 P_0 B - k_1 P_1 B - d_B B \\ \dot{R}_A &= -\rho R_A + \beta R \\ \dot{R} &= \rho c R_A - k_1 P_1 R - d_B R \\ \dot{P}_0 &= b_0 k_0 B P_0 - d_0 P_0 \\ \dot{P}_1 &= b_1 k_1 B P_1 + b_1 k_1 R P_1 - d_1 P_1 \quad .\end{aligned} \tag{A2}$$

Only variables that differ from those in model (A1) are defined in the table below. Parameters are the same as in Table A1.

Table A2. New variables for model (A2).

Notation	Description	Units
Variables (Functions of Time)	**Description**	**Units**
R_A	density of resistant bacteria in aggregates	/mL
R	density of resistant, planktonic bacteria	/mL

Parameter values used in Figure 2 are the same as for Figure 1 except: $k_1 = 1 \times 10^{-9}$, $d_0 = d_1 = 0.006$, $d_B = 0.009$, $c = 2.2$, $\rho = 0.018$, $\beta = 5 \times 10^{-3}$. Initial bacterial densities are: $B(1) = 2 \times 10^6$, $B_A(1) = 8 \times 10^5$, $R[1] = R_A[1] = 10$.

References

1. Brüssow, H. Phage therapy for the treatment of human intestinal bacterial infections: Soon to be a reality? *Expert Rev. Gastroenterol. Hepatol.* **2017**, *11*, 785–788. [CrossRef] [PubMed]
2. Abedon, S.T. Use of phage therapy to treat long-standing, persistent, or chronic bacterial infections. *Adv. Drug Deliv. Rev.* **2018**. [CrossRef] [PubMed]
3. Schmidt, C. Phage therapy's latest makeover. *Nat. Biotechnol.* **2019**, *37*, 581–586. [CrossRef] [PubMed]
4. Kortright, K.E.; Chan, B.K.; Koff, J.L.; Turner, P.E. Phage therapy: A renewed approach to combat antibiotic-resistant bacteria. *Cell Host Microbe* **2019**, *25*, 219–232. [CrossRef] [PubMed]
5. Schooley, R.T.; Biswas, B.; Gill, J.J.; Hernandez-Morales, A.; Lancaster, J.; Lessor, L.; Barr, J.J.; Reed, S.L.; Rohwer, F.; Benler, S.; et al. Development and use of personalized bacteriophage-based therapeutic cocktails to treat a patient with a disseminated resistant Acinetobacter baumannii infection. *Antimicrob. Agents Chemother.* **2017**, *61*. [CrossRef] [PubMed]
6. Schooley, R.T.; Biswas, B.; Gill, J.J.; Hernandez-Morales, A.; Lancaster, J.; Lessor, L.; Barr, J.J.; Reed, S.L.; Rohwer, F.; Benler, S.; et al. Erratum for Schooley et al., "Development and use of personalized bacteriophage-based therapeutic cocktails to treat a patient with a disseminated resistant Acinetobacter baumannii infection". *Antimicrob. Agents Chemother.* **2018**, *62*, e02221-18. [CrossRef]
7. Dedrick, R.M.; Guerrero-Bustamante, C.A.; Garlena, R.A.; Russell, D.A.; Ford, K.; Harris, K.; Gilmour, K.C.; Soothill, J.; Jacobs-Sera, D.; Schooley, R.T.; et al. Engineered bacteriophages for treatment of a patient with a disseminated drug-resistant Mycobacterium abscessus. *Nat. Med.* **2019**, *25*, 730–733. [CrossRef]
8. Chan, B.K.; Turner, P.E.; Kim, S.; Mojibian, H.R.; Elefteriades, J.A.; Narayan, D. Phage treatment of an aortic graft infected with Pseudomonas aeruginosa. *Evol. Med. Public Health* **2018**, *2018*, 60–66. [CrossRef]
9. Rhoads, D.D.; Wolcott, R.D.; Kuskowski, M.A.; Wolcott, B.M.; Ward, L.S.; Sulakvelidze, A. Bacteriophage therapy of venous leg ulcers in humans: Results of a phase I safety trial. *J. Wound Care* **2009**, *18*, 237–243. [CrossRef]
10. Sarker, S.A.; Sultana, S.; Reuteler, G.; Moine, D.; Descombes, P.; Charton, F.; Bourdin, G.; McCallin, S.; Ngom-Bru, C.; Neville, T.; et al. Oral phage therapy of acute bacterial diarrhea with two coliphage preparations: A randomized trial in children from Bangladesh. *EBioMedicine* **2016**, *4*, 124–137. [CrossRef]

11. Jault, P.; Leclerc, T.; Jennes, S.; Pirnay, J.P.; Que, Y.A.; Resch, G.; Rousseau, A.F.; Ravat, F.; Carsin, H.; Le Floch, R.; et al. Efficacy and tolerability of a cocktail of bacteriophages to treat burn wounds infected by Pseudomonas aeruginosa (PhagoBurn): A randomised, controlled, double-blind phase 1/2 trial. *Lancet Infect. Dis.* **2019**, *19*, 35–45. [CrossRef]
12. Smith, H.W.; Huggins, M.B. Successful treatment of experimental *Escherichia coli* Infect. Mice Using Phage: Its Gen. Super. Antibiot. *J. Gen. Microbiol.* **1982**, *128*, 307–318. [PubMed]
13. Henry, M.; Lavigne, R.; Debarbieux, L. Predicting in vivo efficacy of therapeutic bacteriophages used to treat pulmonary infections. *Antimicrob. Agents Chemother.* **2013**, *57*, 5961–5968. [CrossRef] [PubMed]
14. Arnold, F.H. Innovation by evolution: Bringing new chemistry to life (Nobel Lecture). *Angew. Chem. (Int. Ed. Engl.)* **2019**. [CrossRef] [PubMed]
15. D'Herelle, F. *Immunity in Natural Infectious Disease*, Authorized English ed.; Smith, G.H., Ed.; Williams & Wilkins Co.: Baltimore, MD, USA, 1924.
16. McEwen, S.; Collignon, P. Antimicrobial resistance: A One Health perspective. *Microbiol Spectr.* **2018**, *6*, ARBA–0009–2017. [CrossRef] [PubMed]
17. Bull, J.J.; Levin, B.R.; DeRouin, T.; Walker, N.; Bloch, C.A. Dynamics of success and failure in phage and antibiotic therapy in experimental infections. *BMC Microbiol.* **2002**, *2*, 35. [CrossRef]
18. Bull, J.J.; Otto, G.; Molineux, I.J. In vivo growth rates are poorly correlated with phage therapy success in a mouse infection model. *Antimicrob. Agents Chemother.* **2012**, *56*, 949–954. [CrossRef]
19. Merril, C.R.; Biswas, B.; Carlton, R.; Jensen, N.C.; Creed, G.J.; Zullo, S.; Adhya, S. Long-circulating bacteriophage as antibacterial agents. *Proc. Natl. Acad. Sci. USA* **1996**, *93*, 3188–3192. [CrossRef]
20. Sutherland, I.W.; Hughes, K.A.; Skillman, L.C.; Tait, K. The interaction of phage and biofilms. *FEMS Microbiol. Lett.* **2004**, *232*, 1–6. [CrossRef]
21. Lu, T.K.; Collins, J.J. Dispersing biofilms with engineered enzymatic bacteriophage. *Proc. Natl. Acad. Sci. USA* **2007**, *104*, 11197–11202. [CrossRef]
22. Chan, B.K.; Abedon, S.T. Phage therapy pharmacology: Phage cocktails. In *Advances in Applied Microbiology*; Laskin, A.I., Sariaslani, S., Gadd, G.M., Eds.; Academic Press: San Diego, CA, USA, 2012; Volume 78, pp. 1–23. [CrossRef]
23. Gladstone, E.G.; Molineux, I.J.; Bull, J.J. Evolutionary principles and synthetic biology: Avoiding a molecular tragedy of the commons with an engineered phage. *J. Biol. Eng.* **2012**, *6*, 13. [CrossRef] [PubMed]
24. Adams, M.H. *Bacteriophages*; Interscience Publishers: New York, NY, USA, 1959.
25. Campbell, A. Conditions for the existence of bacteriophage. *Evolution* **1961**, *15*, 143–165. [CrossRef]
26. Levin, B.R.; Stewart, F.M.; Chao, L. Resource—Limited growth, competition , and predation: A model and experimental studies with bacteria and bacteriophage. *Am. Nat.* **1977**, *977*, 3–24. [CrossRef]
27. Roach, D.R.; Leung, C.Y.; Henry, M.; Morello, E.; Singh, D.; Di Santo, J.P.; Weitz, J.S.; Debarbieux, L. Synergy between the host immune system and bacteriophage is essential for successful phage therapy against an acute respiratory pathogen. *Cell Host Microbe* **2017**, *22*, 38–47.e4. [CrossRef] [PubMed]
28. Abedon, S.T. Bacteriophage-mediated biocontrol of wound infections, and ecological exploitation of biofilms by phages. In *Recent Clinical Techniques, Results, and Research in Wounds*; Springer: Cham, Switzerland: 2018; pp. 1–38.
29. Darch, S.E.; Kragh, K.N.; Abbott, E.A.; Bjarnsholt, T.; Bull, J.J.; Whiteley, M. Phage inhibit pathogen dissemination by targeting bacterial migrants in a chronic infection model. *mBio* **2017**, *8*. [CrossRef]
30. Bull, J.J. Optimality models of phage life history and parallels in disease evolution. *J. Theor. Biol.* **2006**, *241*, 928–938. [CrossRef]
31. Heineman, R.H.; Springman, R.; Bull, J.J. Optimal foraging by bacteriophages through host avoidance. *Am. Nat.* **2008**, *171*, E149–E157. [CrossRef]
32. Westwater, C.; Kasman, L.M.; Schofield, D.A.; Werner, P.A.; Dolan, J.W.; Schmidt, M.G.; Norris, J.S. Use of genetically engineered phage to deliver antimicrobial agents to bacteria: An alternative therapy for treatment of bacterial infections. *Antimicrob. Agents Chemother.* **2003**, *47*, 1301–1307. [CrossRef]
33. Bull, J.J.; Regoes, R.R. Pharmacodynamics of non-replicating viruses, bacteriocins and lysins. *Proc. Biol. Sci. R. Soc.* **2006**, *273*, 2703–2712. [CrossRef]
34. Hodyra-Stefaniak, K.; Lahutta, K.; Majewska, J.; Kaźmierczak, Z.; Lecion, D.; Harhala, M.; Kęska, W.; Owczarek, B.; Jończyk-Matysiak, E.; Kłopot, A.; et al. Bacteriophages engineered to display foreign peptides may become short-circulating phages. *Microb. Biotechnol.* **2019**, *12*, 730–741. [CrossRef]

35. Sutherland, I.W.; Wilkinson, J.F. Depolymerases for bacterial exopolysaccharides obtained from phage-infected bacteria. *J. Gen. Microbiol.* **1965**, *39*, 373–383. [CrossRef] [PubMed]
36. Sutherland, I.W. Polysaccharide lyases. *FEMS Microbiol. Rev.* **1995**, *16*, 323–347. [CrossRef] [PubMed]
37. Hughes, K.A.; Sutherland, I.W.; Clark, J.; Jones, M.V. Bacteriophage and associated polysaccharide depolymerases–novel tools for study of bacterial biofilms. *J. Appl. Microbiol.* **1998**, *85*, 583–590. [CrossRef] [PubMed]
38. Hanlon, G.W.; Denyer, S.P.; Olliff, C.J.; Ibrahim, L.J. Reduction in exopolysaccharide viscosity as an aid to bacteriophage penetration through Pseudomonas aeruginosa biofilms. *Appl. Environ. Microbiol.* **2001**, *67*, 2746–2753. [CrossRef] [PubMed]
39. Azeredo, J.; Sutherland, I.W. The use of phages for the removal of infectious biofilms. *Curr. Pharm. Biotechnol.* **2008**, *9*, 261–266. [CrossRef] [PubMed]
40. Bull, J.J.; Vimr, E.R.; Molineux, I.J. A tale of tails: Sialidase is key to success in a model of phage therapy against K1-capsulated Escherichia coli. *Virology* **2010**, *398*, 79–86. [CrossRef]
41. Mushtaq, N.; Redpath, M.B.; Luzio, J.P.; Taylor, P.W. Prevention and cure of systemic Escherichia coli K1 infection by modification of the bacterial phenotype. *Antimicrob. Agents Chemother.* **2004**, *48*, 1503–1508. [CrossRef]
42. Mushtaq, N.; Redpath, M.B.; Luzio, J.P.; Taylor, P.W. Treatment of experimental Escherichia coli infection with recombinant bacteriophage-derived capsule depolymerase. *J. Antimicrob. Chemother.* **2005**, *56*, 160–165. [CrossRef]
43. Lin, T.L.; Hsieh, P.F.; Huang, Y.T.; Lee, W.C.; Tsai, Y.T.; Su, P.A.; Pan, Y.J.; Hsu, C.R.; Wu, M.C.; Wang, J.T. Isolation of a bacteriophage and its depolymerase specific for K1 capsule of Klebsiella pneumoniae: Implication in typing and treatment. *J. Infect. Dis.* **2014**, *210*, 1734–1744. [CrossRef]
44. Lin, H.; Paff, M.L.; Molineux, I.J.; Bull, J.J. Therapeutic application of phage capsule depolymerases against K1, K5, and K30 capsulated E. coli in mice. *Front. Microbiol.* **2017**, *8*, 2257. [CrossRef]
45. Lin, H.; Paff, M.L.; Molineux, I.J.; Bull, J.J. Antibiotic therapy using phage depolymerases: Robustness across a range of conditions. *Viruses* **2018**, *10*, 622. [CrossRef] [PubMed]
46. Cornelissen, A.; Ceyssens, P.J.; T'Syen, J.; Van Praet, H.; Noben, J.P.; Shaburova, O.V.; Krylov, V.N.; Volckaert, G.; Lavigne, R. The T7-related Pseudomonas putida phage ϕ15 displays virion-associated biofilm degradation properties. *PLoS ONE* **2011**, *6*, e18597. [CrossRef] [PubMed]
47. Donlan, R.M.; Costerton, J.W. Biofilms: Survival mechanisms of clinically relevant microorganisms. *Clin. Microbiol. Rev.* **2002**, *15*, 167–193. [CrossRef] [PubMed]
48. Tseng, B.S.; Zhang, W.; Harrison, J.J.; Quach, T.P.; Song, J.L.; Penterman, J.; Singh, P.K.; Chopp, D.L.; Packman, A.I.; Parsek, M.R. The extracellular matrix protects Pseudomonas aeruginosa biofilms by limiting the penetration of tobramycin. *Environ. Microbiol.* **2013**, *15*, 2865–2878. [CrossRef] [PubMed]
49. Pei, R.; Lamas-Samanamud, G.R. Inhibition of biofilm formation by T7 bacteriophages producing quorum-quenching enzymes. *Appl. Environ. Microbiol.* **2014**, *80*, 5340–5348. [CrossRef] [PubMed]
50. Bárdy, P.; Pantůček, R.; Benešíkk, M.; Doškař, J. Genetically modified bacteriophages in applied microbiology. *J. Appl. Microbiol.* **2016**, *121*, 618–633. [CrossRef] [PubMed]
51. Bessler, W.; Fehmel, F.; Freund-Mölbert, E.; Knüfermann, H.; Stirm, S. Escherichia coli capsule bacteriophages. IV. Free capsule depolymerase 29. *J. Virol.* **1975**, *15*, 976–984.
52. Kassa, T.; Chhibber, S. Thermal treatment of the bacteriophage lysate of Klebsiella pneumoniae B5055 as a step for the purification of capsular depolymerase enzyme. *J. Virol. Methods* **2012**, *179*, 135–141. [CrossRef]
53. Schmerer, M.; Molineux, I.J.; Bull, J.J. Synergy as a rationale for phage therapy using phage cocktails. *PeerJ* **2014**, *2*, e590. [CrossRef]
54. Fleming, D.; Chahin, L.; Rumbaugh, K. Glycoside hydrolases degrade polymicrobial bacterial biofilms in wounds. *Antimicrob. Agents Chemother.* **2017**, *61*, e01998-16. [CrossRef]
55. Hashemolhosseini, S.; Holmes, Z.; Mutschler, B.; Henning, U. Alterations of receptor specificities of coliphages of the T2 family. *J. Mol. Biol.* **1994**, *240*, 105–110. [CrossRef] [PubMed]
56. Hashemolhosseini, S.; Montag, D.; Krämer, L.; Henning, U. Determinants of receptor specificity of coliphages of the T4 family. A chaperone alters the host range. *J. Mol. Biol.* **1994**, *241*, 524–533. [CrossRef] [PubMed]
57. Dinsmore, P.K.; Klaenhammer, T.R. Bacteriophage resistance in Lactococcus. *Mol. Biotechnol.* **1995**, *4*, 297–314. [CrossRef] [PubMed]

58. Durmaz, E.; Klaenhammer, T.R. Abortive phage resistance mechanism AbiZ speeds the lysis clock to cause premature lysis of phage-infected Lactococcus lactis. *J. Bacteriol.* **2007**, *189*, 1417–1425. [CrossRef] [PubMed]
59. Labrie, S.J.; Samson, J.E.; Moineau, S. Bacteriophage resistance mechanisms. *Nat. Rev. Microbiol.* **2010**, *8*, 317–327. [CrossRef] [PubMed]
60. Doron, S.; Melamed, S.; Ofir, G.; Leavitt, A.; Lopatina, A.; Keren, M.; Amitai, G.; Sorek, R. Systematic discovery of antiphage defense systems in the microbial pangenome. *Science* **2018**, *359*. [CrossRef]
61. Oechslin, F. Resistance development to bacteriophages occurring during bacteriophage therapy. *Viruses* **2018**, *10*, 351. [CrossRef]
62. Rostøl, J.T.; Marraffini, L. (Ph)ighting phages: How bacteria resist their parasites. *Cell Host Microbe* **2019**, *25*, 184–194. [CrossRef]
63. Levin, B.R. Frequency-dependent selection in bacterial populations. *Philos. Trans. R. Soc. London. Ser. B Biol. Sci.* **1988**, *319*, 459–472. [CrossRef]
64. Bohannan, B.J.M.; Lenski, R.E. Linking genetic change to community evolution: Insights from studies of bacteria and bacteriophage. *Ecol. Lett.* **2000**, *3*, 362–377. [CrossRef]
65. Mizoguchi, K.; Morita, M.; Fischer, C.R.; Yoichi, M.; Tanji, Y.; Unno, H. Coevolution of bacteriophage PP01 and Escherichia coli O157:H7 in continuous culture. *Appl. Environ. Microbiol.* **2003**, *69*, 170–176. [CrossRef] [PubMed]
66. Gómez, P.; Buckling, A. Bacteria-phage antagonistic coevolution in soil. *Science* **2011**, *332*, 106–109. [CrossRef] [PubMed]
67. Díaz-Muñoz, S.L.; Koskella, B. Bacteria-phage interactions in natural environments. *Adv. Appl. Microbiol.* **2014**, *89*, 135–183. [CrossRef] [PubMed]
68. Fortuna, M.A.; Barbour, M.A.; Zaman, L.; Hall, A.R.; Buckling, A.; Bascompte, J. Coevolutionary dynamics shape the structure of bacteria-phage infection networks. *Evol. Int. J. Org. Evol.* **2019**, *73*, 1001–1011. [CrossRef] [PubMed]
69. Ershova, A.S.; Rusinov, I.S.; Spirin, S.A.; Karyagina, A.S.; Alexeevski, A.V. Role of restriction-modification systems in prokaryotic evolution and ecology. *Biochem. Biokhimiia* **2015**, *80*, 1373–1386. [CrossRef] [PubMed]
70. Iordanescu, S.; Surdeanu, M. Two restriction and modification systems in Staphylococcus aureus NCTC8325. *J. Gen. Microbiol.* **1976**, *96*, 277–281. [CrossRef] [PubMed]
71. Korona, R.; Levin, B.R. Phage-mediated selection and the evolution and maintenance of restriction-modification. *Evol. Int. J. Org. Evol.* **1993**, *47*, 556–575. [CrossRef] [PubMed]
72. Korona, R.; Korona, B.; Levin, B.R. Sensitivity of naturally occurring coliphages to type I and type II restriction and modification. *J. Gener. Microbiol.* **1993**, *139*, 1283–1290. [CrossRef]
73. Jiang, W.; Maniv, I.; Arain, F.; Wang, Y.; Levin, B.R.; Marraffini, L.A. Dealing with the evolutionary downside of CRISPR immunity: Bacteria and beneficial plasmids. *PLoS Genet.* **2013**, *9*, e1003844. [CrossRef]
74. Paez-Espino, D.; Sharon, I.; Morovic, W.; Stahl, B.; Thomas, B.C.; Barrangou, R.; Banfield, J.F. CRISPR immunity drives rapid phage genome evolution in Streptococcus thermophilus. *mBio* **2015**, *6*, e00262-15. [CrossRef]
75. Weissman, J.L.; Holmes, R.; Barrangou, R.; Moineau, S.; Fagan, W.F.; Levin, B.; Johnson, P.L.F. Immune loss as a driver of coexistence during host-phage coevolution. *ISME J.* **2018**, *12*, 585–597. [CrossRef] [PubMed]
76. Gurney, J.; Pleška, M.; Levin, B.R. Why put up with immunity when there is resistance: An excursion into the population and evolutionary dynamics of restriction-modification and CRISPR-Cas. *Philos. Trans. R. Soc. Lond. Ser. B Biol. Sci.* **2019**, *374*, 20180096. [CrossRef] [PubMed]
77. Palmer, K.L.; Gilmore, M.S. Multidrug-resistant enterococci lack CRISPR-cas. *mBio* **2010**, *1*, e00227-10. [CrossRef] [PubMed]
78. Kos, V.N.; Déraspe, M.; McLaughlin, R.E.; Whiteaker, J.D.; Roy, P.H.; Alm, R.A.; Corbeil, J.; Gardner, H. The resistome of Pseudomonas aeruginosa in relationship to phenotypic susceptibility. *Antimicrob. Agents Chemother.* **2015**, *59*, 427–436. [CrossRef] [PubMed]
79. Harcombe, W.R.; Bull, J.J. Impact of phages on two-species bacterial communities. *Appl. Environ. Microbiol.* **2005**, *71*, 5254–5259. [CrossRef] [PubMed]
80. Hernandez, C.A.; Koskella, B. Phage resistance evolution in vitro is not reflective of in vivo outcome in a plant-bacteria-phage system. *Evol. Int. J. Org. Evol.* **2019**. [CrossRef]
81. LaVergne, S.; Hamilton, T.; Biswas, B.; Kumaraswamy, M.; Schooley, R.T.; Wooten, D. Phage therapy for a

multidrug-resistant *Acinetobacter baumannii* craniectomy site infection. *Open Forum Infect. Dis.* **2018**, *5*, ofy064. [CrossRef]

82. Yoichi, M.; Abe, M.; Miyanaga, K.; Unno, H.; Tanji, Y. Alteration of tail fiber protein gp38 enables T2 phage to infect *Escherichia coli* O157:H7. *J. Biotechnol.* **2005**, *115*, 101–107. [CrossRef]
83. Mahichi, F.; Synnott, A.J.; Yamamichi, K.; Osada, T.; Tanji, Y. Site-specific recombination of T2 phage using IP008 long tail fiber genes provides a targeted method for expanding host range while retaining lytic activity. *FEMS Microbiol. Lett.* **2009**, *295*, 211–217. [CrossRef]
84. Pouillot, F.; Blois, H.; Iris, F. Genetically engineered virulent phage banks in the detection and control of emergent pathogenic bacteria. *Biosecur. Bioterrorism Biodefense Strateg. Pract. Sci.* **2010**, *8*, 155–169. [CrossRef]
85. Yehl, K.; Lemire, S.; Yang, A.C.; Ando, H.; Mimee, M.; Torres, M.D.T.; de la Fuente-Nunez, C.; Lu, T.K. Engineering phage host-range and suppressing bacterial resistance through phage tail fiber mutagenesis. *Cell* **2019**, *179*, 459–469.e9. [CrossRef] [PubMed]
86. Chan, B.K.; Sistrom, M.; Wertz, J.E.; Kortright, K.E.; Narayan, D.; Turner, P.E. Phage selection restores antibiotic sensitivity in MDR Pseudomonas aeruginosa. *Sci. Rep.* **2016**, *6*, 26717. [CrossRef] [PubMed]
87. Chaudhry, W.N.; Concepción-Acevedo, J.; Park, T.; Andleeb, S.; Bull, J.J.; Levin, B.R. Synergy and order effects of antibiotics and phages in killing Pseudomonas aeruginosa biofilms. *PLoS ONE* **2017**, *12*, e0168615. [CrossRef] [PubMed]
88. Uchiyama, J.; Shigehisa, R.; Nasukawa, T.; Mizukami, K.; Takemura-Uchiyama, I.; Ujihara, T.; Murakami, H.; Imanishi, I.; Nishifuji, K.; Sakaguchi, M.; et al. Piperacillin and ceftazidime produce the strongest synergistic phage-antibiotic effect in Pseudomonas aeruginosa. *Arch. Virol.* **2018**, *163*, 1941–1948. [CrossRef] [PubMed]
89. Segall, A.M.; Roach, D.R.; Strathdee, S.A. Stronger together? Perspectives on phage-antibiotic synergy in clinical applications of phage therapy. *Curr. Opin. Microbiol.* **2019**, *51*, 46–50. [CrossRef] [PubMed]
90. Abedon, S.T. Phage-antibiotic combination treatments: Antagonistic impacts of antibiotics on the pharmacodynamics of phage therapy? *Antibiotics* **2019**, *8*, 182. [CrossRef]
91. Matsuda, T.; Freeman, T.A.; Hilbert, D.W.; Duff, M.; Fuortes, M.; Stapleton, P.P.; Daly, J.M. Lysis-deficient bacteriophage therapy decreases endotoxin and inflammatory mediator release and improves survival in a murine peritonitis model. *Surgery* **2005**, *137*, 639–646. [CrossRef]

2

Phage-Antibiotic Combination Treatments: Antagonistic Impacts of Antibiotics on the Pharmacodynamics of Phage Therapy?

Stephen T. Abedon

Department of Microbiology, The Ohio State University, Mansfield, OH 44906, USA; abedon.1@osu.edu

Abstract: Bacteria can evolve resistance to antibiotics. Even without changing genetically, bacteria also can display tolerance to antibiotic treatments. Many antibiotics are also broadly acting, as can result in excessive modifications of body microbiomes. Particularly for antibiotics of last resort or in treating extremely ill patients, antibiotics furthermore can display excessive toxicities. Antibiotics nevertheless remain the standard of care for bacterial infections, and rightly so given their long track records of both antibacterial efficacy and infrequency of severe side effects. Antibiotics do not successfully cure all treated bacterial infections, however, thereby providing a utility to alternative antibacterial approaches. One such approach is the use of bacteriophages, the viruses of bacteria. This nearly 100-year-old bactericidal, anti-infection technology can be effective against antibiotic-resistant or -tolerant bacteria, including bacterial biofilms and persister cells. Ideally phages could be used in combination with standard antibiotics while retaining their anti-bacterial pharmacodynamic activity, this despite antibiotics interfering with aspects of bacterial metabolism that are also required for full phage infection activity. Here I examine the literature of pre-clinical phage-antibiotic combination treatments, with emphasis on antibiotic-susceptible bacterial targets. I review evidence of antibiotic interference with phage infection activity along with its converse: phage antibacterial functioning despite antibiotic presence.

Keywords: bactericidal; bacteriophage therapy; bacteriolytic; phage productive; phage therapy; productive infection; virion productive

---

1. Introduction

Bacteriophages, or phages, are the viruses of bacteria. A majority of bacteriophages display lytic infection cycles. These involve phages infecting bacteria lethally and, in the process, producing new bactericidal agents, i.e., new phage virions. Phages have been employed clinically to treat bacterial infections for roughly one-hundred years [1,2], and many of these efforts seem to have been successful, e.g., such as in terms of treatment of chronic infections [3,4], wound infections [4–6], or lung-associated infections [7–10]. This 'phage therapy' furthermore has been proven to be efficacious in at least one modern efficacy (phase I/II) clinical trial [11], and recently there have been several well publicized phage therapy case-study successes [12–14]; see also [4,9,10,15–17]. Phages also can be effective against bacterial biofilms, e.g., [18–21], as well as against persister cells [22,23], though phages do not necessarily actively kill bacteria while these cells are still in the low-growth persister state [24]. In general terms [25], phages in phage therapy represent an older category of antibacterial agents that just might be able to address current needs for new antibacterial agents.

Given this history, an important question arises: Why has phage therapy not caught on more broadly as a reasonable alternative to antibiotics, particularly in North America and much of Europe? This question is especially relevant in light of issues associated with standard antibiotic effectiveness, the need for new approaches to treatment of bacterial infections [26], and several advantages inherent to phage use as antibacterial agents [27–32]. I suggest that part of the answer to this question of why not more phage therapy is that insufficient consideration has been placed on integrating phages into standard-of-care treatments of bacterial infections, that is, in terms of developing phage treatments which are concurrent with antibiotic treatments. Recently, however, there has been renewed focus on phage-antibiotic co-treatments in terms of preclinical experimentation [33]. Indeed, including antibiotics in experimental phage treatments could be relevant for reasons of expediting regulatory approval for phage therapy [34], and phages have been used in combination with antibiotics in various published clinical case studies [10,12,13,15–17]. Furthermore, by employing phage-antibiotic combination therapies, a potential can exist—as combination therapies [35–38]—for interfering with bacterial evolution to both phages and antibiotics [39–41]. For consideration of the potential for bacteria to evolve resistance to phages alone, see References [42–45].

Antibiotics are expected to interfere with aspects of bacterial physiology that can be crucial to phage antibacterial activities, e.g., by interfering with bacterial ribosome functioning. Emphasis here therefore is on documenting the impact of antibiotics on phage-infection pharmacodynamic aspects, i.e., retention of phage ability to negatively impact targeted bacteria despite antibiotic co-treatment. These pharmacodynamic properties include a retention, by bacteria-infecting phages, of both gene expression and antibacterial activity, and also of associated in situ—within treated patients—phage virion production. I address in particular the question of whether or to what degree antibiotic treatments may be antagonistic to the activity of phage infections, and this is especially given treatments in which antibiotic concentrations are greater than or equal to MICs (minimum inhibitory concentrations) [46–48] for targeted, especially clinically antibiotic-susceptible bacteria. This emphasis is rather than on considerations of the impact of phage-antibiotic combination therapy on bacterial resistance evolution [41], of phage-antibiotic synergy (PAS) while employing sub-inhibitory (<1× MIC) antibiotic doses [49], explicitly of treatment-order effects such as dosing with phages prior to dosing with antibiotics [33], or with otherwise substantial discussion of phage-antibiotic facilitative, additive, or synergistic interactions [18]. For general overviews of the subject of phage-antibiotic combination treatments, particularly as they relate to phage therapy, see Torres-Barceló and Hotchberg [41] and Tagliaferri et al. [33].

A defining characteristic of the literature concerning phage infection activity in the presence of antibiotics, given bacteria presumptive exposure to ≥1× MIC of antibiotic, is that different studies tend to present only one of two more-or-less opposing perspectives. These are those studies providing evidence or at least a premise that antibiotics will tend to profoundly interfere with phage infection outputs, particularly interfere with phage virion production, versus studies which suggest instead that antibiotic treatment of bacteria will not substantially interfere with phage infection outputs, or at least not interfere to a point where phage antibacterial activity is excessively diminished. It is the evidence underlying the bases of these two contradictory pharmacodynamic, phage-associated viewpoints that I review here. I start by looking at evidence consistent with antibiotic interference with phage infection activities and then consider evidence instead for continued phage infection activity despite antibiotic presence. A tentative overall conclusion is that the more complex the treatment environment, such as especially as found in vivo, then potentially the more compatible that phage therapy may be with antibiotic treatment.

2. Some Preliminary, General Considerations

The bulk of this article serves as a review of pre-clinical experimentation in which phage treatment or phage infection of bacteria is combined with antibiotic treatment. Emphasis is on interpretation of studies especially regarding the potential for phages to display various activities during their infection of bacteria. These activities, in terms of positive phage pharmacodynamic impacts on bacteria, can be differentiated into bactericidal effects, bacteriolytic effects, and also virion production by phage-infected bacteria. Generally, virion production and subsequent release by lytic phages would imply phage-mediated bacterial lysis, which in turn would imply phage-mediated bactericidal effects. Assessing experiments for these effects, as they may occur in the presence of 1× MIC or greater concentrations of antibiotic, however is not always straightforward, as considered in this section.

Firstly, various experiments or controls are useful for assessing antibiotic impact on phage infection activities. First are determinations of MICs for bacterial hosts. Conditions used for testing antibiotic impact on phage infection activity ideally would be equivalent to those conditions used for MIC determinations in terms of use of the same medium, use of the same antibiotic-incubation time frames, use of the same bacterial densities, and use of bacteria found in the same physiological state, such as log- versus stationary-phase. Second is comparing phage infection activities during antibiotic treatments to phage infection activities as occur under antibiotic-minus conditions; such antibiotic-minus infections in principle should allow full phage infection activity. Therefore, phage-only, antibiotic-only, phage-plus-antibiotic, and neither phage nor antibiotic treatments ideally would represent the minimum number of comparisons provided by an experiment. Third, if possible, it can be helpful to compare experiments using antibiotic-susceptible bacteria to equivalent experiments involving antibiotic-resistant host mutants. Phage infections of such bacteria may also allow full phage infection activity.

Exposure of bacteria to an antibiotic to which a bacterium is susceptible can in principle block subsequent phage infection-mediated bacteria killing. This proposed blockage can be due for example to antibiotic-caused interference with phage gene expression. Either with or without phage-mediated bactericidal activity, however, bacteria in the presence of 1× MIC antibiotic should not produce either colonies or turbid cultures. This has the effect of making it difficult to assess phage infection-mediated bactericidal activity, versus bacteriolytic or phage production activities, particularly while phage-infected bacteria are still in the presence of antibiotic, i.e., as measured in terms of reductions in bacterial colony-forming units (CFUs). Phage bactericidal activity might instead be assessed by first diluting antibiotic away from bacteria so that they may produce colonies if still able to, as following phage adsorption, but this would not be proof that phage-mediated bactericidal activity would also be retained while phage infections are still in the presence of antibiotic.

Phage-associated anti-biofilm activity can occur also as a consequence of the presence of biofilm-matrix degrading enzymes [50,51]. Such enzymes can be associated with phage virions and could mimic phage bactericidal activity in the presence of biofilms. That is, reductions in biofilm presence, e.g., in terms of reductions in biofilm biomass or reductions in numbers of constituent bacteria, can occur following phage treatment even without phages actually killing those bacteria. Such issues can arise given assays for phage activity in the presence of antibiotics when such assays are based solely on reductions in biofilm presence, particularly when applying phages at relatively high multiplicity of infections (MOIs; e.g., MOI = 5 or 10) and given biofilm washing prior to the quantification of anti-biofilm effects (i.e., so as to remove biofilm-released CFUs prior to their enumeration). Therefore, simply phage-associated removal of existing biofilm, especially given phage display of biofilm-matrix degrading enzymes, is not always indicative of phage infection bactericidal activity in the presence of an antibiotic.

Delays can exist between antibiotic application and the point of full antibiotic impact on bacterial metabolism, thereby potentially allowing for phage infection activity prior to full antibiotic impact on bacteria. Experiments in which phages and antibiotics are applied simultaneously or in which antibiotics are applied minutes after phage application therefore might provide a false sense of the potential for or degree of phage infection activity in the presence of an antibiotic. In addition, not all antibiotics are rapidly acting, in terms of degrading bacterial metabolic activity, e.g., such as cell-wall synthesis-inhibiting antibiotics for which duration of exposure along with antibiotic concentration are important components of their impact (versus concentration as a sole, key determinant). Phage infection activity thus in principle could occur during experiments prior to substantial antibiotic impact on bacterial functioning.

Antibiotic concentrations can decline over the course of experiments, particularly given long (multi-day) treatments and application of only a single antibiotic dose [47,48]. Such antibiotic decay could allow for phage infection activity that occurs later during experiments rather than earlier, and thereby phage infection activity that is not necessarily concurrent with ≥1× MIC antibiotic concentrations. In addition, phage infection activity if present might not be associated with the same individual bacteria that are substantially affected by antibiotic, such as due to heterogeneity in antibiotic impact on bacterial cultures as might be observed in association with bacterial biofilms. Consider also the occurrence of antibiotic tolerance as can be associated with bacterial growth in biofilms [47,48,52–56]. In addition, given sufficient lengths of treatment, and sufficiently low starting phage numbers (MOI < 1), then substantial phage virion production could occur during infection of antibiotic-*resistant* bacteria, that is, so long as those bacteria have first been allowed to grow to relatively high densities. Any of these scenarios could result in a false impression of occurrence of phage infection activity, such as virion production in the presence of even seemingly substantially antibiotic-impacted populations of antibiotic-susceptible bacteria.

Generally, it also is important to be aware that there is a difference between phage activity as occurs immediately upon infection (i.e., pharmacodynamic effects) versus bacterial resistance evolution as occurs over longer time frames. Not all experimental treatments, particularly ones of long duration and that are assessed only in terms of changes in relative bacterial presence, will necessarily distinguish between these two phenomena. Resistant bacteria, especially given phage and antibiotic treatments of long duration, can by their presence mimic reduced bactericidal activity by individual agents as relative to phage-antibiotic combined treatments (that is, more bacteria may be present after, e.g., two days of incubation given antibiotic-only treatment than with phage-plus-antibiotic treatment, but possibly only because the latter inhibits bacterial resistance evolution better than the former). This potentially false negative phage-mediated bactericidal activity would be due to different likelihoods of bacterial mutation in combination with resistant-bacterium grow back given application to cultures of single versus multiple antibacterial agents. Comparisons of bacterial numbers following, e.g., 24 or more hours of treatment, thus may be less indicative of phage bactericidal activity in the presence of antibiotic than somewhat sooner assessments, i.e., as made prior to substantial resistant-mutant bacterial grow back.

Lastly, phage virion production can be inferred, within more complex experimental systems such as those consisting of biofilms, from measurements of bacteria-killing activity. Doing so requires knowledge of initial ratios of added phages to bacterial numbers and is based on Poisson distributions [57]. For example, an MOI of 1 without additional phage population growth would be expected to kill at most $1 - e^{-MOI} = 1 - e^{-1} = 63\%$ of bacteria present. Therefore, any bacteria killing that is in excess of 63%, particularly killing that is attributable to phage action, could in this example be indicative of excessive virion numbers and thereby of in situ phage virion production following dosing [58]. The likelihood that virion production has occurred as based on such analyses would be greater the lower the starting phage MOI and the greater the difference, in terms of bacterial removal, between antibiotic-only treatment and phage-plus-antibiotic treatment.

3. Antibiotic Interference with Phage Pharmacodynamics

Antibacterial agents can be distinguished into those which are bacteriostatic versus those which are bactericidal [59]. A general expectation is that bacteriostatic agents may interfere with the action of bactericidal agents [60,61], and this is so particularly to the extent that the latter are more effective against fully metabolically active bacteria rather than bacteria which are less metabolically active [62,63]. The same situation may be present with phages, also as bactericidal agents, as phages too tend to display less activity given reduced bacterial metabolic activity [64–66]. A difference, however, is that individual phage types can generate multiple activities in association with target bacteria. Depending on circumstances, these activities can range from phage gene expression, to bactericidal or bacteriolytic activities, to production of new phage virions, or indeed and typically all of the above.

That antibiotics might interfere with phage infection activity is not a new idea, e.g., as documented by Adams [67]. Indeed, there are many bacterial components that are essential for bacteria to function and essential also for phage infections to function. The most obvious but not only such component is the bacterial ribosome, against which several antibiotics act, e.g., clindamycin, erythromycin, linezolid, and tetracycline. In considering the potential for phage therapy to work in the course of co-treatments with antibiotics, against antibiotic-susceptible bacteria, it therefore is critical to question to what degree antibiotics used in association with phages might interfere especially with phage bactericidal activity, and associated virion production activities. The retention of phage functionality furthermore should be tested at antibiotic concentrations that meet or exceed antibiotic MICs for targeted bacteria, as these are the antibiotic levels that are both expected and desired in vivo during antibiotic treatments. Our expectation, on the other hand, is that sub-MIC antibiotic concentrations may not interfere with phage antibacterial activity. Such continued functioning in the presence of sub-inhibitory antibiotic concentrations in fact represents a central tenet of the PAS literature [33,49]. As noted, however, PAS as a phenomenon is not being considered in detail here.

By way of example, regarding antibiotic interference with phage infection activity, Matsui et al. [68] describe four phages of *Ralstonia solanacearum*—ΦRSF1, ΦRSL1, ΦRSL2, and ΦRSB1—for which phage virion production is fully blocked given bacterial exposure to 5 μg/mL rifampin (20 min incubation prior to phage infection). Here the calculated MIC for this host was 3 μg/mL, and thus phage virion-production was inhibited given exposure to ~2× MIC. Furthermore, as Tagliaferri et al. [33] suggest (p. 10), "Negative interference [of antibiotics with phages] might be more common [than] as assumed, and it is possible that such experimental outcomes in the laboratory are less frequently reported than the positive ones." Notwithstanding this Tagliaferri et al. concern, a great deal of published evidence is consistent with the Matsui et al. result, particularly involving *Mycobacterium tuberculosis* as host. In this section, I summarize experiments indicating a potential for antibiotics to interfere with such phage infection activities. As follows, CFU stands for Colony-Forming Units and PFU stands for Plaque-Forming Units. As throughout this review, I both summarize the results of individual studies and provide my interpretations of those results, presenting the material in ascending author-date order. See Table 1 for summary of the studies presented in this section.

Table 1. Studies suggesting inhibition of phage infection activity in the presence of antibiotics [1,2].

Subsection	Host	Phage	Antibiotic	GE	BC	BL	VP	LT	Ref
Section 3.1	*R. solanacearum*	various [3]	rifampin				–		[68]
Section 3.1.1	*M. tuberculosis*	TM4	various [4]	–					[69]
Section 3.1.2	*M. tuberculosis*	D29	various [5]				–		[70]
Section 3.1.3	*M. tuberculosis*	D29	rifampin				–		[71]
Section 3.1.4	*M. tuberculosis*	D29	rifampin				–		[72]
Section 3.1.5	*M. tuberculosis*	D29	various [6]				–		[73]
Section 3.2	*P. aeruginosa*	LUZ19	rifampin				–		[74]
Section 3.2.1	*B. subtilis*	SPO1	rifamycin			–	–		[75]
Section 3.2.2	*B. subtilis*	β22	rifampin				–		[76]
Section 3.2.3	*E. coli*	λvir	rifampin				–	–	[77]
Section 3.2.4	*E. coli*	T2	rifampin				–		[78]
Section 3.2.5	*E. coli*	T5	rifampin				–		[79]
Section 3.2.6	*E. coli*	Mu	rifampin				–		[80]
Section 3.2.7	*Pseudomonas*	PM2	rifampin				–		[81]
Section 3.2.8	*Pseudomonas*	various [7]	rifampin				–		[82]
Section 3.3.1	*E. coli*	various [8]	nalidixic acid				–		[83]
Section 3.3.2	*E. coli*	various [9]	nalidixic acid				–		[84]
Section 3.3.3	*E. coli*	ECA2	various [10]		–		–		[85]

[1] Shown are approximate summaries of primary take-home messages of studies regarding phage activities in the presence of approximately 1× MIC concentrations of antibiotics or higher, where a '–' indicates a relative absence of demonstrated activity with most hosts tested, a '+' a relative presence of activity, and '±' ambiguous or multiple different results in terms of either phage gene expression (GE), phage bactericidal activity (BC), phage bacteriolytic activity (BL), or phage virion production (VP). LT stands for 'lysis timing' where a '–' in this column indicates lysis delay (thus, a '–' across the table tends to indicate negative impacts of antibiotic on phage infection activity). Note that for lytic phages, virion production implies bactericidal as well as bacteriolytic activity, though these properties are not indicated in the table unless they were explicitly measured in a study. [2] Please use this table as a guide-only to what studies are discussed in this review rather than as a definitive indication of phage properties in the presence of antibiotics, as actual results tend to be more complex than can be summarized this concisely. [3] Section 3.1, phages tested individually: ΦRSF1, ΦRSL1, ΦRSL2, and ΦRSB1. [4] Section 3.1.1, antibiotics tested individually: isoniazid, rifampin, or streptomycin. [5] Section 3.1.2, antibiotics tested individually: isoniazid or rifampin. [6] Section 3.1.5, antibiotics tested individually: amikacin, capreomycin, cycloserine, ethambutol, ethionamide, isoniazid, kanamycin, linezolid, moxifloxacin, ofloxacin, para-aminosalicylic acid, rifampin, or streptomycin. [7] Section 3.2.8, phages tested individually: PAK_P3 or PAK_P4. [8] Section 3.3.1, phages tested individually: 10, β, φR, φX174, T2 or T5. [9] Section 3.3.2, phages tested individually: φR, λ, T2, T4, or T5. [10] Section 3.3.3, antibiotics tested individually: chloramphenicol, ciprofloxacin, or tetracycline.

3.1. *Mycobacterium tuberculosis* Studies

M. tuberculosis is both an important human pathogen and an extremely slow growing bacterium. As a consequence of the latter property, diagnosis of antibiotic resistance in *M. tuberculosis* can take far longer than can be clinically desirable. To reduce the duration of this process, such as down to on the order of a few days, a number of groups have explored the use of phages as indicators of *M. tuberculosis* metabolic activity in the presence of antibiotics. Here reduced bacterial metabolic activity, as a consequence of antibiotic exposure, is assumed to correlate with reduced phage infection activity, activity as measured by various means. In this subsection I review a sampling of this literature, which mostly is supportive of and indeed premised upon the idea that antibiotics can be antagonistic to phage infection activities.

3.1.1. Jacobs et al., 1993, *Mycobacterium tuberculosis*, Various Antibiotics

A luciferase-encoding reporter phage was developed by Jacobs et al. [69], based on the *Mycobacterium smegmatis* phage TM4, with a goal of assessing gene expression during infection of *M. tuberculosis* in the presence of antibiotic. They found that after 48 h of antibiotic incubation, luciferase expression is knocked out when the treated bacteria are antibiotic susceptible but not when bacteria instead are antibiotic resistant. In this case, the antibiotics were isoniazid (1 μg/mL), rifampin (2 μg/mL), or streptomycin (6 μg/mL). As this was a luciferase-based test, light output would be dependent not just on reporter-gene expression following phage infection but also on ATP levels within the infected bacteria, levels of both which should positively correlate with phage infection activity (i.e., more phage gene expression and more intracellular ATP should both result in greater phage infection activity). A multiplicity of 1000 was employed and 80-fold greater luminescence was reported without either rifampin (2 μg/mL) or streptomycin (6 μg/mL) present, and ten-fold greater without isoniazid (1 μg/mL), thus indicating substantial inhibitions of phage infection activity by these antibiotics. These results were not correlated in this study with MICs, however.

3.1.2. Wilson et al., 1997, *Mycobacterium tuberculosis*, Isoniazid and Rifampin

Wilson et al. [70] used phage D29 to measure virion production in the presence and absence of antibiotic while infecting *M. tuberculosis*. Phage plaque formation after termination of antibiotic treatment was used as an indicator of phage virion production, with *Mycobacterium smegmatis* serving as the plaquing indicator bacterial strain. Antibiotic treatments prior to phage addition (~10^9 PFU/mL in situ concentration) consisted of three days of incubation in the presence of isoniazid at concentrations of 2 μg/mL or rifampin at concentrations of 4 μg/mL (resistance was defined as an ability to grow in the presence of 2 μg/mL or more and 1 μg/mL or more, respectively). Generally, plaque formation was associated, as expected, with bacterial antibiotic resistance while no plaque formation was seen given antibiotic sensitivity, as was found to be true for 44 of 46 isolates tested. The two outlying *M. tuberculosis* isolates were reportedly rifampin-susceptible but nevertheless able to support phage virion production despite the antibiotic's presence. Equivalent concordance of potential to support plaque formation, and isoniazid resistance versus sensitivity, was seen for 40 of 46 isolates tested: two otherwise resistant strains failed to support plaque growth in the presence of isoniazid, while four susceptible isolates did support plaque growth. Generally, then, prior antibiotic treatment was found to interfere with the ability of antibiotic-susceptible but not antibiotic-resistant bacteria to support the production of at least one phage virion, though with some exceptions. Of possible relevance to these exceptions, standard MIC determinations were done over one- to two-week periods while antibiotic treatment prior to phage infection was for a total of three days.

3.1.3. Galí et al., 2003, *Mycobacterium tuberculosis*, Rifampin

Galí et al. [71] used microtiter plates to treat *M. tuberculosis* isolates with rifampin (5 μg/mL) and then with phage D29 (10^7 PFU/mL). Bacteria were incubated in the presence of antibiotic for 24 h and then in the presence of phages for 90 min at 37 °C. After inactivation of unadsorbed phages, the production of new phages was detected via spot assays (application of 10 μL of potentially phage-containing culture to a growing lawn of *M. smegmatis* [86]). In the presence of rifampin, all rifampin-resistant *M. tuberculosis* isolates supported phage virion production whereas none of the rifampin-susceptible isolates did. This is an indication that antibiotic presence interfered with the ability of antibiotic-susceptible bacteria to support phage virion production. A rifampin-negative, spotting-positive control was performed for each bacterial isolate tested to rule out phage failure to infect independent of rifampin presence. MICs were not reported. See McNerney [87] for a formal protocol of this approach.

3.1.4. McNerney et al., 2007, *Mycobacterium tuberculosis*, Rifampin

McNerney et al. [72] developed a colorimetric, microtiter plate-based approach using 3-(4,5-dimethylthiazol-2-yl)-2,5-diphenyltetrazolium bromide (MTT) dye towards assaying the impact of *M. tuberculosis* exposure to rifampin on phage D29 virion production. In this assay, colorimetrically indicated *M. smegmatis* culture-clearing (in the absence of antibiotic) was the indicator that phage virion-production had previously occurred in association with overnight rifampin-treated *M. tuberculosis*. This broth-based *M. smegmatis* clearing was compared with a plaquing-based determination of virion production, also post antibiotic exposure. In a small fraction of cases, phage virion production was seen given 2 μg/mL rifampin treatment of *M. tuberculosis* but not at 10 μg/mL. In most cases those bacterial strains deemed rifampin-susceptible, as based on genome sequence information, gave rise to blocked phage virion production even at the lower rifampin density (at least 70 out of 85). In one case, however, phage virion production was seen even at the higher rifampin concentration. As with all of the studies so far described, results predominantly were consistent with a lack of phage infection activity given bacteria exposure to antibiotic. MIC for *M. tuberculosis* strains were not reported.

3.1.5. Pholwat et al., 2012, *Mycobacterium tuberculosis*, Various Antibiotics

Pholwat et al. [73] used qPCR to detect phage D29 virion production given *M. tuberculosis* exposure to several different antibiotics: amikacin, capreomycin, cycloserine, ethambutol, ethionamide, isoniazid, kanamycin, linezolid, moxifloxacin, ofloxacin, para-aminosalicylic acid, rifampin, and streptomycin. As part of this analysis, it was found that treatment with rifampin for 3, 6, 24, or 48 h prior to 24 h of phage treatment yielded substantially less phage signal with rifampin-susceptible versus rifampin-resistant bacteria. Equivalent treatment with isoniazid by contrast revealed a delay in impact. That is, 3- and 6-hour pre-incubations yielded similar phage signal as seen with a multidrug-resistant control, but by 24 and 48 h of antibiotic pre-incubation there was substantially less phage signal.

The difference in the impacts of the two drugs is accounted for by differences in their modes of action, with one acting bacterial cell-internally—where drug concentrations tend to be particularly relevant (rifampin inhibits RNA polymerase)—and the other acting by inhibiting cell-wall synthesis, where duration of drug exposure is also a key variable (in addition, bacteria potentially may have been dead before they were reached by phages after 24 or 48 h of antibiotic pre-incubation). Nevertheless, and contrary to the rest of the results reviewed in this section, this observation of delayed effects with isoniazid is consistent with phage production despite substantial antibiotic pre-treatment of susceptible bacteria, which in turn is suggestive that not all combinations of phage types, antibiotic types, antibiotic concentrations, and durations of pre-incubation will necessarily result in blocks on phage antibacterial activity, even if MICs are exceeded.

The antibiotic concentrations used were those provided by the World Health Organization as "critical concentrations", that is, the amount required to observe therapeutic effects in patients given treatment of drug-susceptible bacteria. Experiments with all of the above-listed antibiotics—given 48-h pre-incubation and 24-h phage exposure—were consistent with a strong concordance between qPCR-based predictions of phage propagation and non-phage-based determinations of drug sensitivity versus resistance (concordance was mostly 100% but was 97% for capreomycin and 82% for ethionamide). These data, as with those seen in previous studies and except given insufficient duration of pre-incubation with isoniazid, are consistent with antibiotic-associated inhibition of phage virion production.

3.1.6. Summary of Studies of *Mycobacterium tuberculosis* Phages

Overall, exploration of inhibition of phage infection activity in the presence of antibiotic, particularly employing the antibiotic, rifampin, has been extensive using *M. tuberculosis* as a host. Indeed, in 2010 a meta-analysis based on 31 different studies was published on the subject by Minion and Pai [88]. Limitations of these various studies to the question of whether antibiotic treatment can generally interfere with phage infection activity, however, is their use of *M. tuberculosis* as phage hosts versus additional bacterial types, relatively limited phage choice, and also questions concerning bacterial viability following long pre-incubations with antibiotic. Especially the first two of these limitations are addressed in the following two sub-sections.

3.2. *RNA Polymerase Inhibitors and Non-Mycobacterium Phages*

Because rifampin is an inhibitor of host RNA polymerase, any phages which carry their own RNA polymerase within their virions, deliver this enzyme upon adsorption, and otherwise do not require their host's RNA polymerase during infections may not be susceptible to rifampin treatments of bacteria. Sensitivity would be in terms of rifampin inhibiting virion production ability, and phage resistance would be seen even when host bacteria are rifampin susceptible. In particular, phage φKZ of *Pseudomonas aeruginosa* is able to replicate, producing virions more or less normally in the presence of 400 μg/mL of rifampin, which is a concentration of rifampin that completely inhibits the growth of a different phage, LUZ19 [74]. Phage φKZ also possesses putative phage-encoding RNA polymerase genes and seems to lack host promoter sequences. With *Bacillus subtilis* phage PBS2, equivalent results were seen with rifampin treatment (20 or 100 μg/mL added 2 or 5 min prior to phage infection; MIC ≤ 1 μg/mL) and also with host RNA polymerase-inhibiting streptolydigin and streptovaricin, but not with the DNA-binding, RNA-synthesis inhibiting actinomycin D and lucanthone antibiotics [89]. Missing from these studies, however, are robust indications of the sensitivity of uninfected host bacteria to the same levels of antibiotic as applied to phage infections, i.e., they are lacking formal determinations of MICs. Numerous other phages have been found instead to be susceptible to these various RNA polymerase-inhibiting antibiotics, rifampin, rifamycin, or streptovaricin, including at MIC-level concentrations. These latter phages are considered in this subsection and to a degree in the next section as well. Although several studies explore the impact of these various drugs on RNA- or ssDNA-genomed phages, emphasis here is placed on dsDNA phages.

3.2.1. Geiduschek and Sklar, 1969, *Bacillus subtilis*, Rifamycin

Geiduschek and Sklar [75] found that phage SPO1 of *B. subtilis* fails to lyse or produce new virion particles given exposure to 1 μg/mL rifamycin starting eight min prior to phage addition (MOI = 5). Both lysis and new virion production occurred more or less normally under the same conditions given infection of rifamycin-resistant mutants of the same host. Under these same conditions, the host was found to be unable to synthesize RNA transcripts as measured via incorporation of ^{3}H uridine. Phage replication also could be blocked given a 2-min but not a 6-min delay between phage adsorption and rifamycin addition (phage addition followed by antibiotic addition), implying that sufficient transcription of phage genes had occurred by 6 minutes to allow the phage to carry out the rest of its life cycle. Phage replication thus is highly impacted by levels of rifamycin which also block host RNA synthesis. MICs for either rifamycin-susceptible or -resistant hosts, however, are not provided.

3.2.2. Hemphill et al., 1969, *Bacillus subtilis*, Rifampin

Hemphill et al. [76] looked at burst sizes by phage β22 of *B. subtilis*. These phages were more or less fully inhibited by rifampin (10 μg/mL) when added sooner after the start of phage infection (MOI

= 4) but only partially inhibited by rifampin when added later after the start of phage infection. Burst sizes were less than 1% of those without rifampin addition but increased substantially given rifampin addition at 35 min into infection cycles. MICs were not reported.

3.2.3. Takeda et al., 1969, *Escherichia coli*, Rifampin

Takeda et al. [77] explored the potential for rifampin to interfere with phage λvir infection activity (MOI = 5). *E. coli* was treated with 25 μg/mL rifampin. With a rifampin-susceptible host, "phage growth" was reported as being "<10% of normal" in the presence of rifampin, while "normal" phage growth occurred in rifampin's absence. Of interest, two hosts which are reported as displaying slight growth given exposure to this concentration of rifampin also are indicated as allowing "±" phage growth ("20–50% of normal"). Although not explicitly indicated, I assume that it is phage burst size that is being measured as "phage growth", indicated as determined via single-step growth experiments [90,91], with ± phage growth also associated with "somewhat" delayed lysis. RNA synthesis during phage infection also dramatically declined following addition of 50 μg/mL rifampin 15 min into the infection cycle. These results are indicative of interference by rifampin with phage infection activity. They also indicate intermediate levels of interference in association with intermediate rifampin impact on the replication of host bacteria. The latter is suggestive of these antibiotic concentrations being lower than MIC, at least as approximated under the conditions employed ("slight . . . growth after overnight incubation").

3.2.4. Sokolova et al., 1970, *Escherichia coli*, Rifampin and Streptolydigin

Sokolova et al. [78] explored the impact of rifampin and streptolydigin on phage T2 infection (MOI << 1) of both antibiotic-susceptible and -resistant *E. coli*. Absent either drug, burst size was on the order of 200 in the doubly susceptible bacterium (rifampin and streptolydigin) but only 100 in the doubly resistant bacterium, suggesting existence of costs in phage infection activity associated with host antibiotic resistance. With susceptible bacteria, addition of either drug at 100 μg/mL, immediately after phage adsorption, in amounts which appear to exceed MICs, reduced burst sizes to negligible (1% of no treatment), whereas a 10-min delay in drug addition reduced burst sizes instead to 5% of no treatment.

3.2.5. Beckman et al., 1972, *Escherichia coli*, Rifampin

Beckman et al. [79] determined the impact of rifampin (400 μg/mL, present from the start of phage adsorption) on *E. coli* phage T5 under single-step growth conditions. Burst sizes were reduced from 120 without rifampin down to zero with. Little impact was seen with rifampin-resistant hosts. MICs were not reported.

3.2.6. Toussaint and Lecocq, 1975, *Escherichia coli*, Rifampin

Toussaint and Lecocq [80] induced phage Mu lysogens of *E. coli*, applied rifampin (100 μg/mL), and then assayed for phage virion production. This production was "blocked completely" with addition up to 15 min into the induced infection cycle. Inhibition of phage virion production was not observed, however, with a rifampin-resistant bacterial host. MIC for the *E. coli* host was not determined.

3.2.7. Riveros-Moreno, 1975, *Pseudomonas* BAL-31, rifampin

Riveros-Moreno [81] employed phage PM2 (MOI = 10) of *Pseudomonas* BAL-31 and 0.3 μg/mL rifampin. Burst sizes were reduced to less than 1% given simultaneous (time 0) rifampin addition. The *Pseudomonas* BAL-31 MIC for rifampin is not indicated.

3.2.8. Blasdel et al., 2017, *Pseudomonas aeruginosa*, rifampin

Blasdel et al. [82] found that 100 µg/mL rifampin, added 10 min prior to phages PAK_P3 or PAK_P4 (added at MOI = 1), blocked their "amplification". MIC was not reported.

3.2.9. Summary of Studies of RNA Polymerase Inhibitors and Non-*Mycobacterium* Phages

These various results are consistent with RNA polymerase-inhibiting antibiotics interfering with infections by different non-*M. tuberculosis* phages. Exceptional were certain phages whose virions appear to carry non-host, otherwise not antibiotic-susceptible RNA polymerases into newly infected bacteria. Otherwise, production of new virions often appears to be completely blocked in the presence of these various drugs. Unfortunately, however, it is difficult to correlate most of these phage infection-inhibition results, and associated antibiotic concentrations, with the MICs of host bacteria. Therefore, the major conclusion is that given sufficient concentrations of antibiotic, then phage infection activity can be blocked by rifampin, but it remains uncertain whether incubation, e.g., with 1× MIC, would result in equivalent interference. In addition, simply phage bactericidal activity was not measured in these experiments, also such as at 1× or greater MIC. That is, it is conceivable that phage antibacterial activities could be retained even at antibiotic concentrations that nevertheless are able to interfere with phage virion production.

3.3. *Inhibition of Phage Infection Activity by Other Antibiotics*

3.3.1. Taketo and Watanabe, 1967, *Escherichia coli*, Nalidixic Acid

Taketo and Watanabe [83] reported that nalidixic acid at concentrations that were able to reduce *E. coli* CFUs after 60-min of exposure, and thereby presumably exceeded MIC (50 µg/mL), were also able to nearly or fully prevent the production of virions both by double-stranded phages (T2 and T5) and by single-stranded DNA phages (φR and φX174), but did not prevent the production of virions by RNA phages (β or 10). In these experiments, antibiotic was added 7 min after phages, with bacteria lysed by chloroform 60 min after antibiotic addition and prior to plating. The inhibition of phage T2 was, however, reversible given suspension of phage-infected bacteria into antibiotic-free media. Therefore, nalidixic acid appears to only reversibly inhibit phage bactericidal and indeed virion production ability, at least after 1-hour incubations with the antibiotic. Nalidixic acid, like ciprofloxacin, is an inhibitor of DNA gyrase and topoisomerase. Therefore, these experiments suggest a substantial impact of inhibition of DNA gyrase or topoisomerase on phage replication, though with caveats as well as corroborations as presented by Baird et al. [84], discussed as follows.

3.3.2. Baird et al., 1972, *Escherichia coli*, Nalidixic Acid

Baird et al. [84] adsorbed phages (MOI < 1) for 5 to 7 min before exposing them also to 50 µg/mL nalidixic acid. They observed nearly consistent results with those of Taketo and Watanabe [83] for phage φR and perhaps for phage T5 as well. They also observed complete inhibition of *E. coli* phage T7 also using 50 µg/mL nalidixic acid and over 95% burst-size reduction with 10 µg/mL. The Baird et al. results for phage T2, however, seem to contradict those of Taketo and Watanabe, with burst size 34% of that without antibiotic. A possible explanation for this discrepancy is that of a need for prior equilibration of the antibiotic with bacterial cells, where a 30-min pre-incubation reduced burst sizes of phage T4—which was impacted identically to that of phage T2 given no pre-incubation—to only 2% of the burst without antibiotic treatment.

Inconsistently, no such pre-incubation was employed by Taketo and Watanabe. Baird et al. suggest, however, that adsorption by newly released virions—following lysis but prior to chloroform treatment at 60 min—could explain the loss of phage viability in the Taketo and Watanabe experiments as those authors did not dilute their infective centers in the course of their experiments, with naturally released virions therefore likely to have infected new bacteria, and thus may have been killed upon chloroform treatment. This hypothesis was tested and confirmed by Baird et al. In a separate experiment, the burst size of phage λ following induction was 2.5% that of the no-antibiotic control given dilution into 50 μg/mL nalidixic acid 7 min following the start of induction. This result suggests possibly a complete blockage of virion production given sufficient antibiotic pre-incubation. Although the Baird et al. results are not fully consistent with those of Taketo and Watanabe, they nevertheless are suggestive of a blocking, perhaps in full given sufficient pre-incubation with antibiotic, of virion production by at least some phages by the presence of 50 μg/mL nalidixic acid, though MIC was not determined.

3.3.3. Valério et al., 2017, *Escherichia coli*, Various Antibiotics

Valério et al. [85] observed an absence of either phage-mediated killing of *E. coli* or phage ECA2 (10^7 PFU/mL) population growth while in the presence of chloramphenicol or tetracycline at 1× MIC. They also observed an absence of phage population growth and probably a lack of phage-mediated bacteria killing in the presence of 1× MIC ciprofloxacin. Although these experiments were performed in phosphate-buffered saline, nevertheless phage population growth was substantial (1 log) and bacterial population growth occurred as well (up to 4 log), both in the absence of antibiotic presence. Therefore, the Valério et al. results are consistent with antibiotic interfering with phage infection activity, but possibly some of the observed antibiotic interference with phage infection activity was intensified given the low nutrient conditions that presumably were present during experiments.

3.3.4. Summary of Studies of Inhibition of Phage Infection Activity by Other Antibiotics

The primary take-home message from this subsection are those of Baird et al. [84], finding that nalidixic acid can reduce the burst sizes of dsDNA phages, particularly given sufficient equilibration of antibiotic with bacteria prior to addition of phages. Taketo and Watanabe [83] failed to observe a similar inhibition of RNA phages by nalidixic acid.

3.4. Antibiotic Interference with Phage Pharmacodynamics, Conclusions

Given that phage bactericidal activity in the presence of antibiotics—antibiotics to which targeted bacteria are susceptible—can be difficult assess (Section 2), it is not surprising that there is a tendency among studies to focus instead on antibiotic-mediated diminishment of virion production. It is important to recognize, however, that at a minimum phage therapy efficacy requires only bactericidal activity (for so-called passive treatments) rather than necessarily virion production as well (for so-called active treatments) [92–96] (see Figure 1). Therefore, even evidence of dramatic reductions in phage virion production in the presence of antibiotics does not imply also a phage inability to contribute to the treatment of antibiotic-susceptible bacteria, also in the presence of antibiotic. Furthermore, we can speculate that under more complex treatment scenarios, such as of biofilms as considered in the following section, the bacteria most impacted by phages may be those that simply happen to be least impacted by antibiotics (Section 2). Therefore, we can question to what degree the findings reviewed in this section—that antibiotics can substantially interfere with phage infection activities—are highly relevant to phage therapy efficacy, especially phage therapy as involving application of relatively high phage doses (thereby allowing passive treatment), and particularly so given the lack of associated MIC determinations in many studies.

At the same time, these experiments, as listed in Table 1 and reviewed in this section, point to a utility, towards at least better appreciating potential in situ phage therapy pharmacodynamics, to assessing phage-antibiotic compatibility relatively early during the development of co-treatment protocols. This assessment can be accomplished, for example, by exploring single-step growth-type characteristics [90,91] in the presence of 1× MIC or greater antibiotic concentrations.

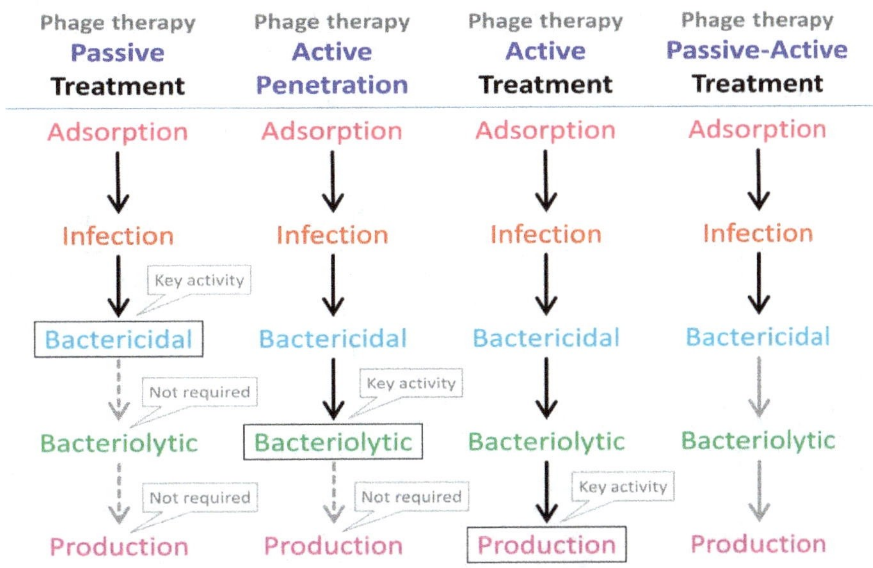

Figure 1. Progression of phage life cycles (top to bottom) and illustration of different phage therapy strategies (left to right) as requiring different degrees of phage infection activity. All terms refer to phage activities rather than antibiotic activities, including phage killing of bacteria (bactericidal), phage lysing of bacteria (bacteriolytic), and phage-infection generation and release of new virion particles (production). Boxes indicate key phage infection activities for a given strategy. Arrows indicate phage infection progressions from top to bottom, i.e., from bacterial adsorption, to bacterial infection, to bacteria killing, to lysing of bacteria, and then to release of new virions (production). Graying of arrows indicates a lack of requirement for this progression (dashed gray arrows) or lack of strict requirement (solid gray arrows) for a given phage therapy strategy (which are named across the top row). Passive treatment (first column) uses bacteria-overwhelming (inundative) phage dosing and thus requires only *bactericidal* activity from phage infections rather than necessarily also bacterial lysis or virion production. Active treatment (third column) does not use bacteria-overwhelming phage dosing so does require in situ phage virion *production*, often in substantial amounts. Active penetration (second column, but not otherwise discussed in the main text) is hypothesized as being involved in phage anti-biofilm activity and as being aided by phage *bacteriolytic* activity; it does not necessarily also require phage virion production. (Mixed) Passive-active treatment (fourth column, and also not otherwise discussed in the main text) is passive treatment that is hypothesized to be aided in its antibacterial activity by increases in phage numbers due to in situ phage virion production (solid gray arrows), which is unlike strictly passive treatments, which by definition do not necessarily involve such activities [94]. See Abedon and Thomas-Abedon [95] and Abedon [96,97] for review and further discussion. This figure is a modification of that presented in Abedon [97].

4. Evidence of Phage-Infection Compatibility with Antibiotic Treatment

It is perhaps a naïve assumption that—at 1× MIC for a given antibiotic—bacterial physiology will be sufficiently negatively affected that support of phage infection activity will always be fully curtailed. MIC determinations, that is, generally involve macroscopic evidence of bacterial growth after a defined length of incubation, i.e., the formation of turbid broth cultures or colonies on agar after some period of incubation [46]. This blocking of macroscopically visible culture growth, however, does not necessarily mean that the affected bacteria are completely inhibited in their metabolism at 1× MIC, nor that phage infection activity therefore should be completely curtailed. Furthermore, MICs are determined under specific experimental conditions that are not necessarily replicated when phage infections are being tested for activity in an antibiotic's presence. Less bacterial metabolic activity also may be required for a phage infection to be bactericidal than for it be bacteriolytic, and likely less metabolic activity to be bacteriolytic than to be virion productive. Therefore, e.g., a bacterial culture that is unable to replicate due to antibiotic presence, particularly antibiotic presence at approximately 1× MIC, might still be able to support, for example, phage-mediated bacteria killing, or even bacterial lysis or phage virion production. This section considers published evidence that one or more-fold MIC of antibiotic can still be compatible with phage infection activity, at least for some antibiotics under some conditions, though often with qualifications including as listed in this paragraph. Considered in this section are broth-culture, biofilm, and in vivo explorations of antibiotic impact on phage infection activities. See Table 2 for summary of the studies presented.

Table 2. Studies suggesting retention of phage infection activity in the presence of antibiotics[1,2].

Subsection	Host	Phage	Antibiotic	BC	BL	VP	LT	CT	Ref
Section 4.1.1	*B. subtilis*	SPO1	nalidixic acid		+	+	−		[98]
Section 4.1.2	*B. subtilis*	various [3]	nalidixic acid		+	+		?	[84]
Section 4.1.3	*B. subtilis*	SPP1	nalidixic acid		+		−	?	[99]
Section 4.1.4	*B. subtilis*	PBS2	nalidixic acid		+	−			[100]
Section 4.1.5	*M. aurum*	D29	various [4]			±		?	[101]
Section 4.1.6	*B. subtilis*	AR9	rifampin			+		?	[102]
Section 4.1.7	*R. solanacearum*	various [5]	rifampin			±		?	[68]
Section 4.1.8	*P. aeruginosa*	cocktail	various [6]			+			[103]
Section 4.1.9	*A. baumannii*	KARL-1	various [7]			+			[104]
Section 4.1.10	*E. coli*	ELY-1	ciprofloxacin			+			[105]
Section 4.2.1	*K. pneumoniae*	unnamed	amoxicillin			+		?	[106]
Section 4.2.2	*K. pneumoniae*	KPO1K2	ciprofloxacin			+		?	[107]
Section 4.2.3	*S. aureus*	SAP-26	various [8]	+					[108]
Section 4.2.4	*E. coli*	T4	tobramycin			+		?	[39]
Section 4.2.4	*P. aeruginosa*	PB-1	tobramycin			−		?	[39]
Section 4.2.5	*S. aureus*	MR-5	linezolid	+				?	[109]
Section 4.2.6	*K. pneumoniae*	KPO1K2	amikacin			±		?	[110]
Section 4.2.7	*P. aeruginosa*	various [9]	various [10]			±		?	[18]
Section 4.2.8	*S. aureus*	SATA-8505	various [11]			±		?	[111]
Section 4.2.9	*P. mirabilis*	vB_PmiS-TH	ampicillin	+					[112]
Section 4.2.10	*P. aeruginosa*	cocktail	ciprofloxacin	+				?	[113]
Section 4.2.11	*S. aureus*	PYO	various [12]			+		?	[34]
Section 4.2.12	*P. aeruginosa*	various [13]	ciprofloxacin			+		?	[114]
Section 4.3.1	*K. pneumoniae*	SS	amikacin			−		?	[115]
Section 4.3.2	*S. aureus*	MR-10	linezolid	−					[116]
Section 4.3.3	*S. aureus*	Sb-1	teicoplanin			+		?	[117]
Section 4.3.3	*P. aeruginosa*	vB_PsaP PAT14	various [14]			+		?	[118]
Section 4.3.4	*S. aureus*	MR-5	linezolid			+		?	[118]
Section 4.3.5	*P. aeruginosa*	cocktail	ciprofloxacin			+		?	[103]
Section 4.3.6	*E. coli*	unnamed	ciprofloxacin						[119]

[1] Shown are approximate summaries of primary take-home messages of studies regarding phage activities in the presence of approximately 1× MIC concentrations of antibiotics or higher. A '−' indicates a relative lack of phage infection activity (meaning a negative impact of antibiotic on phage infection a activity), a '+' indicates relative presence of phage infection activity (relative, that is, to no or very little activity at all; thus a relative lack of highly substantial negative impact of antibiotic on phage infection activity is indicated with a '+'), and '±' indicates multiple different results (some '+' results in combination with some not strictly '+' results, especially as when testing multiple phages or multiple antibiotics). Results are summarized in terms of phage bactericidal activity (BC), phage bacteriolytic activity (BL), and phage virion production (VP), or lysis timing (LT). For the latter, a '−' indicates lysis delay. Therefore, a mark of '−', across the table, tends to indicate negative impacts of antibiotic on phage infection activity. See the main text for relevant caveats regarding these summaries, as indicated in the column marked CT with a '¿. That is, a '?' indicates that relatively low negative impacts of antibiotics on phage infection activities as indicated by a given study may be somewhat debatable, though these caveats do not necessarily apply to all results provided by a given study, and nor have studies lacking an explicit indication of possible caveats necessarily either employed or indicated all possible relevant controls. Note that, for lytic phages, virion production implies bactericidal as well as bacteriolytic activity, though these properties are not indicated in the table unless they were explicitly measured in a study. Not presented in the table are the findings that phage φKZ of *P. aeruginosa* [74] and phage PBS2 of *B. subtilis* [89], both of which appear to be resistant to rifampin along with, for the latter, also other host RNA polymerase-inhibiting antibiotics, for both phages presumably as due to their apparently exclusive use of phage-carried, non-host RNA polymerase enzymes during infections (Section 3.2). [2] Generally, please use this table as a guide-only to what studies are discussed in this review rather than as a definitive indication of phage properties in the presence of antibiotics, as actual results tend to be more complex than can be summarized this concisely. [3] Section 4.1.2, phages tested individually: φ29, SP50, or SP82. [4] Section 4.1.5, antibiotics tested individually: clofazimine, colistin, dapsone, ethambutol, isoniazid, rifampin, or streptomycin. [5] Section 4.1.7, phages tested individually: ΦRP12 or ΦRP31, and also ΦRSB1, ΦRSL1, ΦRSL2, or ΦRPSF1. [6] Section 4.1.8, antibiotics tested individually: ciprofloxacin or meropenem. [7] Section 4.1.9, antibiotics tested individually: ciprofloxacin, colistin, or meropenem. [8] Section 4.2.3, antibiotics tested individually: azithromycin, rifampin, or vancomycin. [9] Section 4.2.7, phages tested individually: NP1 or NP3. [10] Section 4.2.7, antibiotics tested individually: ceftazidime, ciprofloxacin, colistin, gentamycin, or tobramycin. [11] Section 4.2.8, antibiotics tested individually: cefazolin, dicloxacillin, linezolid, tetracycline, or vancomycin. [12] Section 4.2.11, antibiotics tested individually: ciprofloxacin, daptomycin, erythromycin, gentamycin, linezolid, oxacillin, tetracycline, or vancomycin. [13] Section 4.2.12, phages tested individually: ΦPT-18[b], ΦPT-20[a], ΦPT-1S[a], ΦPT-5[a] or ΦPT-2[b]. [14] Section 4.3.3, antibiotics tested simultaneously: amikacin, cilastatin, and imipenem.

4.1. *Broth-Culture Experiments*

Broth-culture experiments have a utility of relative ease of execution, ready phage access to all bacteria present (assuming sufficient broth mixing), and relatively low physiological heterogeneity among those bacteria present. Ideally, experiments will explore the impact of measured 1× MIC or greater antibiotic concentrations on phage infection activity, with reporting of evidence for or against bactericidal, bacteriolytic, or phage virion production activities. Furthermore, characterizations of phage infection activities, at a minimum, should consist of phage single-step growth-like experiments [90,91], i.e., in which phage latent periods and burst sizes are determined, or instead other means by which phage bactericidal or bacteriolytic activities are directly measured. Here, with those issues in mind, I consider published broth-culture experiments that are suggestive of retention of phage pharmacodynamic impacts on bacteria in broth culture given antibiotic presence of 1× MICs or greater.

4.1.1. Gage and Fujita, 1969, *Bacillus subtilis*, Nalidixic Acid

Perhaps equivalent to observations of rifampin-resistant phages (Section 3.2), Gage and Fujita [98] found that *B. subtilis* phage SPO1 (MOI = 6) was able to display bacteriolysis and virion production in the presence of nalidixic acid (50 μg/mL), "at concentrations that drastically inhibited *B. subtilis* DNA synthesis". Latent periods, however, were approximately twice as long as without antibiotic, and burst sizes were reduced by roughly 30%. Consistent with display of this level of infection activity, the rates of DNA synthesis by antibiotic-treated, phage SPO1-infected bacteria were substantially higher than as seen with nalidixic acid treated, phage-uninfected bacteria: 0% vs 75% reductions at 5 μg/mL, respectively, and 30% vs 95% at 50 μg/mL. Nonetheless, and unfortunately, it is not possible from the data presented to conclude that antibiotic concentrations exceeded 1× MIC for the bacterial host.

4.1.2. Baird et al., 1972, *Bacillus subtilis*, Nalidixic Acid

Baird et al. [84] found, similarly to Gage and Fujita [98], that *B. subtilis* phages φ29, SP50, and SP82 displayed burst sizes of 75%, 44%, and 46% that of the no-nalidixic acid controls as well as lysis delays in the presence of 50 μg/mL nalidixic acid. It is possible, though, that this relatively insubstantial reduction in phage virion production in the presence of nalidixic acid is a consequence of delays in equilibration of antibiotic with bacteria, thereby representing less antibiotic impact on phage virion production than might otherwise occur at that concentration. Specifically, Baird et al. also found that phage T4's burst size infecting *E. coli* could be reduced from 34% to 2% of no antibiotic treatment given sooner exposure to antibiotic: delays of 5- to 7-min in antibiotic addition relative to phage addition (phages added first) versus 30 min delays in phage addition relative to antibiotic addition (antibiotic added first), respectively.

Baird et al. [84] also observed virion production activity by several additional phages also in the presence of nalidixic acid (φR, λ, T4, T5, and T7), though burst sizes tended to be somewhat reduced, with lysis delayed by 30 to 100 min. These latter observations come with the same concern as with phage T2—that antibiotic might not have been sufficiently equilibrated with bacteria prior to the start of phage infections to give rise to a full impact on phage infection activity. MICs were not reported.

4.1.3. Pedrini et al., 1972, *Bacillus subtilis*, Nalidixic Acid

Pedrini et al. [99] considered the impact of nalidixic acid on the infection of phage SPP1 of *B. subtilis*. The antibiotic concentrations used was able to "block completely the DNA replication" of that host. As tested, this included 10 μg/mL of the drug, though at least a 10-min incubation was required before DNA replication ceased. An MOI of 1.5 was used and lysis was followed by optical density (OD_{540}). While drops in OD, presumably as phage-induced, were fairly gradual, continuing for over at least a 100-min period, nevertheless with 10 μg/mL nalidixic acid added 10-min prior to phage addition, lysis kinetics were identical to as seen without the antibiotic present, and in the presence of 50 μg/mL nalidixic acid lysis was simply delayed by about 25 min rather than altered in the rate of lysis once begun. Phage SPP1 thus likely remains at least bacteriolytic even given exposure to nalidixic concentrations that are substantially more than that necessary to interfere with bacterial DNA replication. MIC for the host, though, was not reported.

4.1.4. Price and Fogt, 1973, *Bacillus subtilis*, Nalidixic Acid

Price and Fogt [100] observed a reduction in the burst size of *B. subtilis* phage PBS2 (MOI = 5) of approximately 90% in the presence of simultaneously added 50 μg/mL nalidixic acid, but with burst size seemingly further reduced given antibiotic addition 5- or 15-min prior to phage addition. This is suggestive of substantial blocking of phage virion production but also (again) that delays may exist in equilibration of the antibiotic into cells following its addition to cultures. At this concentration of drug, bacterial DNA replication seems to have been blocked in uninfected cells. The same concentration, however, delayed but did not block phage-induced culture lysis, indicating a retention of at least bacteriolytic activity and presumably bactericidal activity as well (and hence the inclusion of this result under evidence of phage-antibiotic compatibility). Burst size, however, appeared to be substantially reduced.

This observation of presumptive bactericidal and/or bacteriolytic activities makes sense to the extent that phage gene expression, and thereby production of lysis-inducing proteins, is able to persist even if phage DNA replication is blocked. Addition of 20 μg/mL of nalidixic acid, described as "low levels", by contrast blocked bacterial DNA replication in uninfected bacteria for over 70 min, but did not block bacterial DNA replication for over 90 min. This lower antibiotic concentration was associated with burst size reductions of about 50% given simultaneous phage and antibiotic addition, or greater reductions (~70%) when phages were added 5- or 15-min after antibiotic, though there was no associated delay in lysis. It is uncertain to what degree antibiotic concentrations of 50 μg/mL may have exceeded MIC. These results nevertheless are consistent with retention of at least some phage antibacterial activity despite nalidixic acid presence, and to a degree even retention of virion production by this phage in the presence of 50 μg/mL of this antibiotic.

4.1.5. David et al., 1980, *Mycobacterium aurum*, Various Antibiotics

David et al. [101] found that the concentration of isoniazid required to reduce phage burst sizes by 50% was over two orders of magnitude greater than the MIC for this drug (*Mycobacterium aurum* as host bacterium and infection by phage D29). This is consistent with cell-wall synthesis inhibitors requiring a fair amount of time before they affect bacterial functioning. For the antibiotic ethambutol, the equivalent ratio to MIC was so high that it was not determinable. This drug too is a cell-wall synthesis inhibitor. Dapsone gave about an order of magnitude greater phage inhibitory value (50% reduction in burst size) than the measured MIC. Although dapsone is not a cell-wall synthesis inhibitor, it is an enzyme inhibitor.

For all other antibiotics tested (clofazimine, colistin, rifampin, and streptomycin), ratios were closer to 1, suggesting indeed an inhibition of at least phage virion production at antibiotic concentrations close to MIC. Of these, colistin and streptomycin had the greatest impacts on phage virion production versus bacterial replication, with the ratio to MIC being 0.78 and 0.54, respectively, e.g., as versus 166 for isoniazid. The colistin result is potentially odd, however, given that this antibiotic too acts on the bacterial cell envelope rather than interfering internally, though then again mycobacteria do not have Gram negative cell envelopes, where Gram-negative pathogens and their outer membranes are the normal targets of colistin. These results are clearly indicative nevertheless of a potential—while infecting this bacterium—for this phage to replicate in the presence of certain antibiotics (dapsone, ethambutol, and isoniazid). A caveat, however, is that drugs were not added until after phage adsorption was considered to have occurred, and thus antibiotic was delayed in its addition, potentially resulting in greater phage infection activity than otherwise might have been seen versus, e.g., given pre-incubation of antibiotic.

4.1.6. Lavysh et al., 2017, *Bacillus subtilis*, Rifampin

Lavysh et al. [102] studied a *B. subtilis* phage, AR9, which displayed incomplete inhibition of phage virion production given infection exposure to rifampin (50 μg/mL). Indeed, in single-step growth experiments an approximately ten-fold reduction in burst size was reported, as representing a total of only about eight virions produced per phage-infected bacterium, though it is not obvious when antibiotic was applied relative to phages. Antibiotic concentrations at 50 μg/mL alone resulted, after 10-min exposure, also in ~100-fold reductions in cell viability. Therefore, the authors suggest that phage AR9 may in fact not be rifampin susceptible, e.g., as potentially due to the phage virion carrying its own RNA polymerase, but with the decrease in phage burst size related instead to cell killing by the antibiotic. This hypothesis would seem to be somewhat consistent with the indicated 1-log drop in pre-burst phage infective centers with rifampin treatment (their Figure S2), and this explanation would be rather than due to more specific inhibition by rifampin of phage functioning during infection.

Inconsistent with the infection death hypothesis, using a ~ten-fold less rifampin-susceptible host, Lavysh et al. [102] still see a roughly ten-fold drop in burst size with rifampin treatment, but without the pre-burst reduction in infective centers (again, their Figure S2). Interpretation of these results in terms of retention by phage AR9 of infection activity in the presence of rifampin therefore would appear to be complicated. Either what is being observed is reduced virion production in the presence of substantial amounts of rifampin, by a rifampin-susceptible phage, or instead a more general failure of host physiology affecting the burst size of an otherwise rifampin-resistant phage. Still, some phage virion production is observed in the presence of rifampin, though MICs for the hosts were not explicitly determined.

4.1.7. Matsui et al., 2017, *Ralstonia solanacearum*, Rifampin

Matsui et al. [68] tested the ability of phages ΦRP12 and ΦRP31 of *R. solanacearum* to replicate in the presence of up to 20 μg/mL of rifampin (MIC = 5 μg/mL). At 1× or 2× MIC, resulting titers were reduced by about one log, whereas at 4× MIC, i.e., 20 μg/mL, they were reduced by roughly 2 logs. The authors suggest that these results are an indication that these phages, like phage PBS2 of *B. subtilis* [89] or phage φKZ of *P. aeruginosa* [74], carry their own RNA polymerases, particularly as other phages they tested, ΦRSB1, ΦRSL1, ΦRSL2, and ΦRPSF1, were completely blocked in terms of phage virion production at 1× MIC. It is notable, however, that phage virion production for phages φKZ and PBS2 was demonstrated at much higher rifampin concentrations, i.e., 100 and 400 μg/mL, respectively, with relatively little decline in virion production, though unfortunately in neither of these latter cases was MIC reported. As no RNA polymerase was demonstrated for the *R. solanacearum* phages—unlike for phage φKZ, for which candidate subunits were identified and for which no bacterial promoters could be identified—it is more difficult to conclude that phages ΦRP12 and ΦRP31 truly carry their own enzyme within virions or instead for some reason are simply in some manner less susceptible to this antibiotic than the other phages tested.

4.1.8. Oechslin et al., 2017, *Pseudomonas aeruginosa*, Ciprofloxacin and Meropenem

Oechslin et al. [103] treated broth cultures of *P. aeruginosa* with combinations of a phage cocktail (10^8 PFU/mL) and either ciprofloxacin or meropenem (both at 2.5× MIC), presumably with each added simultaneously. After six hours of exposure, bacterial numbers were reduced by roughly 6 logs in both cases following either phage-only treatment or combined treatment, versus less than 1-log reductions by antibiotic alone, and approximately 1-log increases without treatment. As the calculated MOI was only 1, the 6-log declines in CFUs are indicative of phage virion production during treatments, both with and without antibiotic presence.

4.1.9. Jansen et al., 2018, *Acinetobacter baumannii*, Ciprofloxacin, Colistin, and Meropenem

Jansen et al. [104] followed broth cultures of *A. baumannii* for 16 h in the presence of phage KARL-1 added at various starting MOIs (all less than 1, the highest being 0.1) and various concentrations of the antibiotics ciprofloxacin, colistin, or meropenem (ranging from less than to more than MIC; the bacterial isolate used is described as multi-drug resistant, but nevertheless antibiotic concentrations used in experiments exceeded MICs, so this study is included here). With antibiotics alone there was substantial resulting culture turbidity at all treatment concentrations, though especially with ciprofloxacin there was some increasing reduction in turbidity with increasing antibiotic concentration. With phage-antibiotic combinations there generally was less turbidity at the end of experiments than with antibiotic alone, even starting with higher antibiotic concentrations (i.e., >MIC) or lower phage MOIs (down to 10^{-7}). Even if differences in end-point turbidities were a consequence of increased likelihoods of mutation to resistance without combination therapy versus with, these results are still suggestive of phage population growth in the presence of antibiotic since phage concentrations would need to exceed MOI = 1 for these combination treatment effects to be observed. What is uncertain, however, is whether this proposed phage population growth occurred in association with antibiotic-susceptible versus antibiotic-resistant bacteria. Their Figure S5, however, is at least suggestive that this latter hypothesis is not correct. Instead, it would appear that experimental conditions might have differed from those that were used to determine MICs such that antibiotic-susceptible bacteria nevertheless were able to at least increase in turbidity over time in the presence of all antibiotic concentrations tested, though mostly with less of an increase than as observed with the untreated control culture (colistin-treated cultures were an exception to this latter point, where increases in culture turbidity without phage treatment, with all but the highest colistin concentrations similar to the untreated control). The lower impact, i.e., higher resulting culture turbidities that were observed with the lowest starting phage MOIs (in combination with treatment with ciprofloxacin or colistin), seems to be due to delays in phage population growth to MOIs of greater than 1, that is, as associated with lower phage starting numbers, thereby resulting in less efficient culture clearing.

4.1.10. Lopes et al., 2018, *Escherichia coli*, Ciprofloxacin

Lopes et al. [105] found evidence of an over 1 log but nonetheless only transient (not long lived) increase in phage ELY-1 numbers in the presence of both 1× MIC ciprofloxacin and *E. coli*. In the same experiments, phage impact on the *E. coli* target in combination with ciprofloxacin was greater, by nearly 1 log, than ciprofloxacin impact alone, though phage-antibiotic combination treatments reduced bacterial numbers somewhat less than phage impact alone. As starting phage titers were only about 10^6 PFU/mL, these results, in combination, are consistent with the occurrence of some phage virion production in the presence of ciprofloxacin, at least at 1× MIC.

No increase in phage numbers was seen with 2× MIC ciprofloxacin, and this was versus an approximately 3-log increase in phage numbers without ciprofloxacin present. No difference in terms of impact on bacterial presence was observed with ciprofloxacin alone versus with phages present as well, also given antibiotic concentrations of 2× MIC. Therefore, overall, at least a small amount of phage virion production appears to be present at 1× MIC ciprofloxacin in this system, but not at 2× MIC.

4.1.11. Summary of Evidence of Phage Infection Activity in Broth in the Presence of Antibiotics

The results presented in this subsection are consistent with at least some phage infection activity in broth bacterial cultures, and specifically phage virion production at antibiotic concentrations of at least 1× MIC. Evidence is also provided that positive phage infection-activity results can be reduced given longer pre-incubations of antibiotic with bacteria prior to phage application. Furthermore, while bacteriolytic activity can be retained in the presence of antibiotic, burst sizes also can be reduced and latent periods extended. Different phages also appear to display different levels of sensitivity to antibiotic presence. In my opinion, the primary take-home messages of this subsection are that antibiotics at concentrations that inhibit bacterial replication do not necessarily also fully interfere with phage infection activity, including in terms of virion production, but that it is important to confirm that this result is retained even given delays between antibiotic addition and subsequent phage addition.

4.2. Biofilm Experiments

A number of studies have been recently published that employ combinations of phages and antibiotics to treat in vitro-grown bacterial biofilms. Interpretation of results of these experiments, in terms of phage-antibiotic interactions and resulting pharmacodynamics, can however be challenging due to the possible heterogeneity of these cultures in terms of the susceptibility of individual bacteria to phages, antibiotic, or both. In addition is the issue of the potential for phages to carry biofilm-matrix degrading enzymes including in association with virions (Section 2). Biofilms also can be notoriously tolerant of even high densities of antibiotic, e.g., [52,54,111], where antibiotic impact in any case can be highly dependent on the conditions a bacterium is experiencing [46,59]. Various phage impacts on the presence of biofilm bacteria are discussed in this subsection in terms of possible retention of phage infection activity despite antibiotic co-treatments.

4.2.1. Bedi et al., 2009, *Klebsiella pneumoniae*, Amoxicillin

Bedi et al. [106] found somewhat greater phage impact in the presence of 2× MIC amoxicillin on *K. pneumoniae* one-day-old biofilms—in terms of reductions in numbers of CFUs—than with either phage or antibiotic treatment alone (the name of the phage used does not appear to have been specified by the authors). This result is suggestive of retention of phage anti-biofilm activity despite antibiotic presence. Given that phage doses were of only MOI = 0.01, this result is consistent also with phage virion production in association with the treated biofilm. Note however the potential for heterogeneity in bacterial physiology or in antibiotic susceptibility within biofilms, or indeed the potential for antibiotic to decay over time, which makes it difficult to tell whether the individual bacteria supporting such phage virion production were also bacteria that at the same time were highly affected by antibiotic. Furthermore, amoxicillin as a cell-wall synthesis-inhibiting antibiotic potentially allows phage infection until bacteria either have been killed or nearly killed by amoxicillin activity.

A concern with experiments in which treatments take place overnight or longer is the potential for regrowth of biofilm by resistant bacteria (Section 2). That is, given a combination of phage and antibiotic application, the likelihood of mutation to resistance to both agents typically would be lower than the likelihood of bacterial mutation to resistance to each agent individually (e.g., 10^{-5} mutations per cell division versus 10^{-10}). As a result, differences in numbers of CFUs between antibiotic-only and phage-plus-antibiotic treatments, particularly for experiments done within relatively small volumes, could be due solely to regrowth of antibiotic-resistant bacteria (e.g., 10^{-5} mutations per cell division) but no regrowth of bacteria that are both phage and antibiotic resistant (e.g., 10^{-10} double mutations per cell division). In other words, differences in numbers of CFUs at the point of bacterial enumeration could be due to one treatment having a greater potential for biofilm elimination to be reversed over time (because of growth of resistant bacteria), and this is rather than due to differences in more immediate pharmacodynamic antibacterial impacts.

Phage population growth and therefore virion production nevertheless still must have occurred in the Bedi et al. [106] experiments given the low initial phage MOI used, that is, for phage numbers to have become sufficiently high to interfere with bacterial resistance evolution in the course of the phage-plus-antibiotic treatment. Therefore, even given the potential for regrowth of bacterial resistance mutants, these results should still be consistent with phage virion production in the presence of what at least initially was 2× MIC amoxicillin. Again, however, it remains uncertain to what degree the individual bacteria supporting this presumed phage virion production were fully affected by the antibiotic treatment, e.g., such as due to antibiotic decay over time.

4.2.2. Verma et al., 2009, *Klebsiella pneumoniae*, Ciprofloxacin

Verma et al. [107] treated 12-hour *K. pneumoniae* biofilms with a combination of phage KPO1K2 (MOI = 1) and ciprofloxacin (10 μg/mL; MIC for planktonic bacteria = 0.625 μg/mL). Ciprofloxacin after 0.5 to 3 h of treatment reduced biofilm CFUs by roughly 1 log. This reduction, however, is relative to the untreated control rather than to bacterial densities that were present at the start of treatments. Ciprofloxacin at this density thus likely was preventing biofilm growth, but otherwise may not have actually reduced bacterial numbers. Reductions associated with phage treatment were roughly 3 to 4 log relative to the bacterial concentrations at the start of treatment, and these amounts were regardless of whether antibiotic was present. Such levels of reduction would appear to be consistent not only with display by this phage of bactericidal activity in the presence of antibiotic, but with phage virion production as well, i.e., as an MOI of 1 alone is insufficient to result in multi-log reductions in bacterial densities.

An alternative hypothesis is that phage presence resulted in reduced resistance by biofilm to removal during washing, with washing preceding enumeration of biofilm bacteria. In particular, phage KPO1K2 was found to give rise to a substantial halo surrounding plaques [120], as is suggestive of phage encoding of biofilm-matrix degrading enzyme. These results, particularly absent explicit documentation of phage population growth in association with ciprofloxacin, thus should be viewed as inconclusive in terms of assessing either phage bactericidal or virion production abilities in the presence of antibiotic.

4.2.3. Rahman et al., 2011, *Staphylococcus aureus*, Azithromycin, Rifampin, and Vancomycin

Rahman et al. [108], using 10× MIC rifampin against 24-h *S. aureus* biofilm, observed approximately 1-log greater biofilm reduction in terms of CFUs with phage SAP-26 presence than without. This difference was seen after 8 h of treatment, but not after 4 h, and continued through 12 and 24 h. As the phage titer appeared to be in excess of 10^8 PFU/mL (and I speculate was in fact 10^9 PFU/mL as 10^8 PFU seem to have been suspended in 100 μL), these results are indicative of phage anti-biofilm activity, and possibly phage bactericidal activity, but not necessarily also phage bacteriolytic or virion production activity.

Greater killing with phages being present than without phages being present, in both cases in the presence of rifampin, was also seen after 24 h of treatment as determined via a 2, 3, 5-triphenyltetrazolium chloride-based assay. Here, however, differences were only about two-fold, i.e., ~72%, ~60%, and ~35% cells living given phage-only, rifampin-only, or phage-plus-rifampin treatments. For azithromycin, these numbers instead are ~72%, ~75%, and ~40%, also suggesting phage activity compatibility with the presence of antibiotic. With vancomycin the numbers instead are ~72%, ~83%, and ~60%, which is less convincing of such compatibility of phage infection activity with antibiotic presence.

4.2.4. Coulter et al., 2014, *Escherichia coli* and *Pseudomonas aeruginosa*, Tobramycin

Coulter et al. [39] found that tobramycin (2 μg/mL) was able to reduce 48-h *E. coli* biofilm bacterial numbers by about 2.5 log relative to an untreated control. In the presence of both phage T4 and the antibiotic, however, an approximately 6.5-log reduction in biofilm bacteria numbers was observed. This result should be indicative of phage population growth since the starting phage MOI was 0.01, which on its own at best should result in a killing of about 1% of the bacteria present (Section 2). An equivalent experiment in the same study with *P. aeruginosa* and phage PB-1 (and 0.5 μg/mL tobramycin), by contrast, yielded somewhat weaker evidence of phage activity in the presence of tobramycin.

4.2.5. Kaur et al., 2014, *Staphylococcus aureus*, Linezolid

Kaur et al. [109] is a prevention of bacterial surface adherence study (*S. aureus*). Phage MR-5 and linezolid were applied to orthopedic-grade stainless steel Kirschner wires, with colony counts of adhered bacteria made after 6-, 24-, and 48-hs of incubation in the presence of bacteria. Both phage and antibiotic were applied to wires within hydroxypropyl methylcellulose hydrogels. Linezolid alone (5% *w/w*) and phages alone (1.5×10^9 PFU/mL) allowed similar levels of bacterial colonization of wires. A combination of the two agents, however, resulted in about 1-log less colonization (all statistically significantly different from colonization of untreated wires). Bacteria which failed to encounter or be affected by linezolid upon attempting to adhere to wire surfaces thus seemingly could instead have encountered a phage, resulting in the additional reduction in CFUs.

The implication of this result is retention of phage bactericidal activity in the presence of the antibiotic. Presumably, however, for phages to contribute to reducing bacterial colonization of wires, then it would have been those bacteria which were least impacted by linezolid that would have been most affected by phages, else those bacteria should have been sufficiently impacted by linezolid that phage infection would not have resulted in excess bacterial losses (that is, a phage cannot be solely responsible for preventing colonization by an individual bacterium if that colonization also has been prevented by linezolid). That interpretation would call into question whether phage activity truly was retained given individual bacteria exposure to at least an MIC of antibiotic, with antibiotic concentration otherwise reported as "much higher than the MIC level". It is also conceivable that phages were able to better gain access to bacteria and/or for subsequent bacteria killing to have occurred in the course of bacterial enumeration [121], i.e., as following biofilm disruption, rather than within hydrogels, again calling into question whether phage bactericidal activity was retained in the presence of substantially antibiotic-affected bacteria. In any case, as wires and bacteria were suspended in phosphate-buffered saline during experiments, presumably phage infection activity, and also antibiotic activity, may not have been robust, regardless, until the enumeration step.

4.2.6. Singla et al., 2016, *Klebsiella pneumoniae*, Amikacin

Singla et al. [110] treated *K. pneumoniae* biofilm grown on microtiter plates with a combination of phage KPO1K2 (MOI = 1 relative to bacterial density found in untreated biofilm) and amikacin (40 μg/mL). Phages were either free or liposome entrapped upon application to biofilms, and biofilms were grown between one and seven days prior to the start treatment. The impact of antibiotic generally was less than that of phages, though not necessarily statistically significantly less, and free phages may have been slightly less effective as anti-biofilm agents than liposome-entrapped phages, depending on the age of the biofilm. That antibiotic treatment alone resulted in reductions in bacterial numbers found in biofilms, however, is suggestive that the dose of amikacin employed exceeded MIC, though MIC was not otherwise determined. Treated biofilms generally had bacterial counts that were closer to those of the negative-treatment controls, the older the treated biofilm, ranging from over 3-log reductions for one-day-old biofilms to roughly 1-log reductions for seven-day-old biofilms (the latter not statistically significant especially in terms of free phage or antibiotic impact).

Experiments by Singla et al. [110] consisting of phage treatment in combination with antibiotic were done without phage-only or antibiotic-only controls. In comparing these experiments with separate individual-treatment experiments (i.e., as discussed in the previous paragraph), it would appear that there was little difference between the impact of free phages and antibiotic added in combination versus acting alone. When treatment phages were entrapped in liposomes, however, then the combination of phages and antibiotic resulted in bacterial counts which were reduced by an additional 1 log or more. This latter result is at least suggestive of phage bactericidal activity. Given that an MOI of 1 should result in at best only 63% of the bacteria initially becoming phage infected (a 0.43 log reduction; Section 2), this result is suggestive also that phage virion production in the presence of antibiotic may have occurred, though the occurrence of such growth was not explicitly determined.

Why this possible phage virion production should have occurred in the presence of antibiotic especially in the case where phages were liposome entrapped, but not without liposome entrapment, is uncertain. This is especially uncertain given that, when phages were employed without antibiotic present, reductions in bacterial numbers ranged, as noted, from 1- to 3-log (differences between results of treatment with and without liposome entrapment in the presence of amikacin was not determined in terms of statistical significance). Therefore, these experiments appear to be consistent with phage bactericidal and possibly also virion production activity in the presence of amikacin (though perhaps less virion production than as seen without antibiotic), but the result is complicated by its dependence on phage entrapment within liposomes. I speculate that the improved pharmacodynamic impact with phage liposome entrapment in the presence of amikacin, however, is a consequence of better phage penetration to bacteria. That is, either for spatial reasons (as consistent with authors' suggestion) or for temporal reasons—as in declines in active antibiotic over time in combination with delayed phage adsorption to bacteria when liposome entrapped—bacteria were less affected by antibiotic at the point of phage encounter given phage liposome entrapment. A further complication is that phage KPO1K2 may encode an anti-biofilm-matrix hydrolase [120] (see Section 4.2.2).

4.2.7. Chaudhry et al., 2017, *Pseudomonas aeruginosa*, Various Antibiotics

Chaudhry et al. [18] determined the number of phages present after 48 h of treatment following their exposure to 48-h *P. aeruginosa* biofilm in the presence of various antibiotics, with phages NP1 and NP3 applied in combination to 10^6 PFU/mL. Specifically, they found that while ciprofloxacin and tobramycin blocked phage production at 8× MIC for these antibiotics, that blockage of phage production was not also seen at 1× MIC. Furthermore, for ceftazidime and colistin, phage production was seen even at 8× MIC, though with gentamycin no phage production was seen even at 1× MIC. This evidence, however, is not fully supportive of the idea that phage infections necessarily will be active in the presence of these antibiotics even at 1× MIC, given the potential for biofilm heterogeneity and antibiotic tolerance (Section 2). In addition, phage numbers were determined after 48 h of incubation, at which point phage-sensitive but antibiotic-resistant bacteria may have arisen, or instead antibiotic over the course of assays may have decayed. Either of these cases could potentially support phage population growth in association with individual bacteria which are less antibiotic affected (in addition, if phages are unable to replicate and are otherwise present starting at low titers, then antibiotic resistance need not evolve at the same time as phage resistance, that is, for some degree of biofilm regrowth to occur in the presence of both agents). It is possible, therefore, that what was observed in these experiments was something other than production of new phage virions during infection of highly antibiotic-impacted bacteria.

Contrasting that conclusion, for ceftazidime and colistin 4-log increases in phage numbers were observed in the presence of biofilm and 8× MIC antibiotic concentrations, which suggests an involvement of all of the bacteria present in the observed phage population growth, i.e., as this was similar to the amount of phage population growth seen without antibiotic presence in a different experiment. This result therefore is highly suggestive of at least some phage population growth in association with fully antibiotic-exposed bacteria. As both antibiotics are externally rather than internally acting, however, this result may not be entirely unexpected, as consistent with the results of David et al. [101], as discussed above. That is, a substantial amount of phage virion production might have taken place prior to bacteria being highly affected by these two antibiotics (though note that David et al. did *not* actually see equivalently enhanced phage virion production given treatment with colistin). In addition, for all five antibiotics at 1× MIC concentrations, phages were able to increase in number roughly 2- to 3-log fold over a 12-hour period following exposure to eight-hour biofilms growing on a layer of epithelial cells.

Clearly phage antibacterial activity or even production of new phage particles does not appear to be blocked absolutely under all circumstances of antibiotic co-treatment, as tested in this study. Nevertheless, for at least some of the experiments presented, questions remain as to the degree that antibiotics were affecting those individual bacteria responsible for supporting phage virion production.

4.2.8. Kumaran et al., 2018, *Staphylococcus aureus*, Vancomycin

Kumaran et al. [111] found that treatment of a 24-h *S. aureus* biofilm with a combination of vancomycin and phage SATA-8505 resulted in roughly a half-log greater reduction in numbers of bacteria versus vancomycin alone. This was seen at vancomycin concentrations of 32, 64, and 128 μg/mL, while less reduction was seen at 256, 512, and 1024 μg/ml (MIC for non-biofilm bacteria was 4 μg/mL). Given that dosing was with only 10^6 PFU/ml, these results are suggestive of a retention of not just phage bactericidal activity but also phage virion production despite vancomycin presence. Similar results, however, were absent in the presence of equivalent quantities of cefazolin, dicloxacillin, linezolid, or tetracycline. As vancomycin is a cell-wall-targeting antibiotic, it is conceivable that suggested phage population growth occurred in these experiments prior to substantial vancomycin impact on bacterial metabolism.

4.2.9. Yazdi et al., 2018, *Proteus mirabilis*, Ampicillin

Yazdi et al. [112] treated *P. mirabilis* biofilm with phage vB_PmiS-TH (MOI = 1 or MOI = 100) and ampicillin (1× or 15× MIC). With MOI = 100, either with or without 1× MIC ampicillin, where 1× MIC ampicillin alone had little impact on biofilm bacteria, there was about 90% removal of biofilm after eight hours, as determined via crystal violet staining, but only 70% removal after 24 h. By contrast, with MOI = 100 and 15× MIC, there was no difference between eight and 24 h given this combined treatment, with 90% removal in both cases. Therefore, with time, and without substantial inhibition of bacterial growth as accomplished via inclusion of 15× MIC ampicillin, there appeared to be grow back of what we can presume are phage-resistant bacteria, i.e., 90% biofilm removal by eight hours, then only 70% biofilm removal by 24 h with MOI = 100 and antibiotic concentrations of either 1× or 0× MIC (that is, from the publication, "MOI 100 + AMP 16 μg/mL" or "MOI 100", respectively) versus MOI = 100 and antibiotic concentration of 15× MIC ("MOI 100 + AMP 246 μg/mL") for which no grow back was observed. In the same experiment, with 15× MIC ampicillin, there was somewhat more biofilm removal after eight hours with MOI = 1 (50%) or MOI = 100 (90%) relative to ampicillin alone (20%). The latter results too are suggestive of phage bactericidal activity in the presence of antibiotic.

4.2.10. Chang et al., 2019, *Pseudomonas aeruginosa*, Ciprofloxacin

Chang et al. [113]—with 24-h treatment of 48-h *P. aeruginosa* biofilms—saw greater reductions in biofilm biomass or biofilm viability with phage treatment (a cocktail, with 10^8 PFU/mL) in combination with 1× MIC ciprofloxacin versus phage-only treatments, the latter which generally had little impact. These results would seem to imply that phages or antibiotic are unable to remove bacteria alone, and presumably thereby phages were unable to display bactericidal or bacteriolytic activity except when the other was also present. An alternative explanation is that with combination therapy then resistant bacteria are unable to reestablish biofilms following biofilm removal due to a low potential for bacteria to mutate simultaneously to both phage and antibiotic resistance (Section 2). This explanation, however, is problematic given that treatment was with a phage cocktail which itself should, at least ideally, interfere with bacterial evolution of phage resistance, and that one-half MIC ciprofloxacin in combination with phages gave similar results to 1× MIC. Although overall it is difficult to infer what might be underlying the results observed in this study, explanations nevertheless would seem to support some sort of phage anti-biofilm activity in the presence of 1× MIC antibiotic. This activity does not necessarily include virion production, however, given the high numbers that phages were dosed with. Indeed, whether this activity was explicitly phage-infection related versus strictly enzymatic in this study is difficult to conclude. An important additional caveat is that these anti-biofilm experiments possibly were conducted in buffer rather than in broth.

4.2.11. Dickey and Perrot, 2019, *Staphylococcus aureus*, Various Antibiotics

Dickey and Perrot [34] tested in total eight antibiotics at 2× and 10× MIC against *S. aureus* biofilm, in combination with a phage they described as "PYO", which they isolated from a Republic of Georgia commercially available phage cocktail of the same name. These antibiotics are ciprofloxacin, daptomycin, erythromycin, gentamycin, linezolid, oxacillin, tetracycline, and vancomycin. Phage titers after 48 h (Table 3) can be compared to those present at the start of experiments (<10^7 PFU/mL). The same caveats about what these increases in phage numbers mean are applicable to these results as to those presented by Chaudhry et al. [18], etc., though there appears again to be strong indication of a potential for phage virion production despite antibiotic presence. Indeed, as measured explicitly in the same experiments, phage infection activity for a majority of the antibiotics tested tended to not be reduced given antibiotic presence at 2× MIC. For daptomycin and oxacillin there also appeared to be phage virion production even at 10× MIC. Therefore, these experiments seem to support a potential for phages in association with biofilm to produce new virions in the presence of a variety of antibiotics, though as above it is uncertain to what degree the bacteria supporting phage population growth are individually affected by the antibiotic present. At the same time, it is clear that 10× MIC for certain antibiotics, notably erythromycin, gentamycin, and linezolid, had substantial antagonistic impacts on phage population growth.

Table 3. Impact of Different Antibiotics on *S. aureus* Biofilm Support of Phage Virion Production [1].

Antibiotic	Log Δ PFUs with 0× MIC	Log Δ PFUs with 2× MIC	Log Δ PFUs with 10× MIC
Ciprofloxacin	2	<2	0
Daptomycin	2	>1	1
Erythromycin	2	<1	−3
Gentamycin	2	0	−4
Linezolid	2	<1	−3
Oxacillin	2	2	1
Rifampin	2	<2	<0
Tetracycline	2	1	<0
Vancomycin	2	1	0

[1] Given simultaneous phage-antibiotic addition, as derived from the results of Dickey and Perrot [34], shown are estimated log change in phage titers within experiments (Log Δ PFUs). For example, 0 indicates no change, 2 indicates a 100-fold increase (thereby indicating phage population growth), −4 indicates a 10,000-fold decrease (the latter presumably because phages adsorbed to bacteria either immediately prior to or following bacterial death). For increased clarity, all numbers are approximations as obtained predominantly from their Figure 3. Roughly, values of 1 or more are indicative of at least moderately robust phage population growth.

4.2.12. Issa et al., 2019, *Pseudomonas aeruginosa*, Ciprofloxacin

Issa et al. [114] applied various phages at a titer of 10^3 PFU/mL along with 1× MIC ciprofloxacin (0.5 μg/mL) and characterized the ability of simultaneously supplied *P. aeruginosa* to form biofilms (as then measured after 24 h of treatment). Approximately half as much biofilm biomass was present for all five tested phages (ΦPT-18[b], ΦPT-20[a], ΦPT-1S[a], ΦPT-5[a] and ΦPT-2[b]) in the presence of ciprofloxacin in comparison with ciprofloxacin alone. No phage-only controls are presented with the shown experiment, but previous experiments indicated that phage-only treatment is less effective than ciprofloxacin treatment alone. Given the low numbers of phages provided, these results are suggestive that phage virion production indeed may have occurred despite ciprofloxacin's presence. That the bacteria formed biofilms at all in the presence of ciprofloxacin, however, is puzzling, perhaps suggesting that it was instead ciprofloxacin-resistant mutants which formed the biofilm, and also ciprofloxacin-resistant mutants which supported the proposed phage population growth.

4.2.13. Summary of Evidence of Phage Infection Activity in Biofilms in the Presence of Antibiotics

The results reviewed in this subsection are highly suggestive that phage infection activity can persist in association with bacterial biofilms despite presence of antibiotic concentrations of 1× MIC or greater. Nevertheless, issues exist concerning the heterogeneity of biofilms and cultures, both spatially and temporally. These are in terms of the degree that constituent bacteria are potentially unevenly impacted by antibiotic while supporting phage infection activity, as well as the potential for antibiotics to decay such as to subinhibitory levels over time. In either case, phage infection activity might be occurring in association with antibiotic not inhibitorily affecting bacterial hosts despite initial antibiotic concentrations at or exceeding 1× MIC. Additional issues are the presence of biofilm-matrix degrading enzymes in at least some phage formulations as may mimic phage bactericidal activity, and also the potential for antibiotic-resistant bacteria to sufficiently grow in number over time to support phage virion production in an antibiotic-unaffected manner. Ideally, therefore, determinations of antibiotic impact on phage infection activity would be corroborated at the very least with simplified, shorter term determinations of phage-antibiotic compatibility such as the above-mentioned single-step growth experiments [90,91].

4.3. *Phage-Antibiotic In Vivo Compatibility*

For phage therapy to be effective, then phages at a minimum need to reach targeted bacteria and then kill those bacteria. Generally, the killing process involves several relatively complex physiological steps that are highly dependent on various target-bacterium-supplied functions, especially as resulting in phage gene expression. In addition, to some degree phage in situ replication can be helpful or even crucial to phage therapy success, resulting in so-called active treatments [92–96]. Phage replication along with virion production, however, generally should be associated with more bacterial metabolic functioning than simply phage bactericidal activity. In this section, I consider animal models of phage therapy in which potentially clinically effective dosings of antibiotics are provided along with phages as co-therapies. Given the greater complexity of these models relative to in vitro studies (Sections 4.1 and 4.2), it can be even more difficult to ascertain degrees of retention of phage infection activity in the presence of antibiotic. Nevertheless, as above, evidence of in situ phage replication, towards greater phage titers than are present immediately following phage application, can serve as evidence for at least some degree of phage infection activity and associated pharmacodynamic impact despite presumed concurrent antibiotic negative impacts on the metabolic functioning of targeted bacteria. The issue of whether antibiotics and phages are together robustly impacting the same individual bacteria, however, can be even more difficult to answer with animal models than with in vitro biofilm studies (the latter, Section 4.2).

4.3.1. Chhibber et al., 2008, *Klebsiella pneumoniae*, amikacin

Chhibber et al. [115], using a mouse, *K. pneumoniae*, lobar-pneumonia model, found no difference in phage SS impact on bacteria with versus without antibiotic presence. A reported 1× MIC amikacin (3.75 mg/25 g) was supplied via intraperitoneal delivery at the same time as phages (10^9 PFU), also intraperitoneally, both in association with a simultaneous intranasal bacterial challenge (5×10^6 CFU). Bacterial counts on Day 5 with phage treatment were 5-logs, or more, lower relative to the no-treatment control. Clearly phage bactericidal activity therefore was retained in this model in association with antibiotic. Antibiotic alone, however, had little impact on bacterial numbers. Evidence also is provided that, in the absence of bacteria, phages could concentrate in lung tissue, up to nearly 10^{12} PFU/g. As a result, it is uncertain whether phage replication may have occurred in the presence of antibiotic to result in observed declines in bacterial presence versus phage concentration to inundative titers in the lungs by other means, or, if phage replication did occur, whether antibiotic concentrations in contact with phage-infected bacteria were still equal to at least 1× MIC at the time of that replication. In addition, measured reductions in bacterial loads relative to untreated controls—given phage-only or combined treatments—did not begin until Day 2 of treatment, and reductions were not substantial, relative to bacterial numbers as present on Day 1, until Day 3 of treatment. Over this time frame, antibiotic concentrations likely would have declined to below 1× MIC, as evidenced by bacterial growth in association with the amikacin-only treatment group by Day 2. Therefore, evidence that phage replication occurred in association with 1× MIC or greater concentrations of amikacin in this study at best is not robust.

4.3.2. Chhibber et al., 2012, *Staphylococcus aureus*, Linezolid

Chhibber et al. [116] treated a *S. aureus* model diabetic foot infection, mouse model, using a combination of phage MR-10 (10^6 phages locally applied but 10^8 PFU/mL) and linezolid (25 mg/Kg, orally dosed), with treatment starting 30-min post bacterial challenge. Evidence of phage virion production in the presence of antibiotic at best is slight as determined by phage titers found locally, as too is evidence of phage replication in terms of reductions in CFUs, also as found locally, where reductions were not substantial relative to likely starting bacterial densities. Combination treatments reduced bacterial densities by about 1-log more than phage- or antibiotic-alone treatments, however. This latter result, particularly as it occurred within one day of the bacterial challenge, and at the start of treatments, is suggestive of phage bactericidal activity in the presence of both antibiotic and reasonably antibiotic-affected bacteria as found in vivo.

4.3.3. Yilmaz et al., 2013, *Staphylococcus aureus* and *Pseudomonas. aeruginosa*, Various Antibiotics

Yilmaz et al. [117], in separate experiments consisting of treatment of rat implant-associated in vitro-established infections, provide convincing evidence of phage anti-biofilm activity in the presence of antibiotic against one pathogen (*S. aureus* and phage Sb-1) but less robust results against a second (*P. aeruginosa* and phage vB_PsaP PAT14). Phages were applied directly to infections by injection, once per day for three days (10^7 PFU/dose), and antibiotics were supplied intraperitoneally once per day for 14 days (20mg/kg teicoplanin for *S. aureus*; 120 mg/kg imipenem and cilastatin plus 25 mg/kg of amikacin for *P. aeruginosa*). With *S. aureus*, numbers were reduced relative to the untreated control by 7 logs given antibiotic-only treatment and by 9 logs with combination treatment (though only by 4 logs with treatment by phages alone). With *P. aeruginosa*, by contrast, 3 log reductions were seen with antibiotic-only treatment, but only 4 log reductions with either phage-only or combination treatments. These results might be consistent with phage virion production in vivo, though without volume or in situ phage titer information this possibility is not necessarily easily corroborated. The results nevertheless should be viewed as consistent with at least phage bactericidal activity particularly against *S. aureus*.

4.3.4. Kaur et al., 2016, *Staphylococcus aureus*, linezolid

Kaur et al. [118] presents an in vivo testing, in mice, of prevention of *S. aureus* surface adherence to orthopedic-grade stainless steel Kirschner wires, i.e., as discussed above in terms of in vitro testing [109] (Section 4.2.5). Hydroxypropyl methylcellulose hydrogels impregnated with a combination of both phages and linezolid appear to have been slightly more effective at preventing bacterial colonization than impregnation with linezolid alone (4% *w/w* of wires), which in turn was slightly more effective than impregnation with phage MR-5 alone (10^9 PFU/mL). Perhaps consistently, a faster drop off in phage titers in vivo was seen with antibiotic present versus without, but still with increases in titers in both cases early on during experiments. The in vivo results overall are suggestive of slightly lower phage activity in the absence of linezolid in comparison to what was observed in vitro [109]. Similar conclusions otherwise can be reached between the two studies, [118] and [109]. Therefore, as with the in vitro study, Kaur et al. [118] provides evidence of phage infection activity, but not necessarily substantial activity against bacteria which also have been substantially impacted by antibiotic.

4.3.5. Oechslin et al., 2017, *Pseudomonas aeruginosa*, Ciprofloxacin

Oechslin et al. [103] explored the impact of a combination of a phage cocktail (dubbed PP1131 and delivered intravenously) and ciprofloxacin (also by injection) in a *P. aeruginosa* rat endocarditis model. After six hours of treatment, started 18 h post bacterial challenge, bacterial loads were reduced by 2–3 logs by either phage or antibiotic treatment, but by roughly 7 logs by combined phage and antibiotic treatment. Phage titers in plasma were approximately 10^8 PFU/mL, but ~10^{10} PFU/g in association with aortic valve vegetations versus ~10^9 CFU/g. Based on Poisson distributions (Section 2), it is difficult to say whether or not these results imply that phage production occurred in situ. This is because this is roughly a 10-fold excess of phages, which could easily give rise to 4-log reductions in bacterial densities by adsorption and resulting bactericidal effects alone. These results therefore are certainly consistent with phage bactericidal activity in the presence of ciprofloxacin but not necessarily with new phage production. On the other hand, the excess in phage numbers per gram of aortic valve vegetations relative to per mL of plasma, i.e., as much as a 100-fold excess, and as much as 1000-fold in excess relative to the phage-only control, are consistent with localized phage virion production in association with these localized high densities of bacteria.

Ciprofloxacin was dosed at 20 mg/kg with a single bolus at the same time as phages were applied and calculated MIC was 0.19 μg/mL. Given the short duration of the experiment as well as the substantial impact that antibiotic alone had on bacterial numbers, it seems reasonable to conclude that this proposed aortic valve vegetation-located phage replication occurred in association with bacteria that at least could have been exposed to 1× MIC or greater ciprofloxacin, as would be consistent with their in vitro, broth results presented in the same study (Section 4.1.8). These results, it should be noted and as the authors point out, may represent phage-antibiotic synergy as a 10^7-fold reduction in bacterial numbers is in excess of $10^3 \times 10^3 = 10^6$ approximate reduction as predicted for additive phage-antibiotic interactions.

4.3.6. Vahedi et al., 2018, *Escherichia coli*, Ciprofloxacin

The results of Vahedi et al. [119], though positive for phage therapy impact on the treated *E. coli* mouse gastrointestinal colonization, neither support nor refute compatibility of phage activity with presence of ciprofloxacin. The phage used was not named and treatment doses were delivered orally by gavage.

4.3.7. Summary of Evidence of Phage Infection Activity In Vivo in the Presence of Antibiotics

Animal experiments, as noted, are highly complex in terms of the state of the bacteria interacting with treatment phages. Therefore, the potential for phages to display infection activity while infecting bacteria that are not substantially affected by antibiotic presence, despite those bacteria being antibiotic susceptible, could be high. That results of these in vivo experiments are supportive of phage infection activity during treatments, and even in certain cases virion production, therefore might not be surprising. It is notable, however, that the more impressive of the animal co-treatment results (Section 4.3.5) is associated also with the most impressive of in vitro phage compatibility with antibiotic presence results (Section 4.1.8) [103]. Tentatively we might speculate that the complexity of treated environments may be an aid to phage compatibility with antibiotics, i.e., in terms of phages impacting especially those individual bacteria which, due to circumstances, are less antibiotic affected. This speculation certainly needs to be more rigorously explored, however.

4.4. Evidence of Phage-Infection Compatibility with Antibiotic Treatment, Conclusions

It is unfortunate that much of the strongest evidence of phage infection activity in the presence of antibiotics comes from the most complex experimental systems: in vitro biofilms or in vivo disease models. On the one hand, the results obtained suggest that there can be substantial latitude in terms of the potential for phages to kill bacteria and/or to produce new virions despite antibiotic presence. In particular, perhaps phages are infecting especially those bacteria which are least affected by antibiotic treatments. On the other hand, the ambiguities associated with the interpretation of many studies are highly suggestive of a utility to better characterizing phage compatibility with antibiotic treatments under more rigorous conditions, e.g., as via single-step growth experiments [90,91] as done in broth in which bacteria have been pre-treated by antibiotic prior to phage addition. Once so defined, it would be interesting to determine whether phage infection activity might in fact improve given greater experimental-system and bacterial heterogeneity during phage treatment in the presence of 1× MIC or higher antibiotic concentrations.

5. General Conclusions

Summers [122], in 2001, differentiated the history of phage therapy—at least in terms of the Western experience—into four periods, corresponding to "early enthusiasm, critical scepticism, abandonment, [and] recent interest and reappraisal". The more modern of these periods arguably began, in the

English-language literature, with the mouse study of Smith and Huggins [123] in 1983 and collections of clinical case studies published by Ślopek et al. from 1983 to 1987 [124–130]. From 1983 to 2016, nearly 40 human phage therapy studies were published, also in the English-language literature [2], including those of Ślopek et al. Many though by no means not all of these studies have involved co-treatment of phages with antibiotics (see also [7,131]), though it has not always been obvious how sensitive the treated bacteria were to the antibiotics being used. Historically, however, phage therapy has often been a response to failures of antibiotic treatment [3,6]. More recently, there also have been several case studies involving both phage therapy following antibiotic failures and continued antibiotic treatment even after phage therapy has begun [10,12,13,15–17]. Therefore, it would seem that the time has come for more rigorous scrutiny of phage activity as may or may not be present given antibiotic co-treatments of especially still antibiotic-susceptible bacteria.

The utility of phage-antibiotic co-treatments thus is being increasingly explored in the pre-clinical phage therapy literature [33,41]. Substantial evidence exists, however, that many antibiotics, when used at otherwise clinically relevant concentrations, particularly at or exceeding measured minimum inhibitory concentrations, can interfere with phage infection activity, and therefore with phage primary pharmacodynamic properties. Therefore, ideally phage infection capabilities in the presence of antibiotics, at those concentrations, would be assessed prior to proceeding to more complex, time-consuming, and expensive experimentation, such as animal testing. This idea of testing phages in vitro for basic infection activity prior to the start of more complex procedures is, of course, not a new concept to phage therapy. As noted by Eaton and Bayne-Jones in 1934 [132], p. 1773, "in vitro lysis of the infecting organism by the bacteriophage should always be demonstrated, preferably before the agent is used in treatment." To fully assess phage infection activity, one may for example employ single-step growth-like experiments [90,91], looking for phage ability to lyse bacteria and produce new virions despite antibiotic presence.

Although phage virion production during phage therapy exists as an ideal, it nevertheless is possible for phages to kill bacteria without necessarily also producing phage progeny, resulting in what are known as abortive infections [42,43]. A complication, though, is that retention of phage bactericidal activity, particularly if absent phage-induced bacterial lysis, can be difficult to measure in the presence of antibiotics, since antibiotics also profoundly affect bacterial physiology. Therefore, assessment of the ability of antibiotic-susceptible bacteria to continue to replicate despite phage adsorption, given concurrent antibiotic exposure especially at or exceeding MIC, can be nonsensical as bacteria will continue to not replicate so long as antibiotic is present at sufficient concentrations. Removing antibiotic to observe phage impact in isolation, however, would represent a changing of conditions such that similarly we no longer can know whether phage bactericidal activity is present while antibiotic is still present. More sophisticated experiments therefore may be necessary to assess explicitly phage bactericidal activity, without associated bacteriolytic or virion production activities, in the presence of antibiotic.

Phages may primarily be used to target those bacterial subpopulations, in situ, which for whatever reason—e.g., poor vascularization, biofilm residence, decay in antibiotic densities over time—are exposed to lower concentrations of antibiotic [37,59]. In this case, phage-antibiotic compatibility may be less of a concern at least to the extent that antibiotics are able to eliminate one fraction of targeted bacteria while phages bactericidally eliminate the rest. This may be achieved particularly to the extent that phages are supplied in sufficient numbers that they can reach those bacteria that are less available to antibiotics without phages also being relied upon to display substantial in situ population growth. Above all, though to date we have a number of hints that 1× MIC or greater antibiotic concentrations will not necessarily completely inhibit phage infection-associated pharmacodynamic properties, perhaps particularly in more complex environments, that ability is not necessarily assured for a given phage, antibiotic, host bacterium, or treatment conditions. It can be useful, therefore, to confirm earlier rather than later during the development of phage-antibiotic co-treatment strategies, that reasonably robust phage antibacterial activity and/or phage virion production can occur in the presence of antibiotics that have been co-supplied at otherwise bacterial-infection inhibitory concentrations.

References

1. Abedon, S.T.; Kuhl, S.J.; Blasdel, B.G.; Kutter, E.M. Phage treatment of human infections. *Bacteriophage* **2011**, *1*, 66–85. [CrossRef] [PubMed]
2. Abedon, S.T. Bacteriophage clinical use as antibactertial "drugs": Utility, precedent. *Microbiol. Spectr.* **2017**, *5*, BAD-0003-2016.
3. Abedon, S.T. Use of phage therapy to treat long-standing, persistent, or chronic bacterial infections. *Adv. Drug Deliv. Rev.* **2019**. [CrossRef]
4. Gupta, P.; Singh, H.S.; Shukla, V.K.; Nath, G.; Bhartiya, S.K. Bacteriophage therapy of chronic nonhealing wound: Clinical study. *Int. J. Low. Extrem. Wounds* **2019**, *18*, 171–175. [CrossRef] [PubMed]
5. Loc-Carrillo, C.; Wu, S.; Beck, J.P. Phage therapy of wounds and related purulent infections. In *Bacteriophages in Health and Disease, Hyman, P., Abedon, S.T., Eds.*; CABI Press: Wallingford, UK, 2012; pp. 185–202.
6. Abedon, S.T. Bacteriophage-mediated biocontrol of wound infections, and ecological exploitation of biofilms by phages. In *Recent Clinical Techniques, Results, and Research in Wounds*; Shiffman, M., Ed.; Springer: Berlin/Heidelberg, Germany, 2018.
7. Abedon, S.T. Phage therapy of pulmonary infections. *Bacteriophage* **2015**, *5*, e1020260. [CrossRef] [PubMed]
8. Chang, R.Y.K.; Wallin, M.; Lin, Y.; Leung, S.S.Y.; Wang, H.; Morales, S.; Chan, H.K. Phage therapy for respiratory infections. *Adv. Drug Deliv. Rev.* **2018**, *133*, 76–86. [CrossRef] [PubMed]
9. Hoyle, N.; Zhvaniya, P.; Balarjishvili, N.; Bolkvadze, D.; Nadareishvili, L.; Nizharadze, D.; Wittmann, J.; Rohde, C.; Kutateladze, M. Phage therapy against *Achromobacter xylosoxidans* lung infection in a patient with cystic fibrosis: A case report. *Res. Microbiol.* **2018**, *169*, 540–542. [CrossRef] [PubMed]
10. Aslam, S.; Courtwright, A.M.; Koval, C.; Lehman, S.M.; Morales, S.; Langlais Furr, C.L.; Rosas, F.; Brownstein, M.J.; Fackler, J.R.; Sisson, B.M.; et al. Early clinical experience of bacteriophage therapy in three lung transplant recipients. *Am. J. Transplant.* **2019**, *19*, 2631–2639. [CrossRef]
11. Wright, A.; Hawkins, C.H.; Anggård, E.E.; Harper, D.R. A controlled clinical trial of a therapeutic bacteriophage preparation in chronic otitis due to antibiotic-resistant *Pseudomonas aeruginosa*; a preliminary report of efficacy. *Clin. Otolaryng.* **2009**, *34*, 349–357. [CrossRef] [PubMed]
12. Schooley, R.T.; Biswas, B.; Gill, J.J.; Hernandez-Morales, A.; Lancaster, J.; Lessor, L.; Barr, J.J.; Reed, S.L.; Rohwer, F.; Benler, S.; et al. Development and use of personalized bacteriophage-based therapeutic cocktails to treat a patient with a disseminated resistant *Acinetobacter baumannii* infection. *Antimicrob. Agents Chemother.* **2017**, *61*, e00954-17. [CrossRef]
13. Chan, B.K.; Turner, P.E.; Kim, S.; Mojibian, H.R.; Elefteriades, J.A.; Narayan, D. Phage treatment of an aortic graft infected with *Pseudomonas aeruginosa*. *Evol. Med. Pub. Health* **2018**, *1*, 60–66. [CrossRef] [PubMed]
14. Dedrick, R.M.; Guerrero-Bustamante, C.A.; Garlena, R.A.; Russell, D.A.; Ford, K.; Harris, K.; Gilmour, K.C.; Soothill, J.; Jacobs-Sera, D.; Schooley, R.T.; et al. Engineered bacteriophages for treatment of a patient with a disseminated drug-resistant *Mycobacterium abscessus*. *Nat. Med.* **2019**, *25*, 730–733. [CrossRef] [PubMed]
15. Ferry, T.; Leboucher, G.; Fevre, C.; Herry, Y.; Conrad, A.; Josse, J.; Batailler, C.; Chidiac, C.; Medina, M.; Lustig, S.; et al. Salvage debridement, antibiotics and implant retention ("DAIR") with local injection of a selected cocktail of bacteriophages: Is it an option for an elderly patient with relapsing *Staphylococcus aureus* prosthetic-joint infection? *Open Forum Infect. Dis.* **2018**, *5*, ofy269. [CrossRef] [PubMed]
16. Aslam, S.; Pretorius, V.; Lehman, S.M.; Morales, S.; Schooley, R.T. Novel bacteriophage therapy for treatment of left ventricular assist device infection. *J. Heart Lung. Transplant.* **2019**, *38*, 475–476. [CrossRef] [PubMed]
17. Law, N.; Logan, C.; Yung, G.; Furr, C.L.L.; Lehman, S.M.; Morales, S.; Rosas, F.; Gaidamaka, A.; Bilinsky, I.; Grint, P. Successful adjunctive use of bacteriophage therapy for treatment of multidrug-resistant *Pseudomonas aeruginosa* infection in a cystic fibrosis patient. *Infection* **2019**, *47*, 665–668. [CrossRef]
18. Chaudhry, W.N.; Concepcion-Acevedo, J.; Park, T.; Andleeb, S.; Bull, J.J.; Levin, B.R. Synergy and order effects of antibiotics and phages in killing *Pseudomonas aeruginosa* biofilms. *PLoS ONE* **2017**, *12*, e0168615. [CrossRef]
19. Henriksen, K.; Rorbo, N.; Rybtke, M.L.; Martinet, M.G.; Tolker-Nielsen, T.; Hoiby, N.; Middelboe, M.;

Ciofu, O.P. *aeruginosa* flow-cell biofilms are enhanced by repeated phage treatments but can be eradicated by phage-ciprofloxacin combination. *Pathog. Dis.* **2019**, *77*, ftz011. [CrossRef]

20. Milho, C.; Andrade, M.; Vilas, B.D.; Alves, D.; Sillankorva, S. Antimicrobial assessment of phage therapy using a porcine model of biofilm infection. *Int. J Pharm.* **2019**, *557*, 112–123. [CrossRef]
21. Yuan, Y.; Qu, K.; Tan, D.; Li, X.; Wang, L.; Cong, C.; Xiu, Z.; Xu, Y. Isolation and characterization of a bacteriophage and its potential to disrupt multi-drug resistant *Pseudomonas aeruginosa* biofilms. *Microb. Pathog.* **2019**, *128*, 329–336. [CrossRef]
22. Tkhilaishvili, T.; Lombardi, L.; Klatt, A.B.; Trampuz, A.; Di, L.M. Bacteriophage Sb-1 enhances antibiotic activity against biofilm, degrades exopolysaccharide matrix and targets persisters of *Staphylococcus aureus*. *Int. J. Antimicrob. Agents* **2018**, *52*, 842–853. [CrossRef]
23. Zhang, G.; Zhao, Y.; Paramasivan, S.; Richter, K.; Morales, S.; Wormald, P.J.; Vreugde, S. Bacteriophage effectively kills multidrug resistant *Staphylococcus aureus* clinical isolates from chronic rhinosinusitis patients. *Int. Forum Allergy Rhinol.* **2018**, *8*, 406–414. [CrossRef] [PubMed]
24. Pearl, S.; Gabay, C.; Kishony, R.; Oppenheim, A.; Balaban, N.Q. Nongenetic individuality in the host-phage interaction. *PLoS Biol.* **2008**, *6*, e120. [CrossRef] [PubMed]
25. Falagas, M.E.; Grammatikos, A.P.; Michalopoulos, A. Potential of old-generation antibiotics to address current need for new antibiotics. *Expert Rev. Anti. Infect. Ther.* **2008**, *6*, 593–600. [CrossRef] [PubMed]
26. Czaplewski, L.; Bax, R.; Clokie, M.; Dawson, M.; Fairhead, H.; Fischetti, V.A.; Foster, S.; Gilmore, B.F.; Hancock, R.E.; Harper, D.; et al. Alternatives to antibiotics-a pipeline portfolio review. *Lancet Infect. Dis.* **2016**, *16*, 239–251. [CrossRef]
27. Kutter, E. Phage therapy: Bacteriophages as natural, self-limiting antibiotics. In *Textbook of Natural Medicine*, 3rd ed.; Pizzorno, W., Ed.; Churchill Livingston: London, UK, 2005; pp. 1147–1161.
28. Häusler, T. *Viruses vs. Superbugs: A Solution to the Antibiotics Crisis*; Macmillan: New York, NY, USA, 2006.
29. Loc-Carrillo, C.; Abedon, S.T. Pros and cons of phage therapy. *Bacteriophage* **2011**, *1*, 111–114. [CrossRef] [PubMed]
30. Curtright, A.J.; Abedon, S.T. Phage therapy: Emergent property pharmacology. *J. Bioanalyt. Biomed.* **2011**, *S3*, 010.
31. Nobrega, F.L.; Costa, A.R.; Kluskens, L.D.; Azeredo, J. Revisiting phage therapy: New applications for old resources. *Trends Microbiol.* **2015**, *23*, 185–191. [CrossRef] [PubMed]
32. Wienhold, S.M.; Lienau, J.; Witzenrath, M. Towards inhaled phage therapy in Western Europe. *Viruses* **2019**, *11*, 295. [CrossRef]
33. Tagliaferri, T.L.; Jansen, M.; Horz, H.P. Fighting pathogenic bacteria on two fronts: Phages and antibiotics as combined strategy. *Front. Cell Infect. Microbiol.* **2019**, *9*, 22. [CrossRef]
34. Dickey, J.; Perrot, V. Adjunct phage treatment enhances the effectiveness of low antibiotic concentration against *Staphylococcus aureus* biofilms in vitro. *PLoS ONE* **2019**, *14*, e0209390. [CrossRef]
35. Bonhoeffer, S.; Lipsitch, M.; Levin, B.R. Evaluating treatment protocols to prevent resistance. *Proc. Natl. Acad. Sci. USA* **1997**, *94*, 12106–12111. [CrossRef] [PubMed]
36. Fischbach, M.A. Combination therapies for combating antimicrobial resistance. *Curr. Opin. Microbiol.* **2011**, *14*, 519–523. [CrossRef] [PubMed]
37. Leekha, S.; Terrell, C.L.; Edson, R.S. General principles of antimicrobial therapy. *Mayo Clin. Proc.* **2011**, *86*, 156–167. [CrossRef] [PubMed]
38. REX Consortium. Heterogeneity of selection and the evolution of resistance. *Trends Ecol. Evol.* **2013**, *28*, 110–118. [CrossRef] [PubMed]
39. Coulter, L.B.; McLean, R.J.; Rohde, R.E.; Aron, G.M. Effect of bacteriophage infection in combination with tobramycin on the emergence of resistance in *Escherichia coli* and *Pseudomonas aeruginosa* biofilms. *Viruses* **2014**, *6*, 3778–3786. [CrossRef]
40. Torres-Barceló, C.; Arias-Sanchez, F.I.; Vasse, M.; Ramsayer, J.; Kaltz, O.; Hochberg, M.E. A window of opportunity to control the bacterial pathogen *Pseudomonas aeruginosa* combining antibiotics and phages. *PLoS ONE* **2014**, *9*, e106628. [CrossRef] [PubMed]
41. Torres-Barceló, C.; Hochberg, M.E. Evolutionary rationale for phages as complements of antibiotics. *Trends Microbiol.* **2016**, *24*, 249–256. [CrossRef]

42. Hyman, P.; Abedon, S.T. Bacteriophage host range and bacterial resistance. *Adv. Appl. Microbiol.* **2010**, *70*, 217–248.
43. Labrie, S.J.; Samson, J.E.; Moineau, S. Bacteriophage resistance mechanisms. *Nat. Rev. Microbiol.* **2010**, *8*, 317–327. [CrossRef]
44. Ormälä, A.M.; Jalasvuori, M. Phage therapy: Should bacterial resistance to phages be a concern, even in the long run? *Bacteriophage* **2013**, *3*, e24219. [CrossRef]
45. Azam, A.H.; Tanji, Y. Bacteriophage-host arm race: An update on the mechanism of phage resistance in bacteria and revenge of the phage with the perspective for phage therapy. *Appl. Microbiol. Biotechnol.* **2019**, *103*, 2121–2131. [CrossRef] [PubMed]
46. Wiegand, I.; Hilpert, K.; Hancock, R.E. Agar and broth dilution methods to determine the minimal inhibitory concentration (MIC) of antimicrobial substances. *Nat. Protoc.* **2008**, *3*, 163–175. [CrossRef] [PubMed]
47. Brauner, A.; Fridman, O.; Gefen, O.; Balaban, N.Q. Distinguishing between resistance, tolerance and persistence to antibiotic treatment. *Nat. Rev. Microbiol.* **2016**, *14*, 320–330. [CrossRef] [PubMed]
48. Brauner, A.; Shoresh, N.; Fridman, O.; Balaban, N.Q. An Experimental Framework for Quantifying Bacterial Tolerance. *Biophys. J.* **2017**, *112*, 2664–2671. [CrossRef] [PubMed]
49. Comeau, A.; Tétart, F.; Trojet, S.A.; Prère, M.-F.; Krisch, H.M. Phage-antibiotic synergy (PAS): B-lactam and quinolone antibiotics stimulate virulent phage growth. *PLoS ONE* **2007**, *2*, e799. [CrossRef]
50. Pires, D.P.; Oliveira, H.; Melo, L.D.; Sillankorva, S.; Azeredo, J. Bacteriophage-encoded depolymerases: Their diversity and biotechnological applications. *Appl. Microbiol. Biotechnol.* **2016**, *100*, 2141–2151. [CrossRef]
51. Latka, A.; Maciejewska, B.; Majkowska-Skrobek, G.; Briers, Y.; Drulis-Kawa, Z. Bacteriophage-encoded virion-associated enzymes to overcome the carbohydrate barriers during the infection process. *Appl. Microbiol. Biotechnol.* **2017**, *101*, 3103–3119. [CrossRef]
52. Ceri, H.; Olson, M.E.; Stremick, C.; Read, R.R.; Morck, D.; Buret, A. The Calgary Biofilm Device: New technology for rapid determination of antibiotic susceptibilities of bacterial biofilms. *J. Clin. Microbiol.* **1999**, *37*, 1771–1776.
53. Jolivet-Gougeon, A.; Bonnaure-Mallet, M. Biofilms as a mechanism of bacterial resistance. *Drug Discov. Today Technol.* **2014**, *11*, 49–56. [CrossRef]
54. Macia, M.D.; Rojo-Molinero, E.; Oliver, A. Antimicrobial susceptibility testing in biofilm-growing bacteria. *Clin. Microbiol. Infect.* **2014**, *20*, 981–990. [CrossRef]
55. Olsen, I. Biofilm-specific antibiotic tolerance and resistance. *Eur. J. Clin. Microbiol. Infect. Dis.* **2015**, *34*, 877–886. [CrossRef] [PubMed]
56. Fisher, R.A.; Gollan, B.; Helaine, S. Persistent bacterial infections and persister cells. *Nat. Rev. Microbiol.* **2017**, *15*, 453–464. [CrossRef] [PubMed]
57. Abedon, S.T.; Katsaounis, T.I. Basic phage mathematics. *Meth. Mol. Biol.* **2018**, *1681*, 3–30.
58. Abedon, S.T. Expected efficacy: Applying killing titer estimations to phage therapy experiments. 2017. Available online: http://www.phage-therapy.org/writings/killing_titers.html (accessed on 8 October 2019).
59. Pankey, G.A.; Sabath, L.D. Clinical relevance of bacteriostatic versus bactericidal mechanisms of action in the treatment of Gram-positive bacterial infections. *Clin. Infect. Dis.* **2004**, *38*, 864–870. [CrossRef] [PubMed]
60. Jawetz, E.; Gunnison, J.B.; Speck, R.S.; Coleman, V.R. Studies on antibiotic synergism and antagonism; the interference of chloramphenicol with the action of penicillin. *AMA Arch. Intern. Med.* **1951**, *87*, 349–359. [CrossRef] [PubMed]
61. Ocampo, P.S.; Lazar, V.; Papp, B.; Arnoldini, M.; Abel Zur, W.P.; Busa-Fekete, R.; Fekete, G.; Pal, C.; Ackermann, M.; Bonhoeffer, S. Antagonism between bacteriostatic and bactericidal antibiotics is prevalent. *Antimicrob. Agents Chemother.* **2014**, *58*, 4573–4582. [CrossRef] [PubMed]
62. Handwerger, S.; Tomasz, A. Antibiotic tolerance among clinical isolates of bacteria. *Annu. Rev. Pharmacol. Toxicol.* **1985**, *25*, 349–380. [CrossRef]
63. Tuomanen, E.; Cozens, R.; Tosch, W.; Zak, O.; Tomasz, A. The rate of killing of *Escherichia coli* by beta-lactam antibiotics is strictly proportional to the rate of bacterial growth. *J. Gen. Microbiol.* **1986**, *132*, 1297–1304.
64. Hadas, H.; Einav, M.; Fishov, I.; Zaritsky, A. Bacteriophage T4 development depends on the physiology of its host *Escherichia coli*. *Microbiology* **1997**, *143*, 179–185. [CrossRef]
65. Miller, R.V.; Day, M. Contribution of lysogeny, pseudolysogeny, and starvation to phage ecology. In *Bacteriophage Ecology*; Abedon, S.T., Ed.; Cambridge University Press: Cambridge, UK, 2008; pp. 114–143.

66. Bryan, D.; El-Shibiny, A.; Hobbs, Z.; Porter, J.; Kutter, E.M. Bacteriophage T4 infection of stationary phase *E. coli*: Life after log from a phage perspective. *Front. Microbiol.* **2016**, *7*, 1391. [CrossRef]
67. Adams, M.H. *Bacteriophages*; InterScience: New York, NY, USA, 1959.
68. Matsui, T.; Yoshikawa, G.; Mihara, T.; Chatchawankanphanich, O.; Kawasaki, T.; Nakano, M.; Fujie, M.; Ogata, H.; Yamada, T. Replications of two closely related groups of jumbo phages show different level of dependence on host-encoded RNA polymerase. *Front. Microbiol.* **2017**, *8*, 1010. [CrossRef] [PubMed]
69. Jacobs, W.R., Jr.; Barletta, R.G.; Udani, R.; Chan, J.; Kalkut, G.; Sosne, G.; Kieser, T.; Sarkis, G.J.; Hatfull, G.F.; Bloom, B.R. Rapid assessment of drug susceptibilities of *Mycobacterium tuberculosis* by means of luciferase reporter phages [see comments]. *Science* **1993**, *260*, 819–822. [CrossRef] [PubMed]
70. Wilson, S.M.; Al Suwaidi, Z.; McNerney, R.; Porter, J.; Drobniewski, F. Evaluation of a new rapid bacteriophage-based method for the drug susceptibility testing of *Mycobacterium tuberculosis*. *Nat. Med.* **1997**, *3*, 465–468. [CrossRef] [PubMed]
71. Gali, N.; Dominguez, J.; Blanco, S.; Prat, C.; Quesada, M.D.; Matas, L.; Ausina, V. Utility of an in-house mycobacteriophage-based assay for rapid detection of rifampin resistance in *Mycobacterium tuberculosis* clinical isolates. *J. Clin. Microbiol.* **2003**, *41*, 2647–2649. [CrossRef] [PubMed]
72. McNerney, R.; Mallard, K.; Urassa, H.M.; Lemma, E.; Donoghue, H.D. Colorimetric phage-based assay for detection of rifampin-resistant Mycobacterium tuberculosis. *J. Clin. Microbiol.* **2007**, *45*, 1330–1332. [CrossRef] [PubMed]
73. Pholwat, S.; Ehdaie, B.; Foongladda, S.; Kelly, K.; Houpt, E. Real-time PCR using mycobacteriophage DNA for rapid phenotypic drug susceptibility results for *Mycobacterium tuberculosis*. *J. Clin. Microbiol.* **2012**, *50*, 754–761. [CrossRef] [PubMed]
74. Ceyssens, P.J.; Minakhin, L.; Van den Bossche, A.; Yakunina, M.; Klimuk, E.; Blasdel, B.; De, S.J.; Noben, J.P.; Blasi, U.; Severinov, K.; et al. Development of giant bacteriophage φKZ is independent of the host transcription apparatus. *J. Virol.* **2014**, *88*, 10501–10510. [CrossRef] [PubMed]
75. Geiduschek, E.P.; Sklar, J. Continual requirement for a host RNA polymerase component in a bacteriophage development. *Nature* **1969**, *221*, 833–836. [CrossRef] [PubMed]
76. Hemphill, H.E.; Whiteley, H.R.; Brown, L.R.; Doi, R.H. The effect of rifampin on the production of b22 phage by *Bacillus subtilis*. *Biochem. Biophys. Res. Commun.* **1969**, *37*, 559–566. [CrossRef]
77. Takeda, Y.; Oyama, Y.; Nakajima, K.; Yura, T. Role of host RNA polymerase for lambda phage development. *Biochem. Biophys. Res. Commun.* **1969**, *36*, 533–538. [CrossRef]
78. Sokolova, E.V.; Ovadis, M.I.; Gorlenko, Z.M.; Khesin, R.B. Localization of streptolydigin resistant mutation in *E. coli* chromosome and effect of streptolydigin on T2 phage development in *stl-r* and stl-s strains of *E. coli*. *Biochem. Biophys. Res. Commun.* **1970**, *41*, 870–876. [CrossRef]
79. Beckman, L.D.; Witonsky, P.; McCorguodale, D.J. Effect of rifampin on the growth of bacteriophage T5. *J. Virol.* **1972**, *10*, 179–186. [PubMed]
80. Toussaint, A.; Lecocq, J.P. Sensitivity of bacteriophage Mu-1 development to rifampicin and streptolydigin. *Mol. Gen. Genet.* **1974**, *129*, 185–188. [CrossRef] [PubMed]
81. Riveros-Moreno, V. Effect of rifampicin on bacteriophage PM2 biogenesis. *FEBS Lett.* **1975**, *51*, 249–252. [CrossRef]
82. Blasdel, B.G.; Chevallereau, A.; Monot, M.; Lavigne, R.; Debarbieux, L. Comparative transcriptomics analyses reveal the conservation of an ancestral infectious strategy in two bacteriophage genera. *ISME J.* **2017**, *11*, 1988–1996. [CrossRef] [PubMed]
83. Taketo, A.; Watanabe, H. Effect of nalidixic acid on the growth of bacterial viruses. *J. Biochem.* **1967**, *61*, 520–522. [CrossRef] [PubMed]
84. Baird, J.P.; Bourguignon, G.J.; Sternglanz, R. Effect of nalidixic acid on the growth of deoxyribonucleic acid bacteriophages. *J. Virol.* **1972**, *9*, 17–21. [PubMed]
85. Valerio, N.; Oliveira, C.; Jesus, V.; Branco, T.; Pereira, C.; Moreirinha, C.; Almeida, A. Effects of single and combined use of bacteriophages and antibiotics to inactivate *Escherichia coli*. *Virus Res.* **2017**, *240*, 8–17. [CrossRef] [PubMed]
86. Kutter, E. Phage host range and efficiency of plating. *Meth. Mol. Biol.* **2009**, *501*, 141–149.
87. McNerney, R. Micro-well phage replication assay for screening mycobacteria for resistance to rifampin and streptomycin. *Methods Mol. Med.* **2001**, *48*, 21–30. [PubMed]

88. Minion, J.; Pai, M. Bacteriophage assays for rifampicin resistance detection in *Mycobacterium tuberculosis*: Updated meta-analysis. *Int. J. Tuberc. Lung Dis.* **2010**, *14*, 941–951. [PubMed]
89. Price, A.R.; Frabotta, M. Resistance of bacteriophage PBS2 infection to rifampicin, an inhibitor of *Bacillus subtilis* RNA synthesis. *Biochem. Biophys. Res. Commun.* **1972**, *48*, 1578–1585. [CrossRef]
90. Hyman, P.; Abedon, S.T. Practical methods for determining phage growth parameters. *Meth. Mol. Biol.* **2009**, *501*, 175–202.
91. Kropinski, A.M. Practical advice on the one-step growth curve. *Methods Mol. Biol.* **2018**, *1681*, 41–47. [PubMed]
92. Payne, R.J.H.; Phil, D.; Jansen, V.A.A. Phage therapy: The peculiar kinetics of self-replicating pharmaceuticals. *Clin. Pharmacol. Ther.* **2000**, *68*, 225–230. [CrossRef] [PubMed]
93. Payne, R.J.H.; Jansen, V.A.A. Understanding bacteriophage therapy as a density-dependent kinetic process. *J. Theor. Biol.* **2001**, *208*, 37–48. [CrossRef] [PubMed]
94. Payne, R.J.H.; Jansen, V.A.A. Pharmacokinetic principles of bacteriophage therapy. *Clin. Pharmacokinet.* **2003**, *42*, 315–325. [CrossRef]
95. Abedon, S.T.; Thomas-Abedon, C. Phage therapy pharmacology. *Curr. Pharm. Biotechnol.* **2010**, *11*, 28–47. [CrossRef]
96. Abedon, S. Phage therapy pharmacology: Calculating phage dosing. *Adv. Appl. Microbiol.* **2011**, *77*, 1–40.
97. Abedon, S.T. Phage therapy: Eco-physiological pharmacology. *Scientifica* **2014**, *2014*, 581639. [CrossRef]
98. Gage, L.P.; Fujita, D.J. Effect of nalidixic acid on deoxyribonucleic acid synthesis in bacteriophage SPO1-infected Bacillus subtilis. *J. Bacteriol.* **1969**, *98*, 96–103. [PubMed]
99. Pedrini, A.M.; Geroldi, D.; Falaschi, A. Nalidixic acid does not inhibit bacterial transformation. *Mol. Gen. Genet.* **1972**, *116*, 91–94. [CrossRef] [PubMed]
100. Price, A.R.; Fogt, S.M. Effect of nalidixic acid on PBS2 bacteriophage infection of *Bacillus subtilis*. *J. Virol.* **1973**, *12*, 405–407. [PubMed]
101. David, H.L.; Clavel, S.; Clement, F.; Moniz-Pereira, J. Effects of antituberculosis and antileprosy drugs on mycobacteriophage D29 growth. *Antimicrob. Agents Chemother.* **1980**, *18*, 357–359. [CrossRef] [PubMed]
102. Lavysh, D.; Sokolova, M.; Slashcheva, M.; Forstner, K.U.; Severinov, K. Transcription Profiling of *Bacillus subtilis* cells infected with AR9, a giant phage encoding two multisubunit RNA polymerases. *MBio* **2017**, *8*. [CrossRef] [PubMed]
103. Oechslin, F.; Piccardi, P.; Mancini, S.; Gabard, J.; Moreillon, P.; Entenza, J.M.; Resch, G.; Que, Y.A. Synergistic interaction between phage therapy and antibiotics clears *Pseudomonas aeruginosa* infection in endocarditis and reduces virulence. *J. Infect. Dis.* **2017**, *215*, 703–712. [CrossRef]
104. Jansen, M.; Wahida, A.; Latz, S.; Kruttgen, A.; Hafner, H.; Buhl, E.M.; Ritter, K.; Horz, H.P. Enhanced antibacterial effect of the novel T4-like bacteriophage KARL-1 in combination with antibiotics against multi-drug resistant *Acinetobacter baumannii*. *Sci. Rep.* **2018**, *8*, 14140. [CrossRef]
105. Lopes, A.; Pereira, C.; Almeida, A. Sequential combined effect of phages and antibiotics on the inactivation of *Escherichia coli*. *Microorganisms* **2018**, *6*, 125. [CrossRef]
106. Bedi, M.S.; Verma, V.; Chhibber, S. Amoxicillin and specific bacteriophage can be used together for eradication of biofilm of *Klebsiella pneumoniae* B5055. *World J. Microbiol. Biotechnol.* **2009**, *25*, 1145–1151. [CrossRef]
107. Verma, V.; Harjai, K.; Chhibber, S. Restricting ciprofloxacin-induced resistant variant formation in biofilm of *Klebsiella pneumoniae* B5055 by complementary bacteriophage treatment. *J. Antimicrob. Chemother.* **2009**, *64*, 1212–1218. [CrossRef]
108. Rahman, M.; Kim, S.; Kim, S.M.; Seol, S.Y.; Kim, J. Characterization of induced *Staphylococcus aureus* bacteriophage SAP-26 and its anti-biofilm activity with rifampicin. *Biofouling* **2011**, *27*, 1087–1093. [CrossRef] [PubMed]
109. Kaur, S.; Harjai, K.; Chhibber, S. Bacteriophage mediated killing of *Staphylococcus aureus* in vitro on orthopaedic K wires in presence of linezolid prevents implant colonization. *PLoS ONE* **2014**, *9*, e90411. [CrossRef] [PubMed]
110. Singla, S.; Harjai, K.; Katare, O.P.; Chhibber, S. Encapsulation of bacteriophage in liposome accentuates its entry in to macrophage and shields it from neutralizing antibodies. *PLoS ONE* **2016**, *11*, e0153777. [CrossRef] [PubMed]
111. Kumaran, D.; Taha, M.; Yi, Q.; Ramirez-Arcos, S.; Diallo, J.S.; Carli, A.; Abdelbary, H. Does treatment order

matter? Investigating the ability of bacteriophage to augment antibiotic activity against *Staphylococcus aureus* biofilms. *Front. Microbiol.* **2018**, *9*, 127. [CrossRef] [PubMed]

112. Yazdi, M.; Bouzari, M.; Ghaemi, E.A. Isolaion and characterization of a lytic bacteriophage (vB_PmiS-TH) and its application in combination with ampicillin against planktonic and biofilm forms of *Proteus mirabilis* isolated from urinary tract infection. *J. Mol. Microbiol. Biotechnol.* **2018**, *28*, 37–46. [CrossRef] [PubMed]
113. Chang, R.Y.K.; Das, T.; Manos, J.; Kutter, E.; Morales, S.; Chan, H.K. Bacteriophage PEV20 and ciprofloxacin combination treatment enhances removal of *Pseudomonas aeruginosa* biofilm isolated from cystic fibrosis and wound patients. *AAPS J.* **2019**, *21*, 49. [CrossRef]
114. Issa, R.; Chanishvili, N.; Caplin, J.; Kakabadze, E.; Bakuradze, N.; Makalatia, K.; Cooper, I. Antibiofilm potential of purified environmental bacteriophage preparations against early stage *Pseudomonas aeruginosa* biofilms. *J. Appl. Microbiol.* **2019**, *126*, 1657–1667. [CrossRef]
115. Chhibber, S.; Kaur, S.; Kumari, S. Therapeutic potential of bacteriophage in treating *Klebsiella pneumoniae* B5055-mediated lobar pneumonia in mice. *J. Med. Microbiol.* **2008**, *57*, 1508–1513. [CrossRef]
116. Chhibber, S.; Kaur, T.; Sandeep, K. Co-therapy using lytic bacteriophage and linezolid: Effective treatment in eliminating methicillin resistant *Staphylococcus aureus* (MRSA) from diabetic foot infections. *PLoS ONE* **2013**, *8*, e56022. [CrossRef]
117. Yilmaz, C.; Colak, M.; Yilmaz, B.C.; Ersoz, G.; Kutateladze, M.; Gozlugol, M. Bacteriophage therapy in implant-related infections: An experimental study. *J. Bone Joint Surg. Am.* **2013**, *95*, 117–125. [CrossRef]
118. Kaur, S.; Harjai, K.; Chhibber, S. In vivo ssessment of phage and linezolid based implant coatings for treatment of methicillin resistant *S. aureus* (MRSA) mediated orthopaedic device related infections. *PLoS ONE* **2016**, *11*, e0157626. [CrossRef] [PubMed]
119. Vahedi, A.; Dallal, M.M.S.; Douraghi, M.; Nikkhahi, F.; Rajabi, Z.; Yousefi, M.; Mousavi, M. Isolation and identification of specific bacteriophage against enteropathogenic *Escherichia coli* (EPEC) and in vitro and in vivo characterization of bacteriophage. *FEMS Microbiol. Lett.* **2018**, *365*, fny136. [CrossRef] [PubMed]
120. Verma, V.; Harjai, K.; Chhibber, S. Characterization of a T7-like lytic bacteriophage of *Klebsiella pneumoniae* B5055: A potential therapeutic agent. *Curr. Microbiol.* **2009**, *59*, 274–281. [CrossRef] [PubMed]
121. Chibeu, A.; Balamurugan, S. Application of a virucidal agent to avoid overestimation of phage kill during phage decontamination assays on ready-to-eat meats. *Methods Mol. Biol.* **2018**, *1681*, 97–105. [PubMed]
122. Summers, W.C. Bacteriophage therapy. *Ann. Rev. Microbiol.* **2001**, *55*, 437–451. [CrossRef]
123. Smith, H.W.; Huggins, M.B. Effectiveness of phages in treating experimental *Escherichia coli* diarrhoea in calves, piglets and lambs. *J. Gen. Microbiol.* **1983**, *129*, 2659–2675. [CrossRef] [PubMed]
124. Ślopek, S.; Durlakova, I.; Weber-Dąbrowska, B.; Kucharewicz-Krukowska, A.; Dąbrowski, M.; Bisikiewicz, R. Results of bacteriophage treatment of suppurative bacterial infections. I. General evaluation of the results. *Arch. Immunol. Ther. Exp.* **1983**, *31*, 267–291.
125. Ślopek, S.; Durlakova, I.; Weber-Dąbrowska, B.; Kucharewicz-Krukowska, A.; Dabrowski, M.; Bisikiewicz, R. Results of bacteriophage treatment of suppurative bacterial infections. II. Detailed evalulation of the results. *Arch. Immunol. Ther. Exp.* **1983**, *31*, 293–327.
126. Ślopek, S.; Durlakowa, I.; Weber-Dąbrowska, B.; Dąbrowski, M.; Kucharewicz-Krukowska, A. Results of bacteriophage treatment of suppurative bacterial infections. III. Detailed evaluation of the results obtained in further 150 cases. *Arch. Immunol. Ther. Exp.* **1984**, *32*, 317–335.
127. Ślopek, S.; Kucharewicz-Krukowska, A.; Weber-Dąbrowska, B.; Dąbrowski, M. Results of bacteriophage treatment of suppurative bacterial infections. IV. Evaluation of results obtained in 370 cases. *Arch. Immunol. Ther. Exp.* **1985**, *33*, 219–240.
128. Ślopek, S.; Kucharewicz-Krukowska, A.; Weber-Dąbrowska, B.; Dąbrowski, M. Results of bacteriophage treatment of suppurative bacterial infections. V. Evaluation of the results obtained in children. *Arch. Immunol. Ther. Exp.* **1985**, *33*, 241–259.
129. Ślopek, S.; Kucharewicz-Krukowska, A.; Weber-Dąbrowska, B.; Dąbrowski, M. Results of bacteriophage treatment of suppurative bacterial infections. VI. Analysis of treatment of suppurative staphylococcal infections. *Arch. Immunol. Ther. Exp.* **1985**, *33*, 261–273.
130. Ślopek, S.; Weber-Dąbrowska, B.; Dąbrowski, M.; Kucharewicz-Krukowska, A. Results of bacteriophage treatment of suppurative bacterial infections in the years 1981–1986. *Arch. Immunol. Ther. Exp.* **1987**, *35*, 569–583.

131. Chanishvili, N. *A Literature Review of the Practical Application of Bacteriophage Research*; Nova Publishers: Hauppauge, New York, NY, USA, 2012.
132. Eaton, M.D.; Bayne-Jones, S. Bacteriophage therapy: Review of the principles and results of the use of bacteriophage in the treatment of infections (I). *J. Am. Med. Assoc.* **1934**, *103*, 1769–1776. [CrossRef]

3

Characterization of vB_SauM-fRuSau02, a Twort-Like Bacteriophage Isolated from a Therapeutic Phage Cocktail

Katarzyna Leskinen [1], Henni Tuomala [1,2], Anu Wicklund [1,2], Jenni Horsma-Heikkinen [1], Pentti Kuusela [2], Mikael Skurnik [1,2] and Saija Kiljunen [1,2,*]

1 Department of Bacteriology and Immunology, Medicum, Research Programs Unit, Immunobiology Research Program, University of Helsinki, Helsinki 00290, Finland; katarzyna.leskinen@helsinki.fi (K.L.); henni.tuomala@helsinki.fi (H.T.); anumaria.wicklund@gmail.com (A.W.); jenni.horsma@helsinki.fi (J.H.-H.); mikael.skurnik@helsinki.fi (M.S.)

2 Division of Clinical Microbiology, HUSLAB, University of Helsinki and Helsinki University Hospital, Helsinki 00290, Finland; pentti.kuusela@hus.fi

* Correspondence: saija.kiljunen@helsinki.fi

Academic Editors: Harald Brüssow and Eric Freed

Abstract: *Staphylococcus aureus* is a commensal and pathogenic bacterium that causes infections in humans and animals. It is a major cause of nosocomial infections worldwide. Due to increasing prevalence of multidrug resistance, alternative methods to eradicate the pathogen are necessary. In this respect, polyvalent staphylococcal myoviruses have been demonstrated to be excellent candidates for phage therapy. Here we present the characterization of the bacteriophage vB_SauM-fRuSau02 (fRuSau02) that was isolated from a commercial *Staphylococcus* bacteriophage cocktail produced by Microgen (Moscow, Russia). The genomic analysis revealed that fRuSau02 is very closely related to the phage MSA6, and possesses a large genome (148,464 bp), with typical modular organization and a low G+C (30.22%) content. It can therefore be classified as a new virus among the genus *Twortlikevirus*. The genome contains 236 predicted genes, 4 of which were interrupted by insertion sequences. Altogether, 78 different structural and virion-associated proteins were identified from purified phage particles by liquid chromatography-tandem mass spectrometry (LC-MS/MS). The host range of fRuSau02 was tested with 135 strains, including 51 and 54 *Staphylococcus aureus* isolates from humans and pigs, respectively, and 30 coagulase-negative *Staphylococcus* strains of human origin. All clinical *S. aureus* strains were at least moderately sensitive to the phage, while only 39% of the pig strains were infected. Also, some strains of *Staphylococcus intermedius*, *Staphylococcus lugdunensis*, *Staphylococcus epidermidis*, *Staphylococcus haemolyticus*, *Staphylococcus saprophyticus* and *Staphylococcus pseudointer* were sensitive. We conclude that fRuSau02, a phage therapy agent in Russia, can serve as an alternative to antibiotic therapy against *S. aureus*.

Keywords: *Staphylococcus aureus*; bacteriophage; phage therapy; vB_SauM-fRuSau02; *Twortlikevirus*

1. Introduction

Staphylococcus aureus is a commensal and pathogenic bacterium that causes opportunistic infections in humans and animals. Approximately 20% of humans have persistent and 30% sporadic nasal *S. aureus* colonization [1]. As a pathogen, *S. aureus* causes a broad spectrum of infections in humans ranging from simple abscesses to fatal sepsis, including pneumonia, endocarditis, meningitis, mastitis, food poisoning, and toxic shock syndrome [2]. Currently the antibiotic resistance of this species poses a threat to public health. Even though the incidence of severe infections caused by methicillin-resistant *S. aureus* (MRSA) is decreasing [3], MRSA still is an important cause of nosocomial infections worldwide [4,5]. The emergence of multidrug resistance results in difficulties in eradication of the pathogen with the use of conventional therapies and thus requires development of alternatives to antibiotic-based therapies.

One promising alternative to treat infections caused by antibiotic resistant bacteria is phage therapy, where the natural predators of bacteria (bacteriophages, phages) are used to kill the pathogens [6–8]. The history of phage therapy has been extensively reviewed elsewhere [9,10] and is not discussed here. To be considered safe, phage therapy has to meet a number of criteria: phages used for therapeutic purposes need to be strictly lytic and they should not carry known genes coding for toxins or other harmful substances [11]. Furthermore, the host bacteria used for phage production should have as few prophages as possible and the therapeutic phage preparation should not contain high concentration of bacterial toxins.

All known *S. aureus* phages belong to order *Caudovirales*, i.e., they are tailed phages with an icosahedral capsid that surrounds the double-stranded DNA genome [12,13]. Staphylococcal phages can be classified into three categories: (1) podoviruses with <20 kb genomes; (2) siphoviruses with ~40 kb genomes; and (3) myoviruses with >125 kb genomes [12]. Of these phage groups, staphylococcal siphoviruses are generally temperate and often carry genes promoting bacterial virulence [13], which makes them inappropriate for therapeutic applications. Staphylococcal podoviruses, on the other hand, are strictly lytic but extremely rare and difficult to find [14]. From therapeutic point of view, myoviruses are considered the most interesting staphylococcal phages [14,15].

Many of the staphylococcal myoviruses are classified into the genus *Twortlikevirus* of the *Spounavirinae* subfamily and are related at genetic and proteomic level [16]. The *Twortlikevirus* genus consists of phages with genomes of 127–141 kb, low G+C content (30–31%), and 183 to 217 open reading frames (ORFs) [17]. Currently, this genus contains over 25 members, including phage Twort, G1 [18], K [19], MSA6 [20], GH15 [21], Romulus, and Remus [17]. A typical feature for Twort-like viruses is the presence of long terminal repeats (LTRs), several thousand base pair-long direct repeats at the ends of the genome. The nucleotide sequence and length of LTR regions differ among the representatives of the genus and may influence the host range [15]. Twort-like viruses are also known for their broad host range. This phenomenon is mainly accounted to the presence of multiple receptor binding proteins in the viral capsid that allow them to utilize at least two adsorption apparatuses and recognize different structures [22]. This feature, together with their strictly lytic life cycle, makes Twort-like viruses particularly suitable for clinical applications [15].

In this paper, we report the isolation and analysis of a Twort-like *S. aureus* phage, vB_SauM-fRuSau02 (fRuSau02). The phage was isolated from a therapeutic bacteriophage product from Microgen Company (Moscow, Russia). The product was purchased in a pharmacy in Saint Petersburg, Russia, and was meant to treat infections typically caused by *S. aureus*. However, no information about the phage composition or the efficacy of the phage cocktail was available. Phage fRuSau02 was the only phage we were able to isolate from this product. Here, we show the analysis of fRuSau02 at a genetic and proteome level, the latter of which allowed us to identify the majority of the phage structural proteins. Additionally, we provide an insight into the reasons why this phage might be well-suited for clinical applications by testing its growth efficiency and host range with a broad range of human and porcine isolates. We also present an evaluation of the fRuSau02 production in different host strains, with intention to select an optimal producer strain for clinical applications.

2. Materials and Methods

2.1. Bacterial Strains, Phages and Media

The bacterial strains used in this work are described in Table S1. The collection of human isolates used in this study was provided by The Hospital District of Helsinki and Uusimaa Laboratories

(HUSLAB), Finland. All staphylococcal and phage incubations were done at 37 °C using Luria Broth (LB) [23] medium. Soft agar medium included additionally 0.35 or 0.4% (*w*/*v*) agar (Becton Dickinson, Franklin Lakes, NJ, USA), and LB agar plates were solidified with 1.5% (*w*/*v*) of agar. fRuSau02 was isolated using a clinical *S. aureus* strain 13KP (Table S1) as a host, and the same strain was then used as a standard host strain for the phage. The phage lysates were produced from semiconfluent soft-agar plates as described elsewhere [23].

2.2. Phage Purification

The fRuSau02 lysate (5×10^{10} plaque-forming units (PFU)/mL) was ultrafiltrated with Amicon Ultra-4 (100 kDa) Centrifugal Filter Units (Merck Millipore, Billerica, MA, USA) to one quarter of the initial volume. Three volumes of chromatography buffer A (20 mM Tris-Cl, pH 7.5) were added and the ultrafiltration was repeated. The volume was adjusted with buffer A. The ultrafiltrated phage sample was then purified with ion exchange chromatography (IEX) using Äkta Purifier (GE Healthcare, Chicago, IL, USA) and a CIM QA-1 tube monolithic column with a 6-μm pore size (BIA Separations, Ajdovščina, Slovenia). The sample was injected to the column in buffer A, washed with buffer A containing 350 mM NaCl and eluted with buffer A with 450 mM NaCl. The phage-containing fractions of two purification batches were pooled, and an Amicon Ultra was used to concentrate the product and to change the buffer to TM (50 mM Tris, pH 7.5–10 mM Mg_2SO_4). Purified phage samples were stored at 4 °C.

2.3. Electron Microscopy

IEX-purified phage lysate was pelleted by centrifugation at 16,000× *g*, 4 °C, for 2 h and resuspended into 0.1 M ammonium acetate. Subsequently, the phage particles were allowed to sediment on 200 mesh pioloform-coated copper grids for 1 min and stained negatively using 3% uranyl acetate. Samples were examined with a JEOL JEM-1400 transmission electron microscope JEOL Ltd., Tokyo, Japan) under 80 kV at the Electron Microscopy Unit (Institute of Biotechnology, University of Helsinki, Helsinki, Finland). Pictures were taken using Gatan Orius SC 1000B bottom-mounted Charged Coupled Device (CCD)-camera (Gatan Inc., Pleasanton, CA, USA). Ten virions were measured and data were used to calculate mean values and standard deviations.

2.4. Infection Growth Curves

Overnight bacterial cultures of *S. aureus* 13KP were diluted to a ratio of 1:100 in fresh LB medium, and 180-μL aliquots were distributed into honeycomb plate wells (Growth Curves Ab Ltd., Helsinki, Finland), where they were mixed with 20-μL aliquots of different fRuSau02 phage stock dilutions. The phage stock and bacterial culture were mixed to achieve multiplicity of infection (MOI) values ranging between 5×10^{-7} and 500. A negative control was obtained by mixing 20 μL of phage stock with 180 μL of LB, whereas the positive control consisted of 180 μL of bacterial culture and 20 μL of fresh LB medium. The growth experiment was carried out at 37 °C using a Bioscreen C incubator (Growth Curves Ab Ltd.) with continuous shaking. The optical density at 600 nm (OD_{600}) of the cultures was measured every 1 h. The averages were calculated from values obtained for the bacteria grown in five parallel wells.

2.5. DNA Isolation and Phage Genome Sequencing

fRuSau02 DNA was isolated from crude phage lysate with Invisorb Spin Virus DNA Mini Kit (Stratec Biomedical, Birkenfeld, Germany). Sequencing was performed at the Institute for Molecular Medicine Finland (FIMM) Technology Centre Sequencing Unit [24]. For next-generation sequencing, the DNA library was constructed with Nextera sample prep kit (Illumina, San Diego, CA, USA). Paired-end sequencing was done using Illumina MiSeq PE300 sequencer (Illumina, San Diego, CA, USA) with the read length of 300 nucleotides. TheA5 (Andrew And Aaron's Awesome Assembly)-miseq integrated pipeline for de novo assembly of microbial genomes was used to obtain the genome sequence [25]. fRuSau02 sequence was submitted to GenBank with accession number MF398190.

2.6. Determination of Physical Ends of the Phage Genome

To determine the physical ends of the phage genome, the approximate positions of the terminal repeats were estimated based on the sequence read numbers using the Integrative Genomics Viewer (IGV) [26,27]. The genome was manually edited according to the estimated physical ends and subjected to virtual digestions with several restriction endonucleases. Two enzymes (NheI and PstI), yielding identifiable end fragments, were used to digest the fRuSau02 DNA, and the resulting fragment distributions were compared to the virtual digestions. The NheI fragments corresponding to the physical ends of the phage genome were isolated from a preparative agarose gel and ligated to pUC19 digested with XbaI and SmaI. The ligation mixtures were used as a template for PCR reaction with pUC19—specific primers Puc19-F (CCTCTTCGCTATTACGCCAG) and pUC19-R (CAACGCAATTAATGTGAGTTAGCT). The PCR products corresponding to the sizes of the genome end fragments (2.7 kb and 4.5 kb for left and right ends, respectively) were isolated from a preparative agarose gel and sequenced with ABI3730XL DNA Analyzer (Applied Biosystems, Foster City, CA, USA) capillary sequencer with primers Puc19-F and Puc19-R at FIMM [24]. The sequence information was used to deduce the actual sequence of the genome ends and terminal repeats.

2.7. In Silico Analysis of Phage Genome

The phage genome was autoannotated using Rapid Annotation Using Subsystem Technology (RAST [28] and proofread manually. Promoters and terminators were predicted using PePPER [29] and ARNold [30,31], respectively, with subsequent manual verification. The promoter consensus sequence was analyzed using MEME [32]. A comparative genome figure was generated using CGView [33]. The genome-wide comparison of bacteriophages was conducted with EMBOSS Stretcher [34].

Phylogeny analysis was conducted with the VICTOR Virus Classification and Tree Building Online Resource [35] using the Genome-BLAST Distance Phylogeny (GBDP) method [36] under settings recommended for prokaryotic viruses [35]. The resulting intergenomic distances (including 100 replicates each) were used to infer a balanced minimum evolution tree with branch support via FASTME including Subtree Pruning and Regrafting (SPR) postprocessing [37] for the formula D0. The tree was rooted at the midpoint [38] and visualized with FigTree [39]. Taxon boundaries at the species, genus and family level were estimated with the OPTSIL program [40], the recommended clustering thresholds [35] and an F value (fraction of links required for cluster fusion) of 0.5 [41].

2.8. Proteome Analysis

IEX-purified phages were concentrated by centrifugation for 2 h at 4 °C and 16,000× *g*. Prior to digestion of proteins to peptides with trypsin, the proteins in the samples were reduced with tris(2-carboxyethyl)phosphine (TCEP) and alkylated with iodoacetamide. Tryptic peptide digests were purified by C18 reversed-phase chromatography columns [42] and the mass spectrometry (MS) analysis was performed on an Orbitrap Elite Electron-Transfer Dissociation (ETD) mass spectrometer (Thermo Scientific, Waltham, MA, USA), using Xcalibur version 2.7.1, coupled to an Thermo Scientific nLCII nanoflow High Pressure Liquid Chromatography (HPLC) system. Peak extraction and subsequent protein identification was achieved using Proteome Discoverer 1.4 software (Thermo Scientific). Calibrated peak files were searched against the fRuSau02 and *Staphylococcus aureus* subsp. *aureus* ST398 proteins (ASM188707v1, NCBI) by a SEQUEST search engine. Error tolerances on the precursor and fragment ions were ±15 ppm and ±0.6 Da, respectively. For peptide identification, a stringent cut-off (0.5% false discovery rate) was used. The LC-MS/MS was performed at the Proteomics Unit, Institute of Biotechnology, University of Helsinki.

2.9. Host Range Screening

The fRuSau02 host range was analyzed by spot assay for most of the bacterial stains studied. Some pig isolates failed to grow on soft agar, and their sensitivity was studied by a liquid culture method. For this, bacteria were cultured overnight in Brain Heart Infusion (BHI) medium (Becton, Dickinson and Company, Franklin Lakes, NJ, USA). Cultures were diluted 1:100 in BHI and aliquoted into 200 μL aliquots to 96-well plates. To these, 10 μL of phage fRuSau02 (6.8×10^6 PFU) was added and the plate was incubated at 37 °C with moderate shaking. For non-infected controls, 10 μL of LB was added instead of the phage. Each strain was studied in triplicate wells. Bacterial growth was monitored by measuring OD_{600} with FLUOstar OPTIMA plate reader (BMG LABTECH GmbH, Ortenberg, Germany) at 60 min intervals for 4 h, and the inhibition of growth in phage-infected wells compared to non-infected control wells indicated a sensitive strain.

2.10. Efficiency of Plating and Adsorption Assay

Bacterial strains were checked by the efficiency of plating (EOP), as described earlier [43]. In brief, *S. aureus* strains 13KP, Newman, TB4, and tagO were pre-grown for 2–3 h at 37 °C. Subsequently 300 PFU of phage was mixed with 90 μL/OD_{600} of bacterial culture and 3 mL of soft agar (0.35% LB agar) and poured over an LB plate. Following 24 h incubation at 37 °C, PFUs were counted and the size and morphology of the plaques was evaluated. The experiment was performed in triplicates, and negative controls without the bacteriophages were prepared. To estimate the adsorption of phage particles on the surface of different *S. aureus* strains, a phage adsorption assay was conducted as described earlier [44]. Briefly, approximately 2.5×10^6 PFU of fRuSau02 was mixed with 500 μL of bacterial overnight cultures (OD_{600} = 3.3). The suspension was incubated at room temperature for 5 min, centrifuged at 16,000× *g* for 3 min, and the phage titer remaining in the supernatant was determined. The phage titer in the control supernatant was set to 100%. LB was used as a non-adsorbing control. Each assay was performed in triplicates.

2.11. Staphylococcal Enterotoxin Measurement

Staphylococcal enterotoxins were measured from the phage lysates with the Transia Plate Staphylococcal Enterotoxins assay (BioControl Systems, Inc., Bellevue, WA, USA) using staphylococcal enterotoxin A (Sigma-Aldrich, St. Louis, MO, USA) as standard. Absorbance at 450 nm was recorded with Hidex Sense Microplate Reader (Hidex, Turku, Finland).

3. Results

3.1. Isolation and Morphology

Phage fRuSau02 was isolated from the *Staphylococcus* bacteriophage cocktail produced by the Microgen Company (Moscow, Russia; series: H52, 0813, PN001973/01). Electron microscopy of the negatively-stained fRuSau02 particles revealed that the phage had an icosahedral head with a contractile tail and a basal tuft attached to the tail (Figure 1). The dimensions of the head were 86 nm (vertical) and 83 nm (horizontal), and the tail length without the base plate was 192 nm. Standard deviations were 3.1, 2.8, and 5.3 nm respectively. Only one particle with contracted tail was found (Figure 1b), and the contracted part was 96 nm. Based on the morphological characteristics, phage fRuSau02 belongs to the order *Caudovirales* and the family *Myoviridae* [45,46].

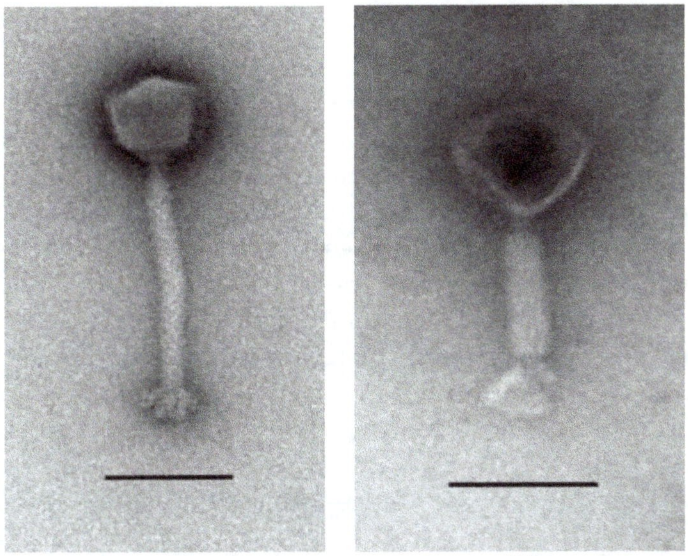

(a) (b)

Figure 1. Electron micrographs of negatively stained vB_SauM-fRuSau02 (fRuSau02) particles. Phage particles with non-contracted (**a**) and contracted (**b**) tails are shown. Bars represent 100 nm.

3.2. *The Efficiency of Infection*

To examine the efficiency of fRuSau02 infection, *S. aureus* 13KP was infected in liquid culture at different MOI values and the bacterial growth was assessed by following the optical density of the culture. The study showed that fRuSau02 is able to efficiently lyse the culture at MOIs above 5×10^{-5} (Figure 2), whereas at MOIs values below this limit there was no lysis observed (data not shown). Additionally, there was no re-growth of the bacterial culture observed within the 24 h time period of the experiment. In coherence, the prolonged incubation of the infected bacteria in the soft agar did not result in emergence of resistance within the first 7 days of incubation indicating low rate of phage-resistance development among the bacteria. Efficient infection and complete lysis of bacterial culture with very low MOI values may be a common feature of twort-like phages, as MOI 1×10^{-4} was earlier shown to be optimal for the production of high-titer lysate of phage MSA6 [20].

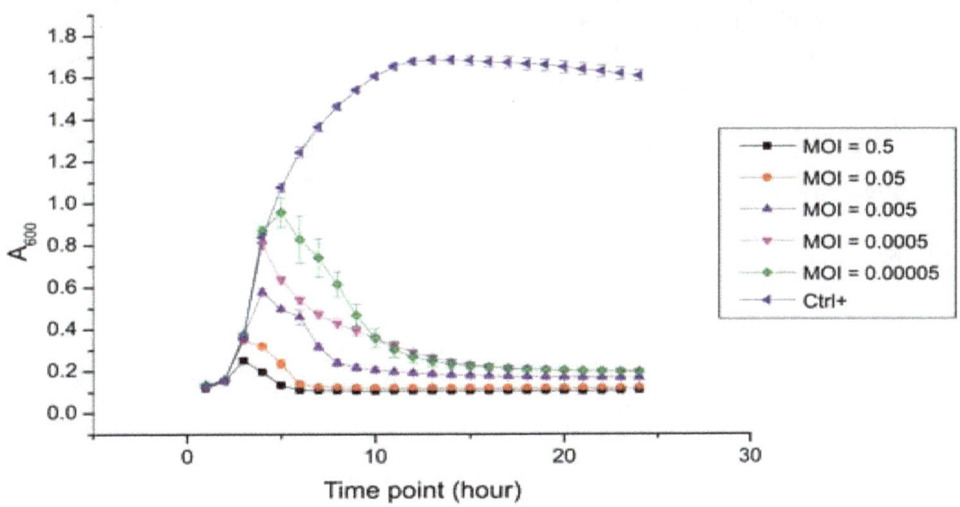

Figure 2. Growth curves of *Staphylococcus aureus* of 13KP infected with fRuSau02. Bacteria were cultured with different concentrations of phage virions in Luria Broth (LB) at 37 °C. Each curve represents the average results for five replicates, error bars represent standard deviation (SD). MOI: multiplicity of infection.

3.3. General Genome Analysis

The linear double-stranded DNA of fRuSau02 comprises 148,464 bp encoding 236 putative ORFs (Figure 3, Table 1). The two terminally redundant 8076 bp long ends encode 20 putative terminal repeat proteins. Sixty-five of the predicted genes are transcribed from the minus strand, including the genes likely to be involved in bacterial cell lysis (holin and numerous putative membrane proteins). Additionally, two single genes from the terminally redundant region, *treI* and *treM*, are also encoded on the minus strand. *In silico* analysis predicted the presence of 43 bacterial promoters and 32 terminators. The analysis failed to identify promoters within the 39,000–66,500 bp range in the fRuSau02 genome where the structural proteins are encoded. The consensus sequence of the promoters was identified (Figure 4 and Table S2). Interestingly, three predicted promoters located in front of spliced or intron encoded genes (*lysK.1*, *ksaI*, *I-MsaI*) presented a distinctive promoter sequence that did not follow the consensus sequence (Table S2). In addition to protein-coding sequences, three functional transfer RNA(tRNA) genes encoding $tRNA^{Met}$, $tRNA^{Phe}$, and $tRNA^{Asp}$ were detected. Additionally, no known genes encoding integrases, lysogeny- or virulence-associated or toxic proteins were identified and therefore this bacteriophage can be considered as virulent and potentially safe for phage therapy. Similarly to phage K, the genome of fRuSau02 completely lacks GATC sites that could be recognized by host-encoded restriction endonucleases [19].

Table 1. The structural proteins of phage fRuSau02 identified using liquid chromatography tandem mass spectrometry (LC-MS/MS).

Locus	Name	No of AA	M_W * [kDa]	pI * (calc.)
RS_018	TreR, terminal repeat encoded protein R	156	17.8	3.78
RS_033	phage structural protein	105	11.8	6.76
RS_036	phage structural protein	64	7.6	4.65
RS_037	phage structural protein	245	28.6	6.58
RS_041	phage structural protein	57	6.8	5.26
RS_042	phage structural protein	160	18.8	4.64
RS_046	putative membrane protein MbpR	91	10.9	5.01
RS_048	phage structural protein	372	42.2	4.84
RS_050	phage structural protein	138	16.0	5.22
RS_051	HmzG, DNA-binding protein	100	11.3	4.91
RS_055	phage structural protein	87	10.1	5.91
RS_059	Lig, putative DNA or RNA ligase	298	35.0	5.57
RS_061	Phr, putative PhoH-related protein	246	28.6	5.29
RS_063	Rbn, phage ribonuclease H	141	15.8	7.27
RS_067	phage structural protein	75	9.2	9.95
RS_070	putative membrane protein MbpS	263	29.3	8.82
RS_072	LysK.1, phage lysin	209	23.1	9.66
RS_074	LysK.2, phage lysin	267	29.8	9.45
RS_075	HolA, phage holin	167	18.1	4.25
RS_078	DmcB	69	8.0	5.97
RS_080	putative membrane protein MbpC	108	13.0	5.54
RS_082	putative membrane protein MbpD	88	10.3	8.31
RS_085	Ter.1, phage terminase	65	7.7	9.60
RS_087	Ter.2, phage terminase	515	59.7	6.10
RS_088	phage structural protein	266	29.8	5.30
RS_094	Prt, portal protein	563	64.0	6.42
RS_095	Pro, prohead protease	257	28.6	5.01
RS_096	phage structural protein	318	35.9	4.46
RS_097	Mcp, major capsid protein	463	51.2	5.24

Table 1. *Cont.*

Locus	Name	No of AA	M_W * [kDa]	pI * (calc.)
RS_098	phage structural protein	98	11.3	9.42
RS_099	phage structural protein	302	34.1	5.24
RS_100	phage structural protein	292	33.7	5.82
RS_101	phage structural protein	206	23.7	10.32
RS_102	phage structural protein	278	31.7	4.79
RS_104	Tsp, major tail sheath protein	587	64.5	4.98
RS_105	TmpA, tail tube protein	142	15.9	5.54
RS_109	phage structural protein	103	12.2	6.13
RS_110	phage structural protein	152	18.1	4.79
RS_111	TmpB, tail morphogenic protein	178	20.9	4.40
RS_112	TmpC, phage DNA transfer protein	1351	143.7	9.11
RS_113	TmpD, tail murein hydrolase	808	91.2	6.74
RS_114	TmpE, putative peptidoglycan hydrolase	295	34.6	4.60
RS_115	Glycerophosphoryl diester phosphodiesterase	848	96.0	4.96
RS_116	phage structural protein	263	29.3	8.19
RS_117	phage structural protein	174	19.9	4.61
RS_118	BmpA, baseplate morphogenetic protein	234	26.6	4.77
RS_119	BmpB, baseplate morphogenetic protein	348	39.2	4.86
RS_120	TmpF, tail morphogenetic protein	1019	116.2	5.08
RS_121	BmpC, baseplate morphogenetic protein	173	19.2	5.39
RS_122	TmpG, tail morphogenetic protein	1152	129.0	5.19
RS_124	receptor binding protein	640	72.6	7.39
RS_126	receptor binding protein	458	50.3	6.27
RS_127	DhlA, DNA helicase	582	67.2	5.85
RS_129	DhlB, DNA helicase	480	54.5	5.72
RS_132	RncB, recombination nuclease B	639	73.4	5.19
RS_133	Asf, anti-sigma factor	198	23.2	6.81
RS_137	phage structural protein	202	23.6	5.72
RS_139	NrdE, ribonucleotide reductase	704	80.1	5.64
RS_140	NrdF, ribonucleotide reductase	349	40.4	4.78
RS_141	phage structural protein	109	12.4	4.68
RS_143	phage structural protein	179	21.1	6.95
RS_152	phage structural protein	423	46.8	4.75
RS_153	Rec.1, phage recombinase	74	7.9	6.61
RS_155	Rec.2, phage recombinase	315	35.7	5.16
RS_157	Sig, sigma factor	220	26.6	5.36
RS_158	phage structural protein	210	23.2	4.84
RS_159	TmpH, phage major tail protein	73	7.9	4.54
RS_160	phage structural protein	86	10.3	5.91
RS_163	putative membrane protein MbpG	122	14.0	5.95
RS_165	phage structural protein	178	20.8	7.47
RS_168	phage structural protein	287	32.3	5.76
RS_169	phage structural protein	243	28.3	5.34
RS_170	phage structural protein	152	17.8	4.98
RS_173	putative membrane protein MbpH	132	15.4	8.94
RS_175	phage structural protein	80	9.4	9.31
RS_181	phage structural protein	98	11.3	7.24
RS_196	phage structural protein	87	9.9	10.05
RS_206	NadV, nicotinamide phosphoribosyltransferase	489	56.1	5.44

* M_W: Molecular weight, pI: Isoelectric point.

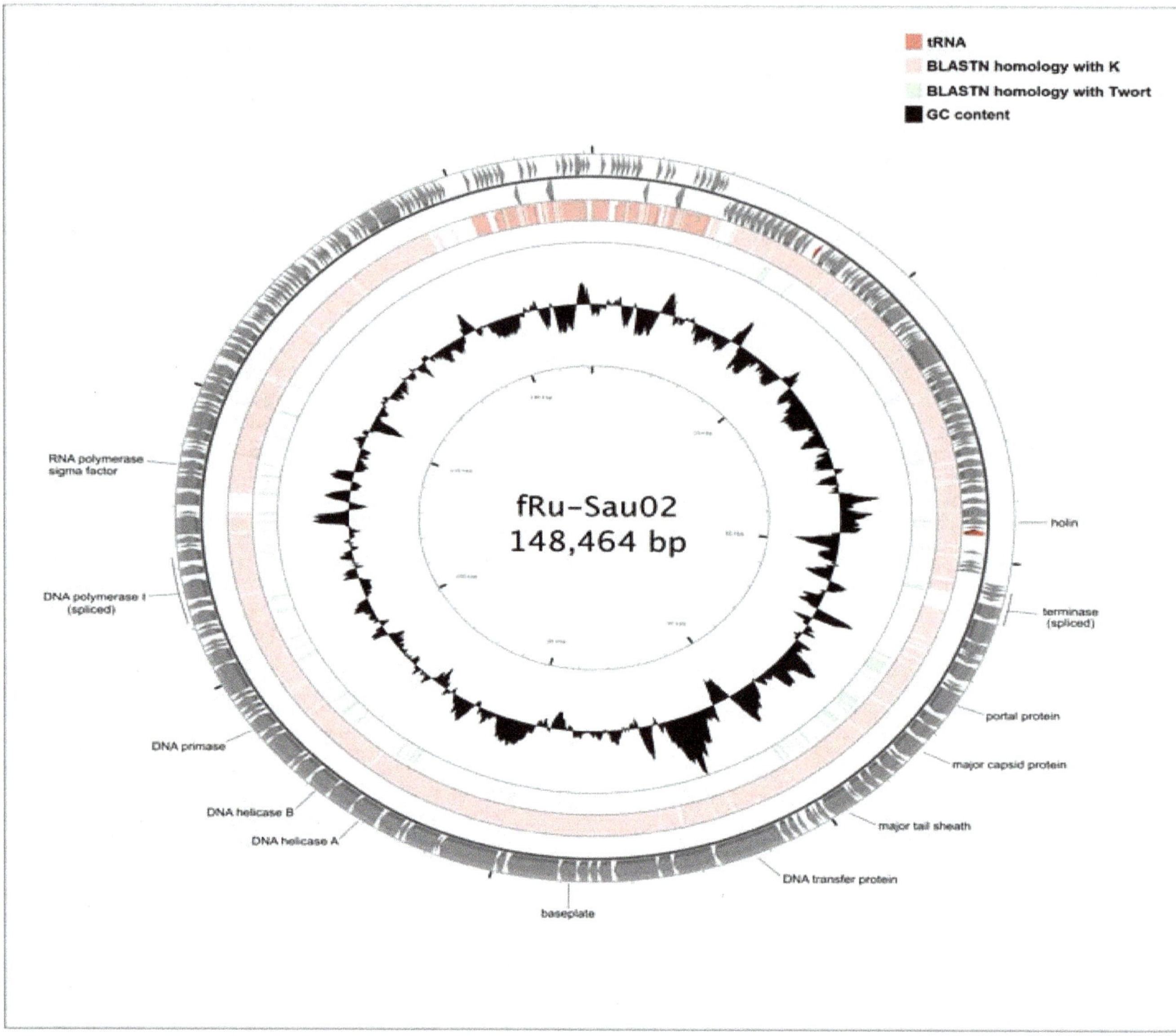

Figure 3. Genome comparison of three Twort-like phages. The outer ring represents the open reading frames (ORFs) of the circularized fRuSau02 phage. The two other rings display the identity between fRuSau02 and K (lavender) and between fRuSau02 and Twort (green). The inner ring shows the GC content of the fRuSau02 genome (black). Selected gene functions are indicated. The figure was generated with CGView [33].

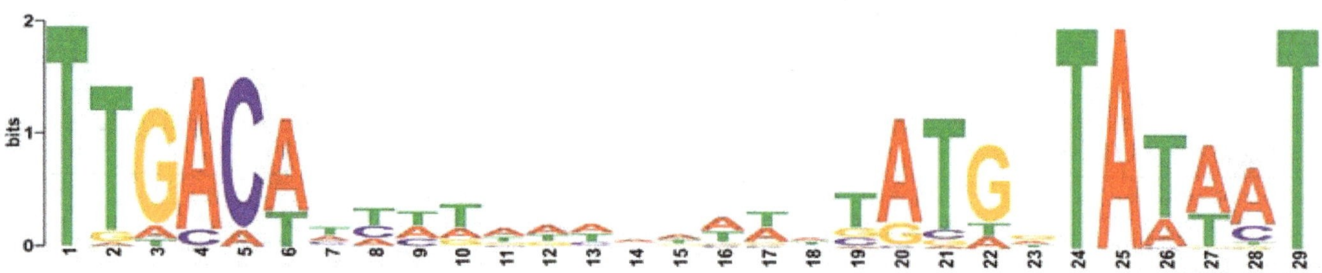

Figure 4. Consensus sequence of the phage fRuSau02 putative promoters. The promoter sequences are listed in supplementary Table S2.

3.4. Comparative Genome Analysis

Bioinformatic analysis of the fRuSau02 genome revealed that the phage has a genome size and organization typical for Twort-like viruses [15]. It is most closely related to phage MSA6 (JX080304), the two viruses showing 99.6% identity at the nucleotide level. The DNA sequence comparison with other Twort-like viruses revealed identity in the range of 39.0–96.0% (Table S3). The highest identity was observed with phages A5W (EU418428)—96.0%, Staph1N (JX080300)—96.0%, and Fi200W (JX080303)—95.1%. The genomic comparison of fRuSau02 with phages K and Twort showed identity rates of 93.5% and 46.5%, respectively. Figure 3 shows a BLASTN comparison of the genomes of phages fRuSau02, K and Twort. The whole-genome level nucleotide phylogeny analysis of fRuSau02 and the 34 phage genomes described in Table S3 showed that fRuSau02 clusters in the same species with A5W, Staph1N, MSA6, Fi200W, and 676Z (Figure 5). The analysis yielded average support of 16% and the OPTSIL clustering resulted altogether to 22, 2, and 1 clusters at species, genus, and family levels, respectively.

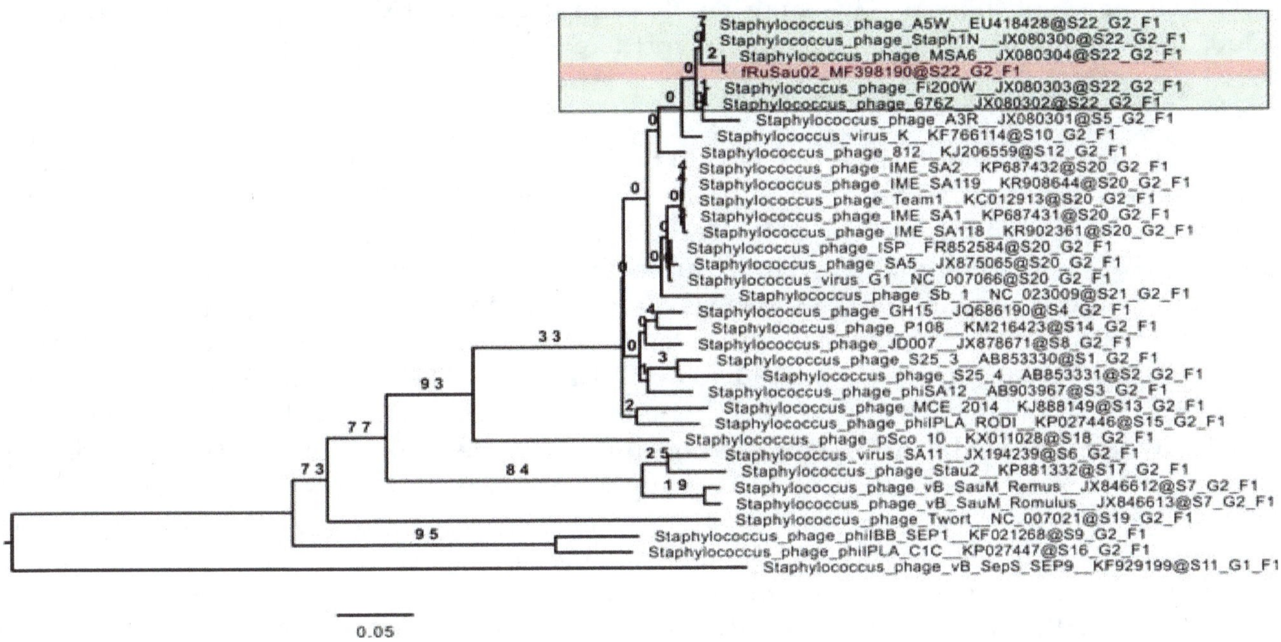

Figure 5. Genome-wide nucleotide phylogeny of 35 Twort-like viruses. The analysis was conducted with VICTOR Virus Classification and Tree Building Online Resource [35] with settings recommended for prokaryotic viruses. The tree was visualized with FigTree [39]. The analysis yielded 22 clusters at species (S1–S22) and two at genus (G1–G2) level, respectively. All the phages clustered to the same family (F1). Phage fRuSau02 is indicated with red box and the phages belonging to the same species with it in the green box.

Most fRuSau02 nucleotide differences to MSA6 were single base pair substitutions or small indels in intergenic regions. There were 25 coding regions having differences to MSA6, eight of which had silent mutations, leading to proteins with 100% amino acid identity with their MSA6 counterparts (terminal repeat encoded protein TreP, phage terminase Ter.2, tail morphogenetic proteins TmpB and TmpG, DNA helicase DhlA, DNA primase/DNA helicase Pri, ribonucleotide reductase NrdE, and intron encoded endonuclease I-MsaI). Ten proteins had difference(s) to the corresponding proteins in MSA6 but showed 100% amino acid identities to their homologs in other Twort-like viruses: terminal repeat encoded protein TreK was identical to phage G1 ORF159 but showed only 87.4% identity to MSA6 TreK. Terminal repeat encoded protein TreG was identical to phage K Gp007, putative membrane protein MbpP to G1 ORF007, hypothetical protein DmcA to Gp122 of phage JD007, putative membrane protein MbpE to phage G1 ORF120, major tail sheath Tsp to phage K Gp166, hypothetical protein RS_209 to Team1 Gp041, putative receptor binding protein RS_126 to SA5 ORF40, terminal repeat encoded protein TreB to A5W TreB and to G1 ORF231, and putative portal protein Prt to G1 ORF014. Each of these proteins had one to two amino acid difference(s) to their MSA6 homologs. Seven proteins had at least one amino acid (according to present knowledge) unique to fRuSau02, i.e., have not been observed in homologous proteins of any other Twort-like virus: putative membrane protein MbpC, tail morphogenetic protein TmpC, putative receptor binding protein RS_124, putative polymerase-associated exonuclease PolA.2, putative RNA polymerase sigma factor Sig, hypothetical protein RS_200, and putative membrane protein MbpI.

Of the "unique" fRuSau02 proteins, RS_124 is of outmost interest. It is 98.1% identical at the amino acid level to the *orf103* gene product of phage *Φ*SA012, shown to be one out of two receptor binding proteins (RBPs) of this phage [22]. Phage fRuSau02 RS_124 has histidine in position 306, where all the other Twort-like viruses sequenced so far have proline. The residue 306 is part of a carbohydrate binding domain, which is formed by amino acids 213–336. Preliminary structural modelling of this region showed that H306 fits nicely into an anti-parallel β-sheet structure, which is completely distorted by H306P change (not shown). This suggests that the structure of the receptor binding protein of fRuSau02 may be different from all the other Twort-like viruses characterized so far.

3.5. Genes Interrupted by Self-Splicing Elements

The presence of mobile splicing elements in the genomes of Twort-like viruses is a characteristic feature of staphylococcal myoviruses [17–19]. In the case of fRuSau02 phage, four protein-encoding genes were found to be interrupted by different insertion sequences (Figure S1): (1) The gene encoding phage lysin (Lys) is fragmented into two by an intron-encoded HNH homing endonuclease gene (*I-KsaI*). (2) The terminase large subunit gene is divided by the intron, encoding I-MsaI, a protein of unknown function. (3) The gene encoding the putative DNA polymerase-associated exonuclease (PolA) contains two introns encoding proteins I-KsaII and I-KsaIII. (4) The gene encoding phage RecA-like recombinase (Rec) contains the intron-encoded endonuclease gene *I-MsaII*. All of the intervening sequences are predicted to be group I introns encoding putative endonucleases. The functionality of the spliced genes was shown by the fact that the presence of full proteins encoded by three out of four spliced genes was observed in the LC-MS/MS analysis. Namely, lysin, terminase large subunit, and phage recombinase were among the proteins identified in the LC-MS/MS analysis of the purified phage particles (Table 1), with peptides present in both the C- and N-terminal parts of the proteins (see below). While this does not conclusively prove that the polypeptides are continuous, this is the most likely option. The gene splicing pattern of lysin and polymerase encoding genes is identical to the one presented by staphylococcal phages G1, K and ISP [19,47,48]. However, fRuSau02 has additional insertions in the terminase large subunit and recombinase genes that were also present in phage Team1. Unlike in the more distant phages Remus/Romulus and Twort, there were no intein domains identified in the fRuSau02 genome [17,49,50].

3.6. Proteomic Analysis of the Phage Structural Proteins

To confirm the identification and expression of the phage structural proteins, a proteomic analysis of the purified phage particles using LC-MS/MS was performed. The comparative analysis of obtained peptide sequences with the sequences of predicted phage proteins allowed for the identification of these structural proteins. To exclude the possibility of obtaining false positive results due to similarity with bacterial proteins that could be carried over from the lysate during the sample preparation, the obtained peptide sequences were compared simultaneously against the phage and bacterial protein sequences. Altogether, 81 phage proteins were identified in the LC-MS/MS analysis, of which 78 fulfilled the inclusion criteria (>2 unique peptides and/or >5% coverage) (Table 1). The analysis of the structural proteome identified the capsid (Mcp) and the tail (Tsp, TmpA, TmpB, TmpC, TmpD, TmpE, TmpF, TmpG, TmpH, BmpA, BmpB, BmpC) proteins, receptor binding proteins (RS_124 and RS_126), the portal protein (Prt), and putative membrane proteins (MbpC, MbpD, MbpG, MbpH, MbpR,

MbpS), as well as phage holin (HolA). Additionally, this study showed the presence of ribonucleotide reductases (NrdE and NrdF), DNA-binding protein (HmzG), putative ligase (Lig), recombination nuclease B (RncB), ribonuclease H (Rbn), and DNA helicases (DhlA and DhlB) as well as sigma and anti-sigma factors (Sig, Asf). Altogether, 33 of the identified proteins were annotated as novel phage structural proteins. As already described above, the LC-MS/MS analysis showed also the presence of three proteins: the phage lysin (LysK), terminase (Ter) and recombinase (Rec) encoded by the genes interrupted by the intervening sequences. The prohead protease Pro was also identified in the LC-MS/MS analysis. The presence of the protease among the structural proteins was described previously for *Lactobacillus delbrueckii*-specific phages [51,52] but may be the result of lack of dissociation from the head after the assembly.

3.7. fRuSau02 Host Range

A collection of 135 *Staphylococcus* strains, including 51 human and 54 porcine *S. aureus* isolates and 30 coagulase-negative *Staphylococcus* strains of human origin were used to assess the host range (Table 2). Of the 50 clinical *S. aureus* strains collected for this study, 35 were methicillin-sensitive and 15 methicillin-resistant (Table S1). Phage fRuSau02 was able to infect 49 (96%) coagulase-positive and 15 (50%) coagulase-negative strains of human origin, whereas the rate of infection of pig isolates was much lower with only 18 (33%) strains infected. The infectivity of *S. aureus* strains did not depend on their response to methicillin. Some of the bacterial strains instead of clear lysis displayed turbid lysis or only slower growth rate. Counting together the clear and turbid lysis, 33 (61%) of pig isolates and 5 (17%) of coagulase-negative strains were resistant to phage infection. Importantly, all *S. aureus* human isolates (including MRSA strains) were at least moderately sensitive to fRuSau02. Further, patient isolates of coagulase-negative *Staphylococcus* strains, including *S. intermedius*, *S. lugdunensis*, *S. epidermidis*, *S. haemolyticus*, *S. saprophyticus* and *S. pseudointer*, showed different rates of infection depending on the strain, however, at least one strain of each species was susceptible to the phage. Further, the coagulase-negative strains and several pig isolates displayed lower efficiency of infection and turbidity of the plaques, while human *S. aureus* isolates were characterized by big (1–3 mm) clear plaques (data not shown).

Table 2. The infectivity of fRuSau02 for different staphylococcal isolates. The details and strain references are listed in supplementary material Table S1.

	fRuSau02 Infectivity					
Bacterial Hosts	**Infected ***		**Intermediate ***		**Resistant ***	
Coagulase-Positive Human Isolates (n = 51)						
S. aureus	49	(96%)	2	(4%)	0	(0%)
Coagulase-Negative Human Isolates (n = 30)						
S. intermedius	0		3		2	
S. lugdunensis	1		4		0	
S. epidermidis	0		1		4	
S. haemolyticus	0		2		3	
S. saprophyticus	1		2		2	
S. pseudointer	0		4		1	
ALL	2	(7%)	16	(53%)	12	(40%)
Coagulase-Positive Porcine Isolates (n = 54)						
S. aureus	18	(33%)	3	(6%)	33	(61%)

* Infected indicates clear lysis or growth inhibition for spot and liquid assays, respectively, intermediate turbid lysis or slower growth rate, and resistant no infection.

3.8. *fRuSau02 Receptor*

Staphylococcal Twort-like phages have been shown to utilize cell wall teichoic acids (WTAs) as their receptors [22]. To test whether this is also the case with fRuSau02, we analyzed the infectivity of fRuSau02 in *S. aureus* strain tagO. This strain carries a mutation in the gene encoding TagO, an enzyme that catalyzes the transfer of *N*-acetylglucosamine to bactoprenol in the first step of teichoic acid biosynthesis [53,54]. As shown in Figure 6A, the phage failed to reproduce in the tagO strain. Furthermore, the adsorption assay revealed that fRuSau02 was not able to adsorb to this strain (Figure 6B). It thus seems that like for other staphylococcal Twort-like phages, WTAs serve as receptors for fRuSau02.

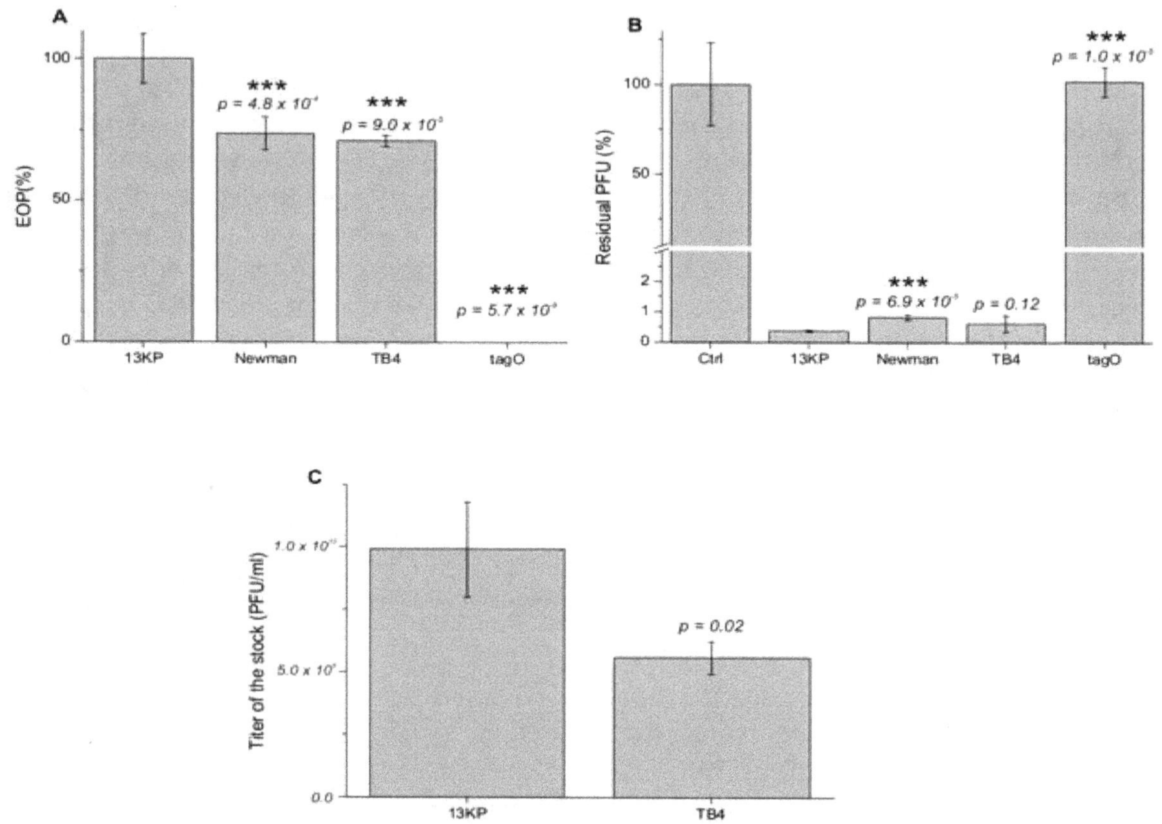

Figure 6. Suitability of host strains for production of fRuSau02. (**A**) The efficiency of plating (EOP) counted as the number of plaque-forming units (PFU) obtained from the same amount of phage lysate for different bacterial strains. The result obtained for the reference strain 13KP was set as 100%; (**B**) Adsorption of fRuSau02 to bacterial surface. Ctrl represents LB as negative control, in which the residual PFU was set to 100%; (**C**) The titer of fRuSau02 lysate produced in strains 13KP and TB4. Error bars indicate SD, *p*-values the level of significance between 13KP and other strains, *** indicates that the difference is statistically significant at the *p*-value < 0.001 level.

3.9. *The Choice of Optimal Host Strain for Therapeutic Phage Production*

In an ideal situation, host strains used for the production of therapeutic phages should be free of prophages. This is because prophages encode virulence factors, such as staphylococcal enterotoxins [55]. In addition, they can be induced from cells during the infection by therapeutic phage and cause genome variations [56]. To study the possibility to produce fRuSau02 in the prophage-free *S. aureus* strain, we compared the efficiency of plating (EOP) in strains 13KP, Newman, and TB4. Of these, 13KP is the strain that was used as a host strain during the phage isolation, and it was used as a control strain with 100% EOP. TB4 is a prophage-free strain [53] and Newman the parental strain for TB4 [57].

The EOP assay showed that both TB4 and Newman had reduced infectivity compared to the reference strain 13KP (Figure 6A). This was not due to the lowered adsorption efficiency of fRuSau2 to these strains, as the adsorption assay did not reveal significant difference between 13KP and TB4. The phage adsorption to Newman was significantly reduced from 13KP, even though the residual PFU even in this strain was only 0.8% (Figure 6B). The potential of TB4 strain for phage production was further studied by preparing phage stocks. Semi-confluent soft-agar overlay plates were prepared using host-strain adjusted amount of fRuSau02 bacteriophage. Phage stocks were prepared in three parallels and titrated (Figure 6C). The results showed that the difference in the amount of phage obtained using 13KP and TB4 as host was statistically significant ($p = 0.020$), however even the titer obtained in TB4 was sufficient for phage production purposes.

As genes for bacterial toxins often reside in prophage genomes, we wanted to analyze whether fRuSau02 lysate produced in TB4 strain contains less toxins than the lysate produced in 13KP or Newman strains. To this end, the staphylococcal enterotoxins were measured from the phage lysates with the Transia Plate Staphylococcal Enterotoxins assay that detects enterotoxins A, B, C, D, and E. The phage lysate produced in 13KP was clearly positive for enterotoxins, with a concentration that approximately corresponded to 320 ng/mL of staphylococcal enterotoxin A. The phage lysate produced in Newman strain had clearly less toxins (~6 ng/mL) and the lysate produced in TB4 remained negative, indicating that the enterotoxin concentration was lower than the detection limit of the assay (~1 ng/mL of enterotoxin A). It should be noted here that the assay is not validated for quantitative analysis, thus the concentrations need to be considered approximates.

To conclude, strain TB4 should be considered as potential bacterial host for the production of bacteriophage preparations for phage therapy, as it does not possess the risk of temperate phage or enterotoxin carry-over.

4. Discussion

This study reports a new bacteriophage, fRuSau02, isolated from a commercial *Staphylococcus* bacteriophage cocktail produced by Microgen. The genomic analysis revealed that fRuSau02 is very closely related to phage MSA6 and many other Twort-like viruses. Bacteriophage fRuSau02 possesses a large genome (148,464 bp) with typical modular organization and a low G+C content and therefore can be classified as a member of the genus *Twortlikevirus*. In coherence, the morphology of the fRuSau02 phage is similar to MSA6 [20], as well as the staphylococcal phage K [19] and *Listeria* phage A511 [58]. The phylogeny analysis of 35 Twort-like phages clustered fRuSau02 and MSA6 in a same species together with A5W, Staph1N, Fi200W, and 676Z. Phage Twort, the type representative of this genus, is more distantly related to fRuSau02, the two phages displaying only 46.5% identity at the nucleotide level. Perhaps the most significant difference between fRuSau02 and MSA6 was the H306P change in the putative receptor binding protein (RS_124 and ORF094 in fRuSau02 and MSA6, respectively). Histidine in position 306 seems unique for fRuSau02, as homologous proteins of other Twort-like viruses analyzed so far, for example G1ORF008 of phage G1, ORF107 of Sb-1, and ORF125 of Team1, all have P306. The preliminary structural modelling indicated the H306P change alters the structure of the carbohydrate-binding region of the RBP, which may have a profound effect on the phage host range.

The in silico analysis revealed the presence of bacterial promoters in the genome of fRuSau02. However, both the presence of genes encoding for the phage sigma and anti-sigma factors and the genomic region of 27.5 kb that does not contain any promoters suggest the existence of phage promoters. Although the performed bioinformatics study failed to reveal any conserved sequences present upstream of the genes of this module, we believe that fRuSau02 possesses two types of promoters. Most likely, in the beginning of the infection process viral genes are transcribed by the bacterial sigma factor. During this step, the sigma and anti-sigma factors encoded by the phage genome are also transcribed. In the later stages of infection, the anti-sigma factor inhibits the activity of the bacterial factor and allows the phage sigma factor to lead the transcription from its own unique promoters. Such a process would allow the bacteriophage to have a high and uniform rate of transcription of late structural genes with a minimal transcription of bacterial genes. Further studies aiming at the recognition of transcriptional starting sites are needed to indicate the possible viral promoters and to validate the annotated bacterial promoters.

The LC-MS/MS analysis revealed 78 phage structural proteins. Due to the high sensitivity of the method, we have to take into consideration the possibility that some of the identified proteins are carried over from the lysate and co-isolated with the phage particles. On the other hand, previous studies showed that some proteins are commonly packed together with the DNA due to their association with nucleic acids [59,60]. For example, the phage sigma and anti-sigma factors (RS_157 and RS_133, respectively) were among the proteins identified, however, it is not likely that they are structural proteins of the phage particles. Earlier studies showed that the primary staphylococcal polymerase σ^{SA}, directs transcription of early genes in Twort-like viruses [47]. In addition, both bacterial RNA polymeras (RNAP) subunits and the sigma factor were among the bacterial proteins identified in the LC-MS/MS study (data not shown) suggesting that these proteins were co-isolated together with the phage particles. It is possible that these proteins show physical properties that make them either more prone to be co-isolated with phage particles during the purification process or they display unspecific binding to the capsid proteins. Similarly, the proteome analysis showed the presence of putative membrane proteins (MbpC, MbpD, MbpG, MbpH, MbpR, MbpS) that can be a part of the structural proteome used during the infection step or during the assembly and lysis. However, due to the fact that they bind to the membranes, it is also possible that they were carryover from the phage lysate.

Phage fRuSau02 was shown to infect a considerable number of human *S. aureus* isolates, however, the rates of infectivity were much lower among the animal isolates. Similar host range pattern has earlier been observed with phage ISP, which also infects efficiently human *S. aureus* isolates but is unable to infect *S. aureus* strains isolated from pigs [48]. The resistance of the pig strains may be due to minor structural differences of WTA between different *S. aureus* strains. It is also plausible that some strains developed phage resistance without the introduction of modifications in the phage receptor structures. For example, the presence of CRISPR sequences in the genome of *S. aureus* allows the bacteria to acquire the immunity against encountered phages [61]. The pig MRSA strains often belong to only few clonal complexes [62], which may explain their different phage profile compared to *S. aureus* stains isolated from other sources. Interestingly, the host profile of fRuSau02 may be somewhat different from ISP, as fRuSau02 was also able to infect some coagulase-negative staphylococcal strains, including *S. haemolyticus* earlier shown to be resistant for ISP [48].

Phages have important potential as antimicrobial agents and may serve as an alternative to antibiotics, especially in case of multi-drug resistant pathogens. Phage therapy is a possible cure for community-acquired and nosocomial infections caused by drug-resistant *Staphylococcus*, as well as a good candidate for prevention of bacterial contamination in industry and animal husbandry [53–67]. Twort-like phages are perhaps the most studied *S. aureus* phage group for clinical applications [15]. For example, phage ISP is one component of a phage therapy cocktail BFC-1, developed for the treatment of burn wound infections [68,69].

To conclude, both our analyses and the fact that fRuSau02 was isolated from a commercial therapeutic phage cocktail suggest that it should be considered as well suited for human phage therapy against coagulase-positive and to some extent also coagulase-negative staphylococcal strains. However, its capacity for the prevention and control of MRSA carriage and/or contamination in the animal husbandry and food industry may be more limited. The efficacy and safety of fRuSau02 as the therapeutic tool is still to be elucidated. Further research that includes pharmacological trials is essential to confirm the possible role of fRuSau02 in the treatment of different forms of MRSA infections in humans.

Table S1: Host range analysis of fRuSau02; Table S2: Putative promoter sequences identified in the fRuSau02 genome; Table S3: Comparative nucleotide analysis between the genomes of fRuSau02 and selected *Staphylococcus* phages; Figure S1: Split genes in the genome of fRuSau02.

Acknowledgments: Helsinki University Hospital special state subsidy for health science research grants, the Academy of Finland (project 1288701) and Jane & Aatos Erkko Foundation are acknowledged for funding (to MS). KL was supported by the Emil Aaltonen Foundation. Annamari Heikinheimo is thanked for providing the porcine *S. aureus* strain collection and Taeok Bae for sharing the TB4 and *tagO* strains. Arnab Bhattacharjee is acknowledged for his help with structural modelling and Joseph Michael Ochieng' Oduor for critically reading the manuscript.

Author Contributions: K.L., A.W., M.S. and S.K. conceived and designed the experiments; K.L., H.T., A.W., J.H.H. and S.K. performed the experiments; K.L., A.W., M.S. and S.K. analyzed the data; P.K. contributed clinical bacterial strains; K.L. and S.K. wrote the paper.

References

1. Gordon, R.J.; Lowy, F.D. Pathogenesis of methicillin-resistant *Staphylococcus aureus* infection. *Clin. Infect. Dis.* **2008**, *46*, S350–S359. [CrossRef] [PubMed]
2. Tong, S.Y.; Davis, J.S.; Eichenberger, E.; Holland, T.L.; Fowler, V.G., Jr. *Staphylococcus aureus* infections: Epidemiology, pathophysiology, clinical manifestations, and management. *Clin. Microbiol. Rev.* **2015**, *28*, 603–661. [CrossRef] [PubMed]
3. Dantes, R.; Mu, Y.; Belflower, R.; Aragon, D.; Dumyati, G.; Harrison, L.H.; Lessa, F.C.; Lynfield, R.; Nadle, J.; Petit, S.; et al. National burden of invasive methicillin-resistant *Staphylococcus aureus* infections, united states, 2011. *JAMA Intern. Med.* **2013**, *173*, 1970–1978. [PubMed]
4. Bal, A.M.; Coombs, G.W.; Holden, M.T.G.; Lindsay, J.A.; Nimmo, G.R.; Tattevin, P.; Skov, R.L. Genomic insights into the emergence and spread of international clones of healthcare-, community- and livestock-associated meticillin-resistant *Staphylococcus aureus*: Blurring of the traditional definitions. *J. Glob. Antimicrob. Resist.* **2016**, *6*, 95–101. [CrossRef] [PubMed]
5. Enright, M.C.; Robinson, D.A.; Randle, G.; Feil, E.J.; Grundmann, H.; Spratt, B.G. The evolutionary history of methicillin-resistant *Staphylococcus aureus* (MRSA). *Proc. Natl. Acad. Sci. USA* **2002**, *99*, 7687–7692. [CrossRef] [PubMed]
6. Chan, B.K.; Abedon, S.T.; Loc-Carrillo, C. Phage cocktails and the future of phage therapy. *Future Microbiol.* **2013**, *8*, 769–783. [CrossRef] [PubMed]
7. Ryan, E.M.; Gorman, S.P.; Donnelly, R.F.; Gilmore, B.F. Recent advances in bacteriophage therapy: How delivery routes, formulation, concentration and timing influence the success of phage therapy. *J. Pharm. Pharmacol.* **2011**, *63*, 1253–1264. [CrossRef] [PubMed]
8. Skurnik, M.; Strauch, E. Phage therapy: Facts and fiction. *Int. J. Med. Microbiol.* **2006**, *296*, 5–14. [CrossRef] [PubMed]
9. Abedon, S.T.; Kuhl, S.J.; Blasdel, B.G.; Kutter, E.M. Phage treatment of human infections. *Bacteriophage* **2011**, *1*, 66–85. [CrossRef] [PubMed]
10. Wittebole, X.; De Roock, S.; Opal, S.M. A historical overview of bacteriophage therapy as an alternative to antibiotics for the treatment of bacterial pathogens. *Virulence* **2014**, *5*, 226–235. [CrossRef] [PubMed]
11. Pirnay, J.P.; Blasdel, B.G.; Bretaudeau, L.; Buckling, A.; Chanishvili, N.; Clark, J.R.; Corte-Real, S.; Debarbieux, L.; Dublanchet, A.; De Vos, D.; et al. Quality and safety requirements for sustainable phage therapy products. *Pharm. Res.* **2015**, *32*, 2173–2179. [CrossRef] [PubMed]
12. Deghorain, M.; Van Melderen, L. The staphylococci phages family: An overview. *Viruses* **2012**, *4*, 3316–3335. [CrossRef] [PubMed]
13. Xia, G.; Wolz, C. Phages of *Staphylococcus aureus* and their impact on host evolution. *Infect. Genet. Evol.* **2014**, *21*, 593–601. [CrossRef] [PubMed]
14. Kazmierczak, Z.; Gorski, A.; Dabrowska, K. Facing antibiotic resistance: *Staphylococcus aureus* phages as a medical tool. *Viruses* **2014**, *6*, 2551–2570. [CrossRef] [PubMed]
15. Lobocka, M.; Hejnowicz, M.S.; Dabrowski, K.; Gozdek, A.; Kosakowski, J.; Witkowska, M.; Ulatowska, M.I.; Weber-Dabrowska, B.; Kwiatek, M.; Parasion, S.; et al. Genomics of staphylococcal Twort-like phages—Potential therapeutics of the post-antibiotic era. *Adv. Virus Res.* **2012**, *83*, 143–216. [PubMed]
16. Lavigne, R.; Darius, P.; Summer, E.J.; Seto, D.; Mahadevan, P.; Nilsson, A.S.; Ackermann, H.W.;

Kropinski, A.M. Classification of *Myoviridae* bacteriophages using protein sequence similarity. *BMC Microb.* **2009**, *9*, 224. [CrossRef] [PubMed]

17. Vandersteegen, K.; Kropinski, A.M.; Nash, J.H.; Noben, J.P.; Hermans, K.; Lavigne, R. Romulus and Remus, two phage isolates representing a distinct clade within the *Twortlikevirus* genus, display suitable properties for phage therapy applications. *J. Virol.* **2013**, *87*, 3237–3247. [CrossRef] [PubMed]
18. Kwan, T.; Liu, J.; DuBow, M.; Gros, P.; Pelletier, J. The complete genomes and proteomes of 27 *Staphylococcus aureus* bacteriophages. *Proc. Natl. Acad. Sci. USA* **2005**, *102*, 5174–5179. [CrossRef] [PubMed]
19. O'Flaherty, S.; Coffey, A.; Edwards, R.; Meaney, W.; Fitzgerald, G.F.; Ross, R.P. Genome of staphylococcal phage K: A new lineage of myoviridae infecting gram-positive bacteria with a low G+C content. *J. Bacteriol.* **2004**, *186*, 2862–2871. [CrossRef] [PubMed]
20. Kwiatek, M.; Parasion, S.; Mizak, L.; Gryko, R.; Bartoszcze, M.; Kocik, J. Characterization of a bacteriophage, isolated from a cow with mastitis, that is lytic against *Staphylococcus aureus* strains. *Arch. Virol.* **2012**, *157*, 225–234. [CrossRef] [PubMed]
21. Gu, J.; Liu, X.; Lu, R.; Li, Y.; Song, J.; Lei, L.; Sun, C.; Feng, X.; Du, C.; Yu, H.; et al. Complete genome sequence of *Staphylococcus aureus* bacteriophage GH15. *J. Virol.* **2012**, *86*, 8914–8915. [CrossRef] [PubMed]
22. Takeuchi, I.; Osada, K.; Azam, A.H.; Asakawa, H.; Miyanaga, K.; Tanji, Y. The presence of two receptor-binding proteins contributes to the wide host range of staphylococcal Twort-like phages. *Appl. Environ. Microbiol.* **2016**, *82*, 5763–5774. [CrossRef] [PubMed]
23. Sambrook, J.; Russell, D.W. *Molecular Cloning, a Laboratory Manual*, 3rd ed.; Cold Spring Harbor Laboratory Press: New York, NY, USA, 2001.
24. FIMM Sequencing Unit. Available online: https://www.fimm.fi/en/services/technology-centre/sequencing/ (accessed on 13 September 2017).
25. Coil, D.; Jospin, G.; Darling, A.E. A5-miseq: An updated pipeline to assemble microbial genomes from Illumina MiSeq data. *Bioinformatics* **2015**, *31*, 587–589. [CrossRef] [PubMed]
26. Robinson, J.T.; Thorvaldsdottir, H.; Winckler, W.; Guttman, M.; Lander, E.S.; Getz, G.; Mesirov, J.P. Integrative Genomics Viewer. *Nat. Biotechnol.* **2011**, *29*, 24–26. [CrossRef] [PubMed]
27. Thorvaldsdottir, H.; Robinson, J.T.; Mesirov, J.P. Integrative Genomics Viewer (IGV): High-performance genomics data visualization and exploration. *Brief. Bioinform.* **2013**, *14*, 178–192. [CrossRef] [PubMed]
28. RAST (Rapid Annotation Using Subsystem Technology). Available online: http://rast.nmpdr.org/ (accessed on 13 September 2017).
29. De Jong, A.; Pietersma, H.; Cordes, M.; Kuipers, O.P.; Kok, J. PePPER: A webserver for prediction of prokaryote promoter elements and regulons. *BMC Genom.* **2012**, *13*, 299. [CrossRef] [PubMed]
30. Gautheret, D.; Lambert, A. Direct RNA motif definition and identification from multiple sequence alignments using secondary structure profiles. *J. Mol. Biol.* **2001**, *313*, 1003–1011. [CrossRef] [PubMed]
31. Macke, T.J.; Ecker, D.J.; Gutell, R.R.; Gautheret, D.; Case, D.A.; Sampath, R. RNAmotif, an RNA secondary structure definition and search algorithm. *Nucl. Acids Res.* **2001**, *29*, 4724–4735. [CrossRef] [PubMed]
32. Bailey, T.L.; Boden, M.; Buske, F.A.; Frith, M.; Grant, C.E.; Clementi, L.; Ren, J.Y.; Li, W.W.; Noble, W.S. MEME suite: Tools for motif discovery and searching. *Nucl. Acids Res.* **2009**, *37*, W202–W208. [CrossRef] [PubMed]
33. Stothard, P.; Wishart, D.S. Circular genome visualization and exploration using GCView. *Bioinformatics* **2005**, *21*, 537–539. [CrossRef] [PubMed]
34. EMBOSS Stretcher. Available online: http://www.ebi.ac.uk/Tools/psa/emboss_stretcher (accessed on 13 September 2017).
35. Meier-Kolthoff, J.P.; Göker, M. Victor: Genome-based phylogeny and classification of prokaryotic viruses. *Bioinformatics* **2017**, 1–9. [CrossRef]
36. Meier-Kolthoff, J.P.; Auch, A.F.; Klenk, H.P.; Goker, M. Genome sequence-based species delimitation with confidence intervals and improved distance functions. *BMC Bioinform.* **2013**, *14*, 60. [CrossRef] [PubMed]
37. Lefort, V.; Desper, R.; Gascuel, O. Fastme 2.0: A comprehensive, accurate, and fast distance-based phylogeny inference program. *Mol. Biol. Evol.* **2015**, *32*, 2798–2800. [CrossRef] [PubMed]
38. Farris, J.S. Estimating phylogenetic trees from distance matrices. *Am. Nat.* **1972**, *106*, 645–668. [CrossRef]
39. FigTree. Available online: http://tree.bio.ed.ac.uk/software/figtree/ (accessed on 13 September 2017).
40. Göker, M.; Garcia-Blazquez, G.; Voglmayr, H.; Telleria, M.T.; Martin, M.P. Molecular taxonomy of phytopathogenic fungi: A case study in *Peronospora*. *PLoS ONE* **2009**, *4*, e6319. [CrossRef] [PubMed]

41. Meier-Kolthoff, J.P.; Hahnke, R.L.; Petersen, J.; Scheuner, C.; Michael, V.; Fiebig, A.; Rohde, C.; Rohde, M.; Fartmann, B.; Goodwin, L.A.; et al. Complete genome sequence of DSM 30083(T), the type strain (U5/41(T)) of *Escherichia coli*, and a proposal for delineating subspecies in microbial taxonomy. *Stand. Genom.Sci.* **2014**, *9*, 2. [CrossRef] [PubMed]
42. Varjosalo, M.; Keskitalo, S.; Van Drogen, A.; Nurkkala, H.; Vichalkovski, A.; Aebersold, R.; Gstaiger, M. The protein interaction landscape of the human CMGC kinase group. *Cell Rep.* **2013**, *3*, 1306–1320. [CrossRef] [PubMed]
43. Kutter, E. Phage host range and efficiency of plating. *Methods Mol. Biol.* **2009**, *501*, 141–149. [PubMed]
44. Leon-Velarde, C.G.; Happonen, L.; Pajunen, M.; Leskinen, K.; Kropinski, A.M.; Mattinen, L.; Rajtor, M.; Zur, J.; Smith, D.; Chen, S.; et al. *Yersinia enterocolitica*-specific infection by bacteriophages TG1 and varphiR1-RT is dependent on temperature-regulated expression of the phage host receptor OmpF. *Appl. Environ. Microbiol.* **2016**, *82*, 5340–5353. [CrossRef] [PubMed]
45. Ackermann, H.W. Bacteriophage observations and evolution. *Res. Microbiol.* **2003**, *154*, 245–251. [CrossRef]
46. Maniloff, J.; Ackermann, H.W. Taxonomy of bacterial viruses: Establishment of tailed virus genera and the order *Caudovirales*. *Arch. Virol.* **1998**, *143*, 2051–2063. [CrossRef] [PubMed]
47. Dehbi, M.; Moeck, G.; Arhin, F.F.; Bauda, P.; Bergeron, D.; Kwan, T.; Liu, J.; McCarty, J.; Dubow, M.; Pelletier, J. Inhibition of transcription in *Staphylococcus aureus* by a primary sigma factor-binding polypeptide from phage G1. *J. Bacteriol.* **2009**, *191*, 3763–3771. [CrossRef] [PubMed]
48. Vandersteegen, K.; Mattheus, W.; Ceyssens, P.J.; Bilocq, F.; De Vos, D.; Pirnay, J.P.; Noben, J.P.; Merabishvili, M.; Lipinska, U.; Hermans, K.; et al. Microbiological and molecular assessment of bacteriophage ISP for the control of *Staphylococcus aureus*. *PLoS ONE* **2011**, *6*, e24418. [CrossRef] [PubMed]
49. Landthaler, M.; Begley, U.; Lau, N.C.; Shub, D.A. Two self-splicing group i introns in the ribonucleotide reductase large subunit gene of *Staphylococcus aureus* phage Twort. *Nucl. Acids Res.* **2002**, *30*, 1935–1943. [CrossRef] [PubMed]
50. Landthaler, M.; Shub, D.A. Unexpected abundance of self-splicing introns in the genome of bacteriophage Twort: Introns in multiple genes, a single gene with three introns, and exon skipping by group I ribozymes. *Proc. Natl. Acad. Sci. USA* **1999**, *96*, 7005–7010. [CrossRef] [PubMed]
51. Casey, E.; Mahony, J.; Neve, H.; Noben, J.P.; Dal Bello, F.; van Sinderen, D. Novel phage group infecting *Lactobacillus delbrueckii* subsp. *Lactis*, as revealed by genomic and proteomic analysis of bacteriophage Ldl1. *Appl. Environ. Microbiol.* **2015**, *81*, 1319–1326. [PubMed]
52. Casey, E.; Mahony, J.; O'Connell-Motherway, M.; Bottacini, F.; Cornelissen, A.; Neve, H.; Heller, K.J.; Noben, J.P.; Dal Bello, F.; van Sinderen, D. Molecular characterization of three *Lactobacillus delbrueckii* subsp. *Bulgaricus* phages. *Appl. Environ. Microbiol.* **2014**, *80*, 5623–5635. [CrossRef] [PubMed]
53. Bae, T.; Baba, T.; Hiramatsu, K.; Schneewind, O. Prophages of *Staphylococcus aureus* Newman and their contribution to virulence. *Mol. Microbiol.* **2006**, *62*, 1035–1047. [CrossRef] [PubMed]
54. Soldo, B.; Lazarevic, V.; Karamata, D. TagO is involved in the synthesis of all anionic cell-wall polymers in *Bacillus subtilis* 168. *Microbiology* **2002**, *148*, 2079–2087. [CrossRef] [PubMed]
55. Betley, M.J.; Mekalanos, J.J. Staphylococcal enterotoxin a is encoded by phage. *Science* **1985**, *229*, 185–187. [CrossRef] [PubMed]
56. Goerke, C.; Wirtz, C.; Fluckiger, U.; Wolz, C. Extensive phage dynamics in *Staphylococcus aureus* contributes to adaptation to the human host during infection. *Mol. Microbiol.* **2006**, *61*, 1673–1685. [CrossRef] [PubMed]
57. Miller, K.D.; Hetrick, D.L.; Bielefeldt, D.J. Production and properties of *Staphylococcus aureus* (strain Newman D2C) with uniform clumping factor activity. *Thromb. Res.* **1977**, *10*, 203–211. [CrossRef]
58. Klumpp, J.; Dorscht, J.; Lurz, R.; Bielmann, R.; Wieland, M.; Zimmer, M.; Calendar, R.; Loessner, M.J. The terminally redundant, nonpermuted genome of *Listeria* bacteriophage A511: A model for the SPO1-like myoviruses of gram-positive bacteria. *J. Bacteriol.* **2008**, *190*, 5753–5765. [CrossRef] [PubMed]
59. Thomas, J.A.; Benitez Quintana, A.D.; Bosch, M.A.; Coll De Pena, A.; Aguilera, E.; Coulibaly, A.; Wu, W.; Osier, M.V.; Hudson, A.O.; Weintraub, S.T.; et al. Identification of essential genes in the *Salmonella* phage SPN3US reveals novel insights into giant phage head structure and assembly. *J. Virol.* **2016**, *90*, 10284–10298. [CrossRef] [PubMed]
60. Thomas, J.A.; Weintraub, S.T.; Wu, W.; Winkler, D.C.; Cheng, N.; Steven, A.C.; Black, L.W. Extensive proteolysis of head and inner body proteins by a morphogenetic protease in the giant *Pseudomonas aeruginosa* phage phiKZ. *Mol. Microbiol.* **2012**, *84*, 324–339. [CrossRef] [PubMed]

61. Yang, S.; Liu, J.; Shao, F.; Wang, P.; Duan, G.; Yang, H. Analysis of the features of 45 identified CRISPR loci in 32 *Staphylococcus aureus*. *Biochem. Biophys. Res. Commun.* **2015**, *464*, 894–900. [CrossRef] [PubMed]
62. Heikinheimo, A.; Johler, S.; Karvonen, L.; Julmi, J.; Fredriksson-Ahomaa, M.; Stephan, R. New dominant spa type t2741 in livestock-associated MRSA (CC398-MRSA-V) in finnish fattening pigs at slaughter. *Antimicrob. Resist. Infect. Control* **2016**, *5*, 6. [CrossRef] [PubMed]
63. Cisek, A.A.; Dabrowska, I.; Gregorczyk, K.P.; Wyzewski, Z. Phage therapy in bacterial infections treatment: One hundred years after the discovery of bacteriophages. *Curr. Microbiol.* **2017**, *74*, 277–283. [CrossRef] [PubMed]
64. Endersen, L.; O'Mahony, J.; Hill, C.; Ross, R.P.; McAuliffe, O.; Coffey, A. Phage therapy in the food industry. *Annu. Rev. Food Sci. Technol.* **2014**, *5*, 327–349. [CrossRef] [PubMed]
65. Gutierrez, D.; Rodriguez-Rubio, L.; Martinez, B.; Rodriguez, A.; Garcia, P. Bacteriophages as weapons against bacterial biofilms in the food industry. *Front. Microbiol.* **2016**, *7*, 825. [CrossRef] [PubMed]
66. Kazi, M.; Annapure, U.S. Bacteriophage biocontrol of foodborne pathogens. *J. Food Sci. Technol.* **2016**, *53*, 1355–1362. [CrossRef] [PubMed]
67. Kutter, E.M.; Kuhl, S.J.; Abedon, S.T. Re-establishing a place for phage therapy in western medicine. *Future Microbiol.* **2015**, *10*, 685–688. [CrossRef] [PubMed]
68. Merabishvili, M.; Pirnay, J.P.; Verbeken, G.; Chanishvili, N.; Tediashvili, M.; Lashkhi, N.; Glonti, T.; Krylov, V.; Mast, J.; Van Parys, L.; et al. Quality-controlled small-scale production of a well-defined bacteriophage cocktail for use in human clinical trials. *PLoS ONE* **2009**, *4*, e4944. [CrossRef] [PubMed]
69. Rose, T.; Verbeken, G.; Vos, D.D.; Merabishvili, M.; Vaneechoutte, M.; Lavigne, R.; Jennes, S.; Zizi, M.; Pirnay, J.P. Experimental phage therapy of burn wound infection: Difficult first steps. *Int. J. Burns Trauma* **2014**, *4*, 66–73. [PubMed]

4

Antibiotic Therapy Using Phage Depolymerases: Robustness Across a Range of Conditions

Han Lin [1], Matthew L. Paff [1,†], Ian J. Molineux [2,3,4,*] and James J. Bull [1,2,5,*]

1 Department of Integrative Biology, University of Texas, Austin, TX 78712, USA; hanl@austin.utexas.edu (H.L.); matthew.paff@utexas.edu (M.L.P.)
2 Institute for Cellular and Molecular Biology, University of Texas, Austin, TX 78712, USA
3 Department of Molecular Biosciences, University of Texas, Austin, TX 78712, USA
4 LaMontagne Center for Infectious Disease, University of Texas, Austin, TX 78712, USA
5 Center for Computational Biology and Bioinformatics, University of Texas, Austin, TX 78712, USA
* Correspondence: molineux@austin.utexas.edu (I.J.M.); bull@utexas.edu (J.J.B.)
† Current address: Nano Vision, 1705 Guadalupe St, Austin, TX 78712, USA.

Abstract: Phage-derived depolymerases directed against bacterial capsules are showing therapeutic promise in various animal models of infection. However, individual animal model studies are often constrained by use of highly specific protocols, such that results may not generalize to even slight modifications. Here we explore the robustness of depolymerase therapies shown to succeed in a previous study of mice. Treatment success rates were reduced by treatment delay, more so for some enzymes than others: K1- and K5 capsule-degrading enzymes retained partial efficacy on delay, while K30 depolymerase did not. Phage were superior to enzymes under delayed treatment only for K1. Route of administration (intramuscular versus intraperitoneal) mattered for success of K1E, possibly for K1F, not for K1H depolymerase. Significantly, K1 capsule-degrading enzymes proved highly successful when using immune-suppressed, leukopenic mice, even with delayed treatment. Evolution of bacteria resistant to K1-degrading enzymes did not thwart therapeutic success in leukopenic mice, likely because resistant bacteria were avirulent. In combination with previous studies these results continue to support the efficacy of depolymerases as antibacterial agents in vivo, but system-specific details are becoming evident.

Keywords: phage therapy; bacterial infection; capsule depolymerase; antibiotic; animal model; bacterial resistance

1. Introduction

In the increasingly urgent search for new treatments against bacterial infections, phages and phage products hold promise [1–3]. Offsetting the now many laboratory studies of phages and phage products showing positive results [4–6], the few clinical phage therapy trials conducted under standards of Western medicine have actually failed [7–9]. The most recent randomized clinical phage therapy trial was also stopped prematurely for lack of efficacy, although small effects were deemed encouraging [10]. The contrasting outcomes between actual trials and laboratory infections raise the possibility that experimental studies poorly represent applications. One obvious concern in generalizing from experimental infections to clinical settings is the potential sensitivity of results to specifics of the experimental protocol. A step toward generality of a therapeutic agent is thus to broaden the experimental protocol and measure the sensitivity of treatment success to experimental variables. Here we evaluate the robustness of phage depolymerase therapies previously demonstrated to rescue mice from experimental infections of capsulated *E. coli* [11].

Several classes of phage proteins have exhibited antibiotic potency, including endolysins [12], viron-associated lysins [13], holins [5], spanins [14] and bacterial polysaccharide depolymerases [15]. Some endolysins are already commercially available and are currently being tested in clinical trials [3,16]. Capsular depolymerases represent an interesting type of antibiotic: they do not kill per se, but merely strip the bacteria of protective polysaccharides and thus expose the bacteria to immune components [17]. They have a potential advantage over endolysins in that they do not lyse the bacteria, thereby minimizing inflammatory responses from endotoxins [18]. In vivo studies of capsule depolymerases are yet limited but appear to generalize across different animal models (Table 1). Furthermore, enzymes that disrupt biofilms, in part by degradation of polysaccharide, but do not kill bacteria are also showing promise [19,20].

Table 1. In vivo studies of capsule depolymerases in animal infection models.

Capsule Depolymerases	Animal Infection Model	References
EndoE (K1E)	*E. coli*; neonatal rats	Mushtaq et al., 2004 [21]; 2005 [22]
CapD; EnvD	*B. anthracis*; mice	Scorpio et al., 2008 [23]; Negus et al., 2015 [24]
K1-ORF34; K64dep	*K. pneumoniae*; mice	Lin et al., 2014 [25]; Pan et al., 2015 [26]
depoKP36	*K. pneumoniae*; moth larvae	Majkowska-Skrobek et al., 2016 [27]
K1F, K1H, K5, K30	*E. coli*; mice	Lin et al., 2017 [11]

Our purpose here is to explore the robustness of capsular depolymerase enzymes in treating experimentally infected mice. The bacteria are *E. coli* with K1, K5 or K30 capsules, and the enzymes were obtained as purified proteins expressed from clones of phage genes. Previous work demonstrated therapeutic success of several enzymes when using (i) simultaneous infection and treatment, (ii) intramuscular administration, and (iii) immunocompetent mice [11]. Here we explore treatment efficacy when relaxing these conditions. By measuring performance of depolymerase treatments under different conditions and with different enzymes, our work also exposes possible realms for improving therapeutic efficacy of depolymerases, as in structure/function properties of the enzymes.

2. Materials and Methods

2.1. Bacterial Strains and Cell Culture

The pathogenic bacterial strains used in this study were K1-capsulated *E. coli* RS218 [28], K5-capsulated ATCC 23506, and K30-capsulated E69 [29]. *E. coli* lab strains used only for phage propagation or cloning were the K1-capsulated K12 strain EV36 [30] and BL21(DE3). Cells were generally grown in LB broth (10 g tryptone, 5 g yeast extract, 10 g NaCl per liter) in 37 °C shakers. Cell density was determined by plating serial cell dilutions on LB agar (1.3% *w*/*v*) plates for colony counts.

Capsule-free isolates of RS218 were selected by culturing RS218 on LB plates containing K1H phage [31]. Colonies that grew on the plates were picked, diluted in LB medium and replated on LB plates containing K1 phage. The colonies grown on these second plates were picked and cultured in LB medium containing K1 phage before mouse injection. The addition of phage was a precaution against any possible revertants to a capsulated state.

2.2. Coliphage Strains and Culture

Phages K1E, K1F and K1H [32] were propagated on host *E. coli* EV36. K1–5 [33] and K30 [34] were grown with host *E. coli* ATCC 23506 and E69, respectively. Phages were purified by equilibrium CsCl-gradient centrifugation and dialyzed into SM buffer (50 mM Tris–HCl, 100 mM NaCl, 8 mM $MgSO_4$, pH 7.5) as previously described [11,35]. Phage titrations were performed by plaque counts on an appropriate host in LB soft agar (0.65%) overlay.

2.3. Plasmids, Protein Expression and Purification

The phage capsule depolymerases were expressed in *E. coli* BL21(DE3) with pET28b constructs containing cloned depolymerase genes as previously described [11]. Proteins were purified with HisPur Ni-NTA resin (Thermo Fisher Scientific, Rockford, IL, USA), and dialyzed into PBS buffer (137 mM NaCl, 2.7 mM KCl, 10 mM Na_2HPO_4, 1.8 mM KH_2PO_4, pH 7.5) with 3.5 kDa MWCO dialysis membranes (Spectrum-Repligen, Houston, TX, USA). Protein concentrations were estimated by absorption at 280 nm with a Nanodrop ND-1000 (Thermo Fisher Scientific, Wilmington, DE, USA).

2.4. Mouse Infection Model

Animal work was performed under NIH guidelines and the University of Texas IACUC protocols (AUP-2015-00035, AUP-2018-00010). Female NIH Swiss outbred mice (Envigo, Somerset, NJ, USA) aged 4–6 weeks with 20–25 g weights were used here in all studies. All intramuscular (IM) inoculations of bacteria used the left thigh; all IM inoculations of enzyme or phage used the right thigh. Mouse survival was monitored twice daily for 5 days.

The following experiments were undertaken.

Delayed treatment of normal mice with enzyme or phage. Mice received an IM injection of 100 μL bacteria, dosed at either 1.2–3.4 $\times$ 10^8 CFU of RS218, 3.1–6.1 $\times$ 10^8 CFU of ATCC 23506, or 1.1–2.8 $\times$ 10^8 CFU of E69 per mouse. Enzyme or phage inoculation in the contralateral thigh followed at 8 h, dosed at 20 μg enzyme in 100 μL PBS or 10^7 pfu phage in 100 μL SM buffer. A dose of 10^7 phage is 10-fold lower than used in the delayed treatment studies of [36], but much higher than doses used in studies with simultaneous treatment [37]. Given the rate of phage amplification in the host [37], 10^7 was expected to be highly effective.

Different administration routes for immediate enzyme treatment. Mice received IM 1.2–2.9 $\times$ 10^8 CFU of RS218 in 100 μL volume, and then 20 μg K1E, 2 μg K1F or 2 μg K1H in 100 μL volume either by contralateral IM or IP (intraperitoneal) inoculation.

The leukopenic mouse model. Mice were rendered leukopenic by IP injection of cyclophosphamide (CP) at 150 mg/kg body weight 4 days prior and then at 100 mg/kg body weight 1 day prior to infection. To determine an approximate lethal dose of bacteria, different mice were inoculated across a range of bacterial doses in 10-fold increments spanning 10^3–10^7 CFU (RS218) or 10^4–10^8 CFU (capsule-free RS218 derivative). Simultaneous enzyme (20 μg K1E, K1H) or phage (K1H 10^7 pfu contralateral) treatment was tested in leukopenic mice infected by RS218 at the lethal dose of 2.2–5.1 $\times$ 10^4 CFU. Delayed enzyme (20 μg K1F, K1H) treatment was also tested in leukopenic mice 8 h after infection.

Mouse survival was analyzed by Kaplan-Meier survival curves using SPSS software, where the cumulative survival probability was plotted over the time course of 5 days and statistically evaluated by log rank test [25,38,39].

2.5. Capsule Isolation and Degradation Assay

Capsules were isolated as previously described [11,40] for degradation assays monitored by gel electrophoresis and Alcian Blue staining. To compare activity of purified K1 enzyme to enzyme activity of intact phage, 10–20 μg K1 capsule was mixed with serial dilutions (0.25–8 μg) of K1E, K1F, K1H enzyme or CsCl-purified cognate phage at the calculated amount of enzyme equivalents at 37 °C for 1 h before gel electrophoresis. Enzyme equivalents of phages were calculated from the molecular weight of each enzyme [41,42] and the fact that these phages contain six depolymerase trimers and thus 18 enzyme molecules per phage particle [35]. 10^{10} phage would thus have ~3 $\times$ 10^{-2} μg enzyme (varying somewhat among different enzymes). This calculation assumes that phage stocks plate at a particle:plaque ratio of 1; a reduced efficiency of plating would underestimate the amount of enzyme in the phage sample.

To compare levels of K1 enzyme activity in mouse blood, 100 μL PBS containing 20 μg K1E, K1F or K1H enzyme or no enyzme (control) was injected to mice by IM or IP. Mice were euthanized at 1 h or 24 h after injection and blood was collected to prepare serum. 10–20 μg K1 capsule was incubated with 10 μL K1E serum or 0.3 μL K1F, K1H serum at 37 °C overnight before gel examination. The volumes of serum used in each reaction were determined in preliminary tests to achieve a dynamic range of degradation differentiable by visual inspection. Reactions with control serum were included as negative control, while reactions with serial dilutions of enzymes added immediately to the control serum were included as positive control.

2.6. Resistance Competition Assay (RCA)

The assay measures the in vivo effects of treatment on bacterial numbers. It works by inoculating mice with a mixture of mostly treatment-sensitive bacteria and a small number of treatment-resistant bacteria [36]. Mice are either treated or not (the latter being controls). Resistant bacteria increase in frequency (relative to controls) to the extent that treatment suppresses the population of sensitive bacteria. For this assay, RS218 was mixed with the K5-capsulated ATCC 23506 (ratio approximately 99:1). Six mice were inoculated in the left thigh with the normal bacteria dose (~2.9×10^8 cells) and either treated simultaneously with contralateral IM of 20 μg K1H enzyme (3 mice) or not treated (3 controls). At 4 h post infection, mice were euthanized. The left thigh was removed, homogenized in 10 mL buffer, and the suspension plated at different dilutions on both LB plates and on LB plates saturated with 10^7 pfu K1H phage. The LB plates support growth of both K1 and K5 bacteria, whereas plates with phage grow only the K5-capsulated strain, allowing a determination of K5 (ATCC 23506) frequency. Calculations of the RCA value used the formula in [36]: $\mathrm{RCA} = \ln [(p_t (1 - p_0))/(p_0(1 - p_t))]/t$, with p_0 as the proportion of resistant bacteria in control mice and p_t as the proportion resistant bacteria in treated mice, both measured at time t (hours of treatment). For an RCA value of R, e^{-R} is the per hour growth of bacteria under treatment relative to growth without treatment.

3. Results

3.1. Delayed Treatment Reduces Efficacy

We reported that phage capsule depolymerases were broadly effective in treating lethal *E. coli* infections in mice [11]. That work applied treatment simultaneously with infection. Here we explored the efficacy of delayed treatment, as a delay might better represent clinical therapeutics.

Delayed treatment is better than no treatment only for some enzymes. The delayed treatments of phage capsule depolymerases given 8 h after infection exhibited reduced efficacy (Figure 1). The delayed treatment with K1F or K1H enzyme resulted in 50–60% survival compared to zero survival in control (Figure 1A), while the simultaneous treatment led to 90–100% survival [11]. K1E did not rescue well in simultaneous treatment, thus the delayed treatment was not tested here. Delayed K5 enzyme treatment showed a 60% survival (Figure 1B) compared to 100% survival when treatment was immediate; both were significantly better than no-treatment controls. Delayed treatment with the least active enzyme K30 gp41 did not significantly improve survival (Figure 1C).

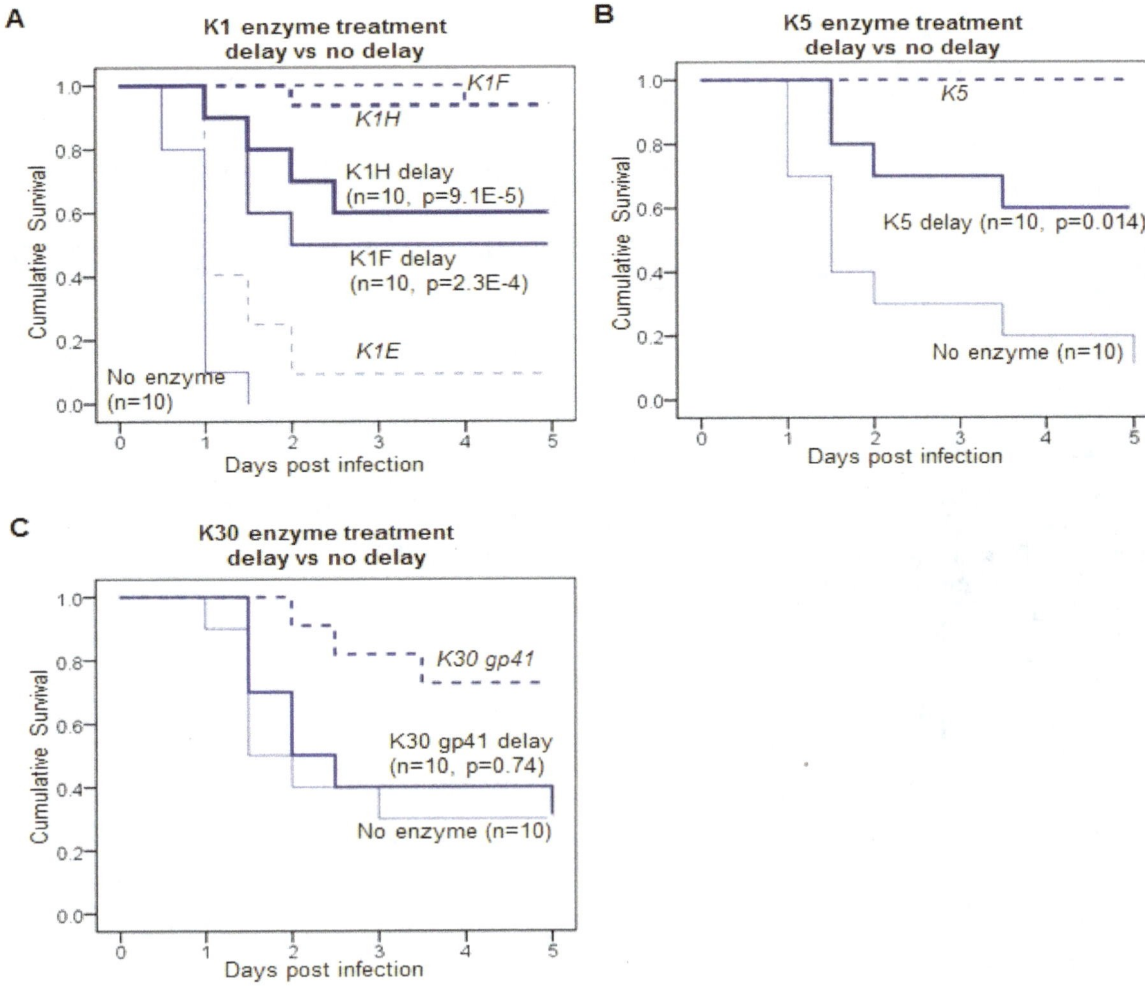

Figure 1. Delayed treatment of infection using capsule depolymerases. (**A**) 1.2–3.4 × 10^8 CFU of K1-capsulated *E. coli* treated with 20 μg of K1F or K1H enzyme; (**B**) 3.1–6.1 × 10^8 CFU of K5-capsulated *E. coli* treated with 20 μg of K5 enzyme; (**C**) 1.1–2.8 × 10^8 CFU of *E. coli* E69 treated with 20 μg of K30 enzyme. All inoculations were IM (intramuscular, thigh); enzyme was administered 8 h after bacteria in the contralateral thigh. Mouse survival was monitored for 5 days and Kaplan-Meier survival curves in solid lines were plotted with the cumulative probability of survival over time for each treatment. Previously reported survival curves of simultaneous enzyme treatments are included for comparison (dashed lines). The mouse number (n) of each treatment is given for each curve. Log rank test: p values are listed for delayed treatments compared to the no-enzyme control.

Phages outperform enzyme only for K1 bacteria. Phages might be expected to outperform enzymes on the grounds that phage have multiple effects: They amplify within the host, they kill, and cell lysis releases free enzyme as unassembled tailspikes. Yet a superiority of phages under delayed treatment was observed only for K1-capsulated bacteria. K1H or K1E phage yielded higher survival rates than K1 enzymes in delayed treatment (Figure 2A). In contrast, K5 or K30 phages were no better than their enzymes in delayed treatment (Figure 2B,C). As a control for the effects of phage amplification, K1F phage, which does not propagate on RS218, had no effect in mice (data not shown), whereas K1F enzyme efficacy was similar to that of K1H (Figure 1A).

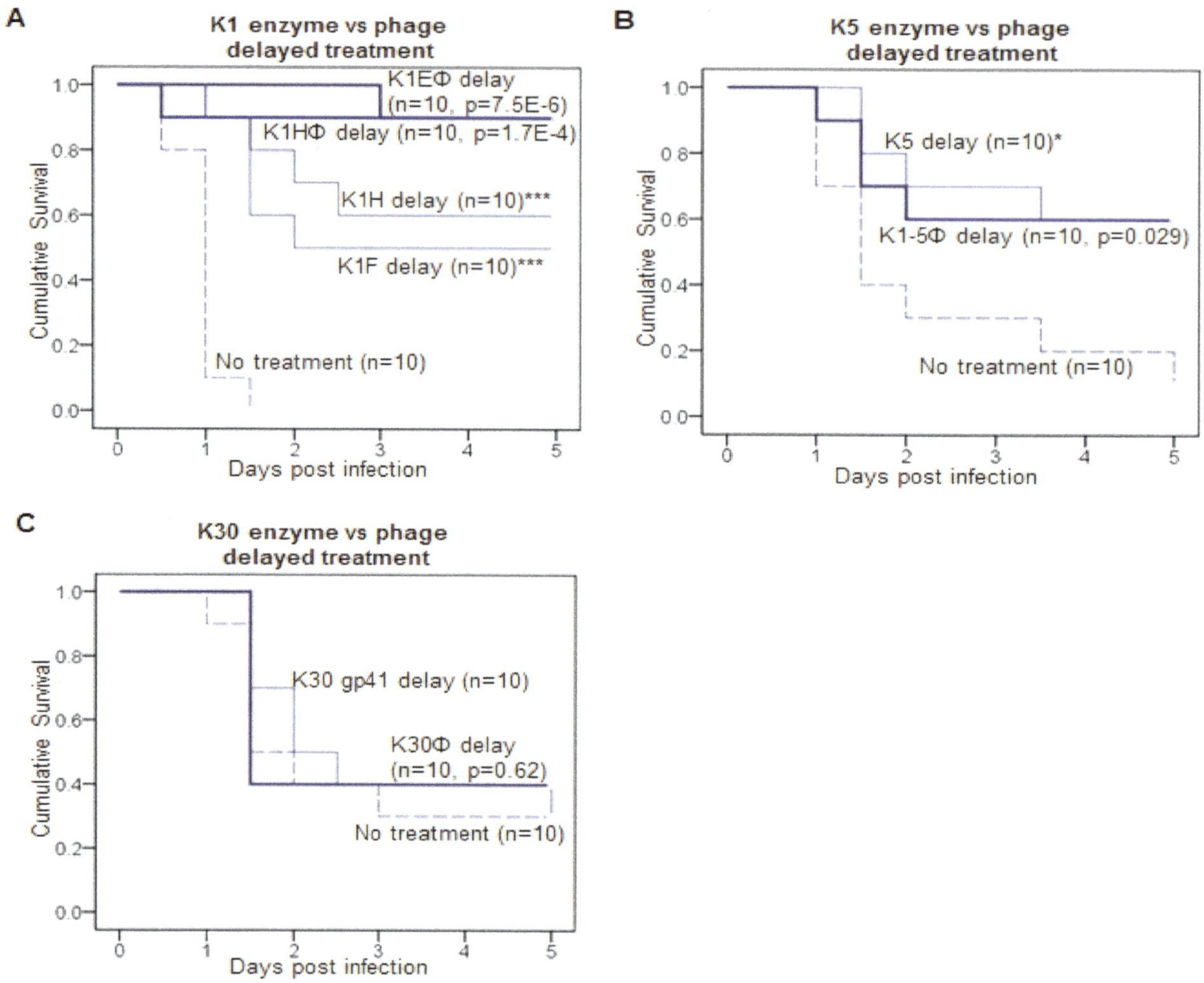

Figure 2. Comparison of depolymerases and cognate phages in treatment. Delayed treatments using phages were carried out in parallel to depolymerase. (**A**) K1E and K1H phage; (**B**) K1-5 phage; (**C**) K30 phage. Depolymerase data are from Figure 1. For phage treatment, mice were infected with intramuscular (IM) inoculations; 8 h later they received ~10^7 pfu phage IM in the contralateral thigh. For comparison to depolymerase treatment, this dose of phage carries about 3×10^{-5} µg of depolymerase (see Methods for calculation). Kaplan-Meier survival curves were plotted as in Figure 1. The mouse number n of each treatment is labeled on each curve. Log rank test: p values for delayed phage treatments compared to the no treatment control are listed, or * $p < 0.05$, *** $p < 0.001$ for delayed enzyme treatment as in Figure 1.

Phages carry active depolymerases as tailspikes that are used in adsorption and penetration of the capsule. It is possible that the activities of the purified enzymes were substantially less than the activities of tailspikes on intact phages. We thus compared the in vitro degrading activities of purified enzyme with activities of intact phages (Figure 3). Degradation by phages was 4–8 fold better than degradation by molar equivalents of purified enzyme. Perhaps surprisingly, in view of the different in vivo performances of the enzymes, in vitro differences among the three K1-specific phages were small.

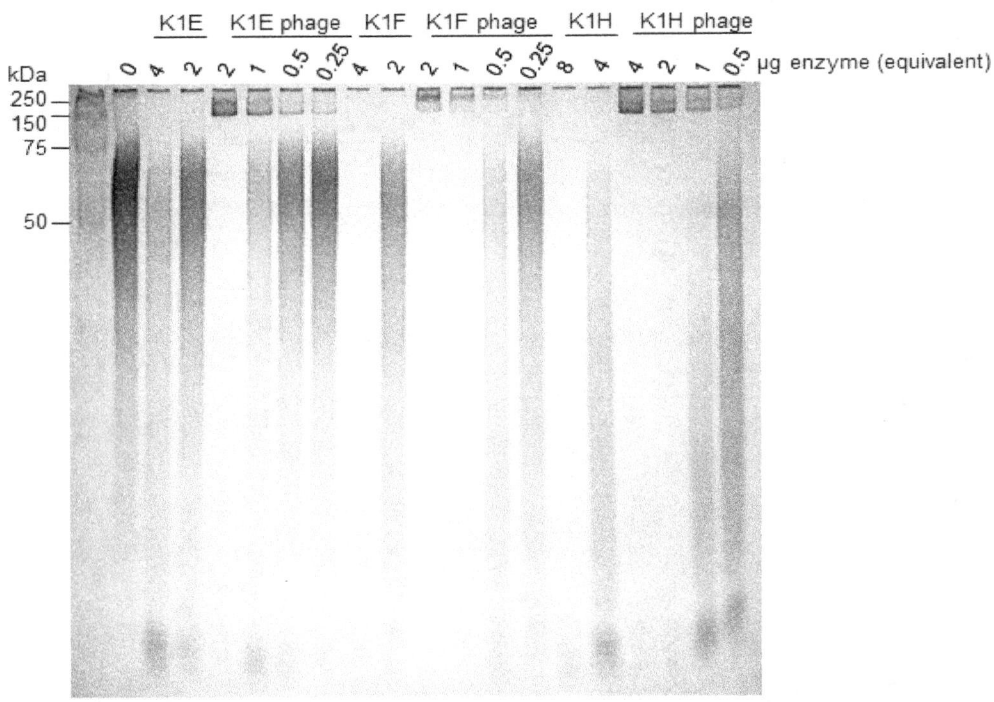

Figure 3. In vitro activity comparison of depolymerases and cognate phages. 10–20 µg of K1 capsule were incubated with serial dilutions of K1E, K1F, K1H depolymerase or phages at the indicated amount of enzyme equivalents (0.25–8 µg). Active enzyme is indicated by loss of signal within the lane; enzyme associated with phages is 4–8 fold more active than free enzyme. Incubation was at 37 °C for 1 h; reactions were fractionated using 12% TBE-PAGE with Alcian Blue staining. Protein standards were loaded in the leftmost lane and their molecular weights indicated.

3.2. Efficacy Varies with Route of Administration and Enzyme

K1E enzyme rescued rat pups by IP inoculation [21,22] but was minimally effective in mice by IM inoculation [11]. It does not appear that our purified K1E enzyme is at fault—its in vitro activity approximately matches that of the other K1 enzymes (Figure 3). Motivated by suggestions that administration routes may affect drug bioavailability [43–45], we compared the efficacy of IM versus IP administration routes of the different K1 enzymes; these studies used immediate treatment.

Different enzyme efficacies in mice by different administration routes. Following an IM inoculation of RS218 bacteria, K1E depolymerase efficacy was significantly higher for IP than for IM inoculation at the high dose of 20 µg (Figure 4A). Using only 2 µg for the more active (in vivo) K1F enzyme (Figure 4B) the opposite pattern is suggested, but the small sample sizes provide little power in significance tests. K1H (2 µg dose) yielded similarly low rescue rates for both routes of administration (Figure 4C).

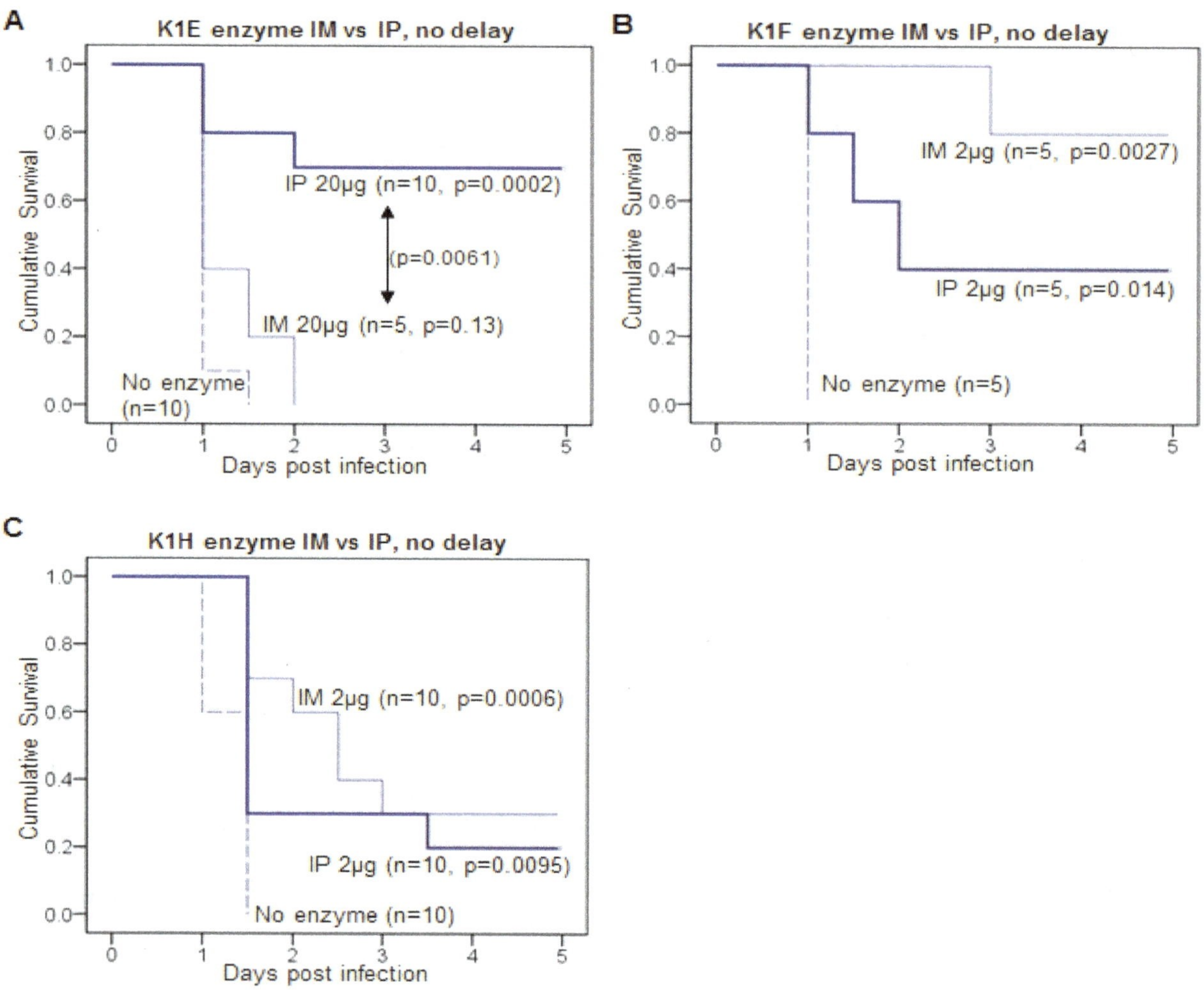

Figure 4. Administration route can affect treatment efficacy. (**A**–**C**) Kaplan-Meier survival curves of depolymerase treatment comparing intramuscular (IM) to intraperitoneal (IP) inoculation in mice. (**A**) Treatment with 20 µg K1E; (**B**) Treatment with 2 µg K1F; (**C**) Treatment with 2 µg K1H. In all mice, 1.2–2.9 × 10^8 CFU of K1-capsulated *E. coli* were injected IM, followed by inoculation of enzyme either IM in the contralateral thigh or IP. Mouse survival was monitored for 5 days and the cumulative probability of survival was plotted for each treatment. The mouse number *n* of each treatment is labeled by each curve. Log rank test: *p* values between enzyme treatment and the no-enzyme control, or significant *p* values between IM and IP treatment are listed.

Basis of the effect of administration route. We tested capsule degradation activity of serum from mice that had been inoculated with enzyme by different routes. If bioavailability of enzyme is affected by route of administration, then serum from mice inoculated by the IP route should have different activity per unit volume than serum from mice inoculated IM. Consistent with treatment efficacy differences, detectable degradation by K1E serum was observed only for the IP route, and then only at 1 h post inoculation (Figure 5A, boxed region). As for K1F and K1H sera, IP delivery resulted in slightly higher capsule degradation activity than IM at 1 h post inoculation, and activity was largely maintained after 24 h exposure (Figure 5B,C). However, both K1F and K1H sera exhibited much higher activities than K1E serum, independent of administration route.

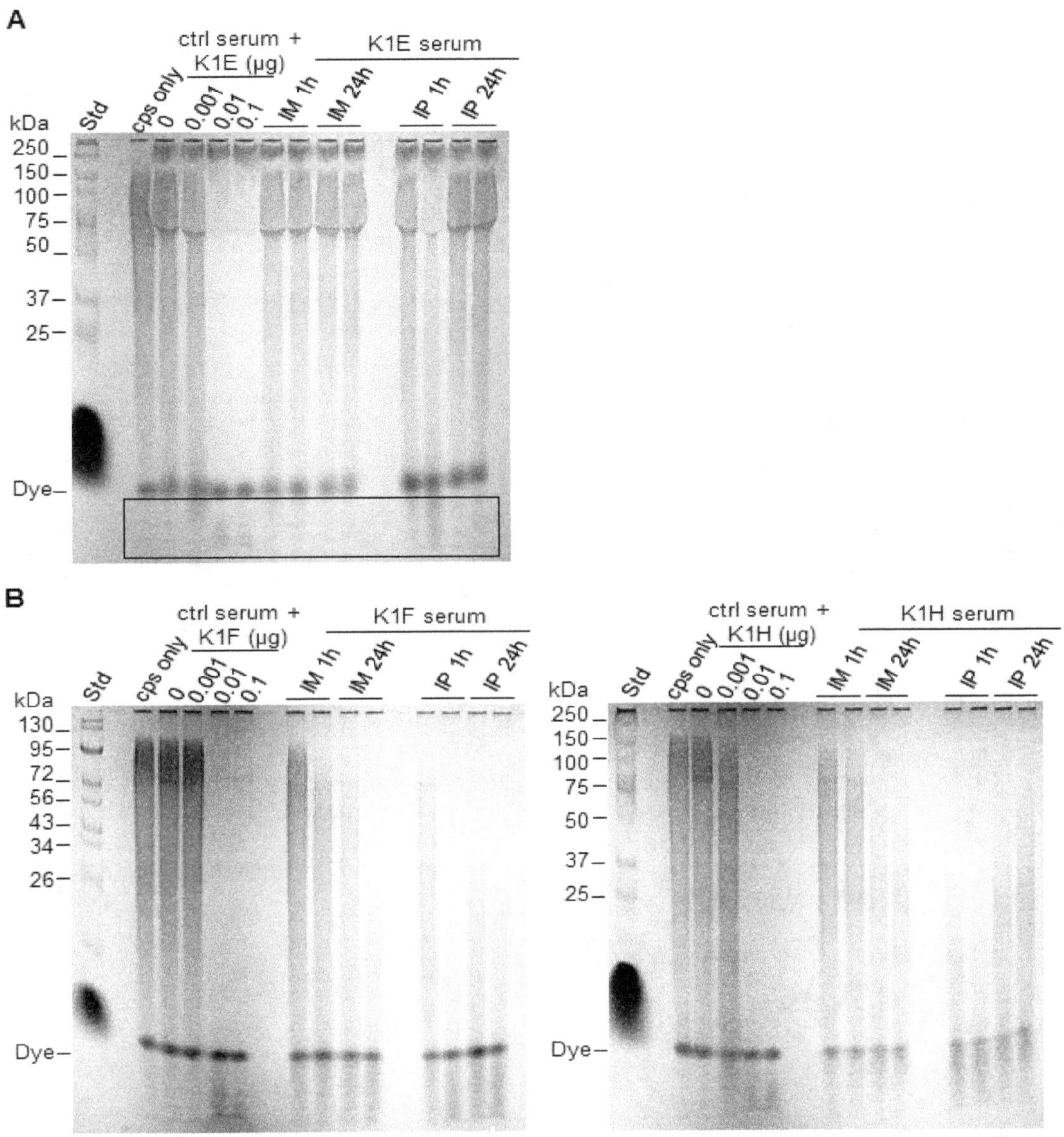

Figure 5. Comparison of depolymerase serum activity using different administration routes. Except for the molecular weight standard ("std") on the left of each panel, each lane fractionates 10–20 ug of K1 capsule ("cps only") or an overnight reaction of capsule incubated with serum and/or enzyme. Lanes with "serum" used serum from mice inoculated with enzyme (**A**) K1E; (**B**) K1F (left) or K1H (right) (IM or IP, 1 mg/kg weight) and sacrificed at 1 or 24 h. Two mice were tested for each route and time point, shown in separate lanes. Lanes with "ctrl serum" had different amounts of free enzyme added to the control serum (from mice not receiving enzyme injection), as the control reactions. Only a slight activity of K1E is evident, and then only for IP 1h (bottom of lane, boxed). In contrast, K1F and K1H both exhibit clear activity by both routes of administration, with a possible effect of route for K1H at 1 h.

3.3. K1: Treatment Is Successful with Leukopenia

The above models used immunocompetent mice, requiring high inocula of bacteria to overwhelm innate immunity. To better represent infections that progress from low to high concentrations of bacteria, we tested mice that had been rendered leukopenic, limiting the studies to K1-capsulated bacteria.

Leukopenic mice are far more susceptible to RS218 than are immune-competent mice (Figure 6). A bacterial inoculum slightly exceeding 10^4 was fatal in the leukopenic mice (Figure 6A), compared to the lethal threshold dose of 10^6–10^7 in immunocompetent mice (Figure 6C). In leukopenic mice, doses above 10^4 cfu reduced survival time, to about a half day shorter using 10^7 bacteria (Figure 6A). Phage and enzyme each rescued the leukopenic mice in most cases, whether with immediate (Figure 7A,B) or delayed treatment (Figure 7C).

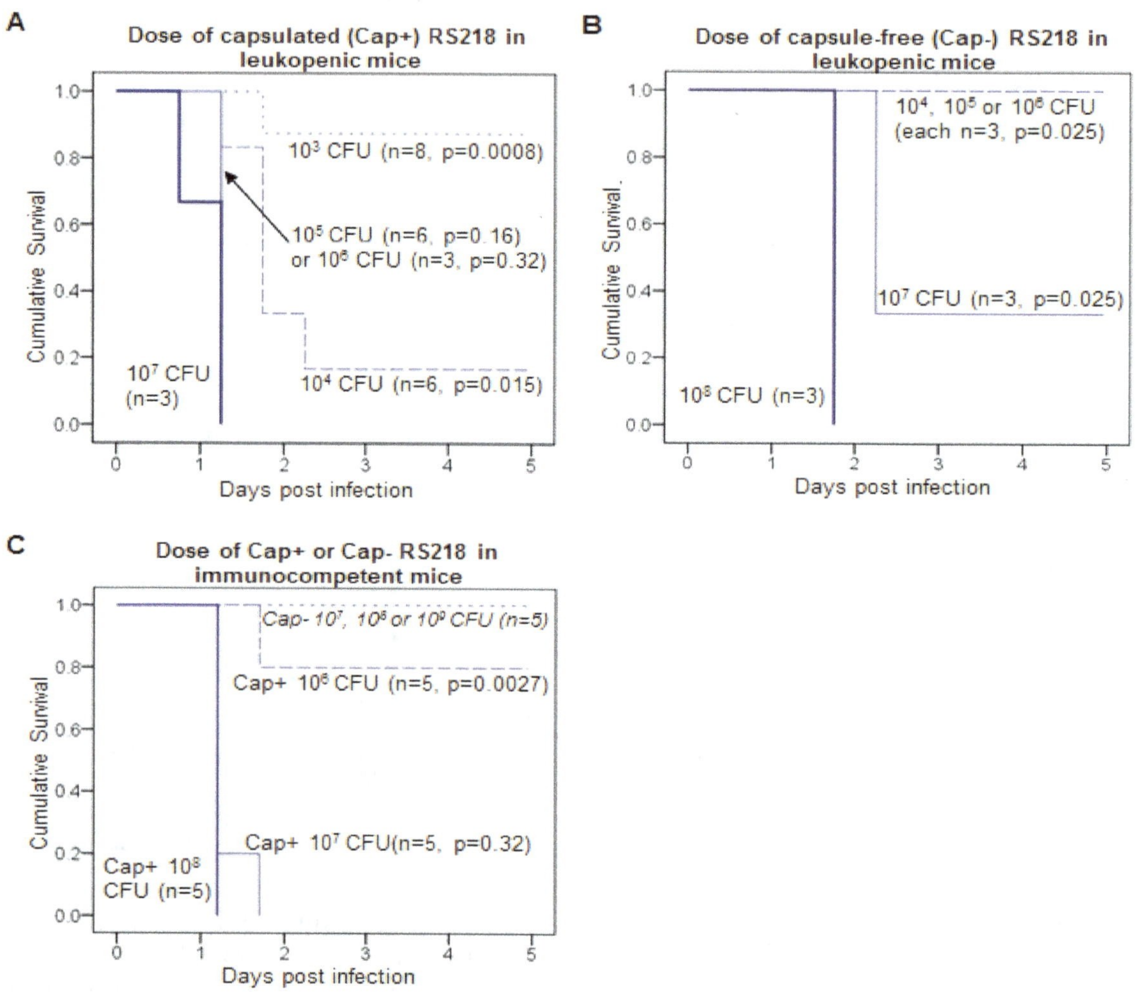

Figure 6. Capsule-free RS218 is avirulent in mice. Kaplan-Meier survival curves of mice per dose of different strains. (**A**) K1-capsulated RS218 (Cap+) in leukopenic mice; (**B**) capsule-free RS218 (Cap−) in leukopenic mice; (**C**) Cap+ and Cap− RS218 in immune competent mice. The median lethal dose is 10^3–10^4 CFU for Cap+ and 10^6–10^7 CFU for Cap- RS218 in leukopenic mice, a difference of 3 orders of magnitude. The median lethal dose in normal mice is 10^6–10^7 CFU for Cap+ RS218, while Cap− RS218 is not lethal at doses as high as 10^9 CFU. Mouse survival was monitored for 5 days and the cumulative probability of survival was plotted for each dose. The mouse number n of each treatment is labeled by each curve. Log rank test: p values are listed for lower doses compared to the highest dose of each strain.

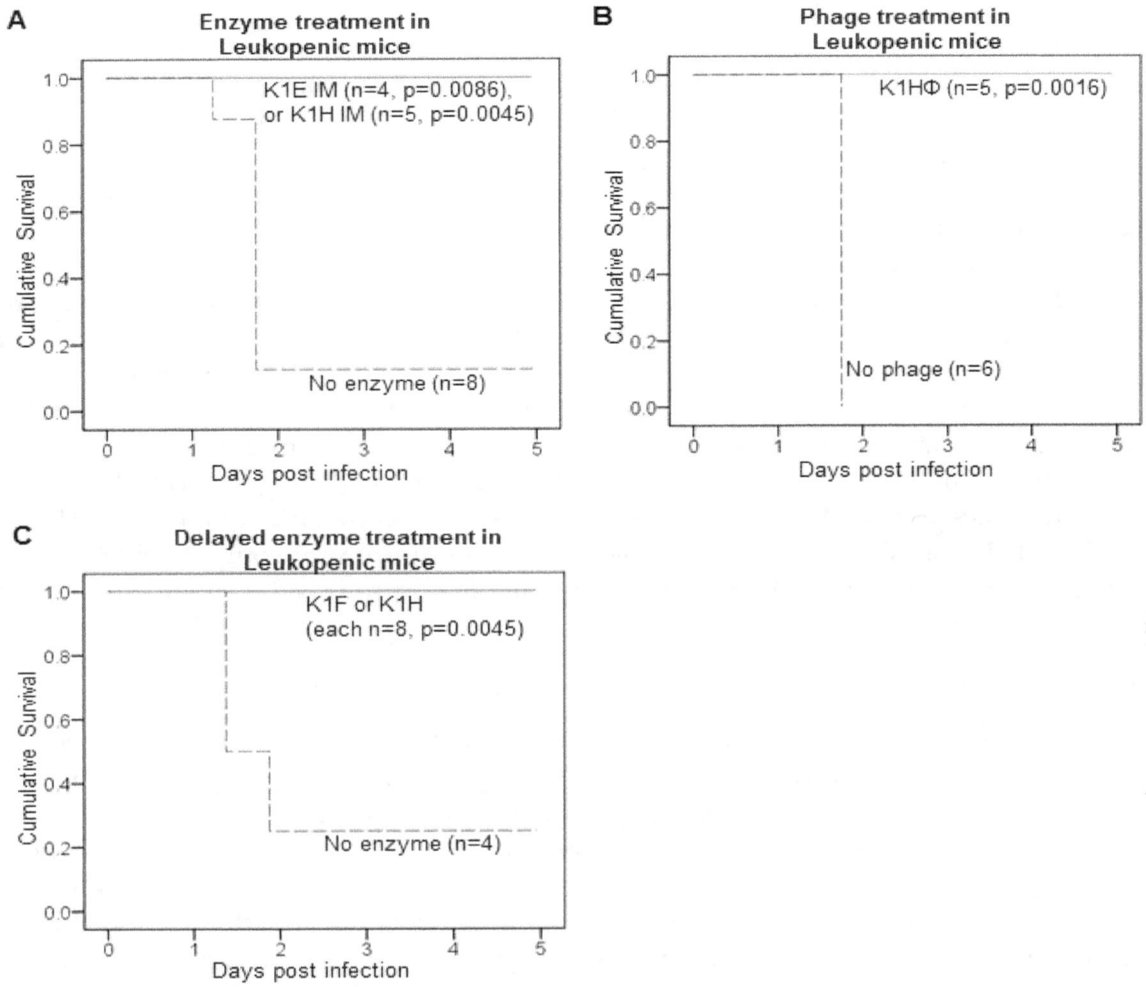

Figure 7. Enzymes and phages rescue infections of leukopenic mice. Total rescue of infections by K1 *E. coli* in leukopenic mice was achieved by simultaneous treatment with (**A**) K1E or K1H depolymerase; (**B**) K1H phage, and by delayed treatment with (**C**) K1F or K1H depolymerase. Each panel shows Kaplan-Meier survival curves with sample sizes given by n. Infection was initiated by intramuscular (IM) inoculations of 2.2–5.1 $\times$ 10^4 CFU of K1 *E. coli* in the left thigh. Treatment was an IM injection of 20 μg enzyme or 10^7 phage in the contralateral thigh. Treatment was administered either (**A**,**B**) immediately at the time of infection or (**C**) 8 h after infection. Mouse survival was monitored for 5 days and the cumulative probability of survival was plotted for each treatment. Log rank test: p values are listed for each treatment compared to no-treatment control.

Avirulence of capsule-free bacteria. Our use of leukopenic mice was motivated to assess the potential for treatment failure via the evolution of treatment-resistant bacteria, as observed in a neutropenic mouse-*Pseudomonas* infection model [39]. Resistance is a potential cause of treatment failure with both phages and antibiotics [39,46–50]. Treatment success in our studies indicates that resistance did not ascend, at least not enough to affect survival (true both for immunocompetent and leukopenice mice). We thus addressed the reason evolution of resistance was not a problem in our system despite its cause of treatment failure in others. In the case of enzyme treatment, the relevant "resistance" phenotype is presumably absence of a capsule, since the enzyme has no substrate on those cells; that phenotype is also resistant to phages encoding K1 enzymes [51]. Therefore, the lethal consequences of a capsule-free RS218 derivative in leukopenic mice was evaluated over a series of inoculum sizes (Figure 6B,C). The capsule-free bacteria are profoundly less virulent: The mice could survive an inoculum 10^3–10^4 times larger of capsule-free bacteria than of capsulated bacteria. Thus, resistant (capsule-free) bacteria are more easily controlled by the immune system than are treatment-sensitive, capsulated bacteria and thus are not a reason for treatment failure. (The same argument applies to cells resistant to treatment with phages that require the capsule.) Smith and Huggins (1982) observed reduced virulence of K1 capsule-free bacteria in immunocomptent mice, so these results generalize across both immunocompetent and immune-compromised mice.

Successful, delayed treatment of leukopenic mice. For immunocompetent mice, immediate treatment was superior to delayed treatment for all enzymes. For K1-capsulated bacteria, delayed treatment was still better than the absence of treatment but not as good as immediate treatment. The inferiority of delayed treatment might stem from an artefact of the infection model, specifically that such a high dose of bacteria must be introduced so that the window of opportunity for treatment is short. From the work presented above of lethal inoculum doses in leukopenic vs immunocompetent mice (Figure 6C), leukopenia increases the dynamic range of bacterial densities in which to evaluate treament efficacy—a lower inoculum can be used and the time available to treat increases. To test this latter premise, we attempted delayed treatment of leukopenic mice using K1 enzymes. The bacterial inoculum was approximately 5×10^4 CFU, and enzyme treatment (20 μg K1F or K1H) was given at 8 h. All 16 treated mice survived, whereas only 1 of the 4 controls survived (Figure 7C). This survival rate is significantly higher than that with delayed treatment of immunocompetent mice, but a direct comparison of delayed treatment between leukopenic and immunocompetent mice is not easily interpreted (see Discussion).

3.4. Measuring the Dynamical Impact of Treatment: Resistance Competition Assay

Survival is an endpoint measure of efficacy but gives little insight to the underlying process of bacterial dynamics. Levin [36] developed a metric of the quantitative impact of treatment on bacterial abundances—the resistance competiton assay (RCA). Mice are inoculated with a mix of two bacterial strains, one sensitive and the other resistant to treatment. In untreated controls, the two strains grow in vivo according to their intrinsic abilities, though not necessarily at the same rate. With treatment, the sensitive strain is specifically inhibited. Relative to controls, the resistant strain thus increases its proportion, and the magnitude of this increase depending on how much the sensitive strain is inhibited or killed. An RCA value greater than 0 indicates that the treatment suppresses the sensitive strain, higher values moreso.

Six mice were used for an RCA measure of K1H enzyme, 3 controls and 3 treatments. The resistant strain was the K5-capsulated strain, one that is virulent in vivo (as opposed to a capsule-free RS218). Initial frequency of the resistant strain in the mix was 0.006. At four hours, the frequencies of resistant cells were significantly higher in the enzyme-treated mice than in the controls (Table 2), and the RCA value was 0.30.

Table 2. Frequencies of resistant bacteria in the Resistance Competition Assay.

Control Mice	Treated Mice [1]	Average RCA
0.001, 0.0008, 0.0029	0.0052, 0.0049, 0.0047	0.30

[1] A *t*-test comparing (logged) frequencies of treated mice versus control mice = 3.3 (4 df), $p = 0.015$ (1-tailed). A non-parametric combinations test of the perfect association of high frequencies in treated mice gives $p = 0.05$.

4. Discussion

This study broadly supports a growing realization that phage depolymerases might be useful therapeutics against particular kinds of bacterial infections. The work here also starts to put bounds on the degree of generality in depolymerase utility. Our study used 3 different capsulated *E. coli* strains and tested 3 enzymes against K1 capsules, one enzyme against K5, and one enzyme against K30. The work presented extends tests of therapeutic efficiency to varying conditions and may thus provide insight to efficacy in clinical infections.

K1 depolymerases that performed well in immunocompetent mice also performed well in immune-compromised, leukopenic mice. As expected, leukopenic mice were far less tolerant of bacteria than were immunocompetent mice. Given the artificiality of mouse infections with high doses of bacteria, leukopenic mice may yield a more realistic infection model than do immunocompetent mice, chiefly by increasing the dynamic range of bacterial densities that overwhelm the immune response. In support of this interpretation, leukopenic mice exhibited a modest increase in survival time (when inoculated with low numbers of bacteria), intramuscular treatment with K1E enzyme was improved with leukopenia (Figure 7A), and leukopenic mice were more easily rescued with delayed treatment than were immunocompetent mice. We caution, however, that differences in treatment efficacy between immunocompetent and leukopenic mice are not easily interpreted because of the many differences in the two model infections. Even so, the greater range of useful inoculum sizes afforded by leukopenia increases the latitude of experimental designs.

In contrast to observations with *Pseudomonas* infections of neutropenic mice treated with phages [39], evolution of resistance to K1 capsular depolymerases did not thwart treatment success in leukopenic mice. The absence of resistance evolution likely stems from the avirulence of capsule-free bacteria. The bacterium's only reasonably accessible evolutionary path to avoid the depolymerase is to lose the capsule (it cannot easily generate a new capsule type). This would leave the resistant cell in the same phenotypic state as an otherwise capsulated cell that was stripped of its capsule by enzyme. Thus resistant bacteria and enzyme-treated bacteria may be functionally equivalent in the mouse.

On the negative side for enzyme therapy, delayed treatment of immune competent mice not only reduced efficacy but the reduction was complete for the K30 depolymerase, which lost all efficacy under delayed treatment. However, K30 was also the enzyme showing the weakest effect under simultaneous treatment (e.g., it required the highest dose of all enzymes to rescue mice; Lin et al., 2017 [11]) so there was a strong *a priori* basis for anticipating the large effect of delay with K30 enzyme. In contrast, delayed administration of two K1 enzymes retained efficacy, albeit at a reduced level. Perhaps significantly, with delayed treatment, the two cognate K1-specific phages achieved higher rescue than enzymes. Although no negative consequence of delayed treatment was observed in leukopenic mice (tested only for K1 depolymerases), the outcome with immune competent mice likely reflects a true negative effect of delayed treatment that would be manifested in other contexts.

To gain additional insight to enzyme efficacy, we conducted a resistance competition assay (RCA). RCA values of 2.1 and 1.7 were reported for immediate treatment with streptomycin and a phage requiring the K1-capsule, both highly effective [36], whereas values ranging from 0.2–0.5 were reported for treatments that were only somewhat effective. The observed RCA value for immediate K1H depolymerase treatment determined here is 0.3; over the course of 10 h, this translates into a 95% reduction of bacterial numbers relative to the no treatment control.

The RCA value for K1H, an enzyme that is highly effective in rescuing mice, is thus somewhat lower than expected from previous results. We can suggest several possible reasons for this discrepancy. First, immediate treatment with enzyme may not be quite as effective as with streptomycin or the K1-dependent phage—all treatments yield near 100% survival, but differences could be masked at this upper limit of the dynamic range; indeed, the enzymes do not invariably rescue [11]. Second, treatment spans a time course, and the RCA is measured at a point in time, so 4 h may not be the best time for comparison (e.g., enzyme may be slower to diffuse than antibiotic). Third, assays with phage treatment risk inflating the RCA by allowing bacterial killing to continue during the thigh-processing step. Finally, in comparison to phages, enzymes do not lyse cells and release toxins, so recovery with enzyme treatment may be feasible with a lower dose of killing than is required with phages. Although we cannot yet suggest whether any of these explanations has merit, the comparisons provide interesting avenues for further study.

A greater therapeutic efficacy of phages than of cognate depolymerase enzyme is not surprising, given that phages amplify on the bacteria, whereas enzyme concentration remains static or, more likely, declines due to inactivation and clearance. However, understanding the basis of greater phage efficacy is non-trivial because phage amplification has several components relevant to treatment—direct bacterial killing from phage infection, release of progeny phage particles that contain fresh enzyme molecules, plus the release of additional free enzyme in the form of unassembled tailspikes at the time of cell lysis. A phage inoculum of 10^7 pfu (used here) carries about 2.5–3 $\times$ 10^{-5} μg enzyme, hence ~1.3 $\times$ 10^{-6} less depolymerase delivered in the phage inoculum than delivered in our enzyme treatment. Even with this profound difference and only 4–8 fold greater activity of phage virion-associated enzyme than of the purified form, K1H or K1E phage still gave rise to better survival rates than purified K1 enzymes. This greater efficacy of phages could speak either to a benefit of direct killing or to possibly orders of magnitude greater enzyme produced as the phage population expands. We of course don't know the balance between these two effects. Yet, whatever argument is put forth for the superiority of K1 phages (except K1F, which does not grow on the K1-capsulated host used here) under delayed treatment, K5 phage or K30 phage did not improve survival rate over their pure enzymes at the doses tested.

Reduced efficacy with delayed treatment of any form is not surprising, especially with infections that are rapidly lethal. However, although it is tempting to interpret the effect of a treatment delay as merely giving the bacteria a "head start" to reach a lethal threshold, previous work using K1 infections of mice showed that the bacteria changed state with time to become recalcitrant to treatment [36]. This change in susceptibility may be due to the bacterial environment suddenly changing from laboratory growth media to mouse tissue, as altered bacterial physiology and community lifestyle could affect phage infection [52] and probably phage product treatment. Thus, the effect of therapeutic treatment delay could be one of the bacteria becoming more difficult to treat than of them being more numerous. The use of leukopenic mice as an experimental infection model may help avoid that complication and yield therapeutic regimes more redily translatable to clinical use.

A surprising result was the effect of route of administration on efficacy, at least for enzyme K1E. It is of course easy to argue that each enzyme has its own biochemical properties that may affect pharmacokinetics. For example, unlike the other K1 enzymes used here, K1E purified under our protocol tends to form 18-mers instead of trimers [11]. The larger enzyme complex might affect in vivo distribution and result in poor IM treatment efficiency, but this can only be argued on a *post facto* basis. Whatever the cause, the result indicates that treatment "failure" by one route does not imply failure by other routes.

By applying modifications of animal models, we have obtained more detailed understanding of how phage biology and enzyme biology complicate the pharmacokinetic and pharmacodynamic properties of phage and enzyme in infection treatment. The complex biological and pharmacological properties of phages is one major reason holding back whole phages from drug development and approval [53]. Phage derived enzymes are more similar to conventional antibiotics and thus more suitable than whole phages for the current drug approval processes even if not necessarily more suitable for treatment efficacy. In contrast to phages, depolymerases do not lyse bacteria and thus do not release endotoxin, so there may be circumstances in which enzymes are superior to phages [54,55]. A better understanding of enzyme structure and enzyme kinetics could greatly advance the development and approval of phage-derived enzymes as a novel class of antibiotics.

Author Contributions: Experiment design and Methodology, H.L., J.J.B. and I.J.M.; Investigation, H.L., M.L.P. and J.J.B.; Data Validation and Analysis, H.L., and J.J.B.; Writing, H.L., J.J.B. and I.J.M.

References

1. Lewis, K. Platforms for antibiotic discovery. *Nat. Rev. Drug Discov.* **2013**, *12*, 371–387. [CrossRef] [PubMed]
2. Drulis-Kawa, Z.; Majkowska-Skrobek, G.; Maciejewska, B. Bacteriophages and phage-derived proteins—Application approaches. *Curr. Med. Chem.* **2015**, *22*, 1757–1773. [CrossRef] [PubMed]
3. Cooper, C.J.; Koonjan, S.; Nilsson, A.S. Enhancing whole phage therapy and their derived antimicrobial enzymes through complex formulation. *Pharmaceuticals (Basel)* **2018**, *11*, 34. [CrossRef] [PubMed]
4. Pires, D.P.; Cleto, S.; Sillankorva, S.; Azeredo, J.; Lu, T.K. Genetically Engineered Phages: A Review of Advances over the Last Decade. *Microbiol. Mol. Biol. Rev.* **2016**, *80*, 523–543. [CrossRef] [PubMed]
5. Roach, D.R.; Donovan, D.M. Antimicrobial bacteriophage-derived proteins and therapeutic applications. *Bacteriophage* **2015** *5*, e1062590. [CrossRef] [PubMed]

6. Abedon, S.T.; García, P.; Mullany, P.; Aminov, R. Editorial: Phage Therapy: Past, Present and Future. *Front. Microbiol.* **2017**, *8*. [CrossRef] [PubMed]
7. Vandenheuvel, D.; Lavigne, R.; Brussow, H. Bacteriophage Therapy: Advances in Formulation Strategies and Human Clinical Trials. *Annu. Rev. Virol.* **2015**, *2*, 599–618. [CrossRef] [PubMed]
8. Rhoads, D.D.; Wolcott, R.D.; Kuskowski, M.A.; Wolcott, B.M.; Ward, L.S.; Sulakvelidze, A. Bacteriophage therapy of venous leg ulcers in humans: Results of a phase I safety trial. *J. Wound Care* **2009**, *18*, 237–238, 240–243. [CrossRef] [PubMed]
9. Sarker, S.A.; Sultana, S.; Reuteler, G.; Moine, D.; Descombes, P.; Charton, F.; Bourdin, G.; McCallin, S.; Ngom-Bru, C.; Neville, T.; et al. Oral Phage Therapy of Acute Bacterial Diarrhea with Two Coliphage Preparations: A Randomized Trial in Children from Bangladesh. *EBioMedicine* **2016**, *4*, 124–137. [CrossRef] [PubMed]
10. Jault, P.; Leclerc, T.; Jennes, S.; Pirnay, J.P.; Que, Y.-A.; Resch, G.; Rousseau, A.F.; Ravat, F.; Carsin, H.; Le Floch, R.; et al. Efficacy and tolerability of a cocktail of bacteriophages to treat burn wounds infected by *Pseudomonas aeruginosa* (PhagoBurn): A randomised, controlled, double-blind phase 1/2 trial. *Lancet Infect. Dis.* **2018**. [CrossRef]
11. Lin, H.; Paff, M.L.; Molineux, I.J.; Bull, J.J. Therapeutic Application of Phage Capsule Depolymerases against K1, K5, and K30 Capsulated *E. coli* in Mice. *Front. Microbiol.* **2017**, *8*, 2257. [CrossRef] [PubMed]
12. Briers, Y.; Lavigne, R. Breaking barriers: Expansion of the use of endolysins as novel antibacterials against Gram-negative bacteria. *Future Microbiol.* **2015**, *10*, 377–390. [CrossRef] [PubMed]
13. Oliveira, H.; Sao-Jose, C.; Azeredo, J. Phage-Derived Peptidoglycan Degrading Enzymes: Challenges and Future Prospects for in vivo Therapy. *Viruses* **2018**, *10*, 292. [CrossRef] [PubMed]
14. Song, J.; Xia, F.; Jiang, H.; Li, X.; Hu, L.; Gong, P.; Lei, L.; Feng, X.; Sun, C.; Gu, J.; et al. Identification and characterization of HolGH15: The holin of Staphylococcus aureus bacteriophage GH15. *J. Gen. Virol.* **2016**, *97*, 1272–1281. [CrossRef] [PubMed]
15. Latka, A.; Maciejewska, B.; Majkowska-Skrobek, G.; Briers, Y.; Drulis-Kawa, Z. Bacteriophage-encoded virion-associated enzymes to overcome the carbohydrate barriers during the infection process. *Appl. Microbiol. Biotechnol.* **2017**, *101*, 3103–3119. [CrossRef] [PubMed]
16. Fischetti, V.A. Development of Phage Lysins as Novel Therapeutics: A Historical Perspective. *Viruses* **2018**, *10*, 310. [CrossRef] [PubMed]
17. Roberts, I.S. The biochemistry and genetics of capsular polysaccharide production in bacteria. *Annu. Rev. Microbiol.* **1996**, *50*, 285–315. [CrossRef] [PubMed]
18. Azeredo, J.; Sutherland, I.W. The use of phages for the removal of infectious biofilms. *Curr. Pharm. Biotechnol.* **2008**, *9*, 261–266. [CrossRef] [PubMed]
19. Fleming, D.; Chahin, L.; Rumbaugh, K. Glycoside Hydrolases Degrade Polymicrobial Bacterial Biofilms in Wounds. *Antimicrob. Agents Chemother.* **2017**, *61*. [CrossRef] [PubMed]
20. Fleming, D.; Rumbaugh, K.P. Approaches to Dispersing Medical Biofilms. *Microorganisms* **2017**, *5*, 15. [CrossRef] [PubMed]
21. Mushtaq, N.; Redpath, M.B.; Luzio, J.P.; Taylor, P.W. Prevention and cure of systemic *Escherichia coli* K1 infection by modification of the bacterial phenotype. *Antimicrob. Agents Chemother.* **2004**, *48*, 1503–1508. [CrossRef] [PubMed]
22. Mushtaq, N.; Redpath, M.B.; Luzio, J.P.; Taylor, P.W. Treatment of experimental *Escherichia coli* infection with recombinant bacteriophage-derived capsule depolymerase. *J. Antimicrob. Chemother.* **2005**, *56*, 160–165. [CrossRef] [PubMed]
23. Scorpio, A.; Tobery, S.A.; Ribot, W.J.; Friedlander, A.M. Treatment of experimental anthrax with recombinant capsule depolymerase. *Antimicrob. Agents Chemother.* **2008**, *52*, 1014–1020. [CrossRef] [PubMed]
24. Negus, D.; Vipond, J.; Hatch, G.J.; Rayner, E.L.; Taylor, P.W. Parenteral Administration of Capsule Depolymerase EnvD Prevents Lethal Inhalation Anthrax Infection. *Antimicrob. Agents Chemother.* **2015**, *59*, 7687–7692. [CrossRef] [PubMed]
25. Lin, T.L.; Hsieh, P.F.; Huang, Y.T.; Lee, W.C.; Tsai, Y.T.; Su, P.A.; Pan, Y.J.; Hsu, C.R.; Wu, M.C.; Wang, J.T. Isolation of a bacteriophage and its depolymerase specific for K1 capsule of Klebsiella pneumoniae: Implication in typing and treatment. *J. Infect. Dis.* **2014** *210*, 1734–1744. [CrossRef] [PubMed]
26. Pan, Y.J.; Lin, T.L.; Lin, Y.T.; Su, P.A.; Chen, C.T.; Hsieh, P.F.; Hsu, C.R.; Chen, C.C.; Hsieh, Y.C.; Wang, J.T. Identification of capsular types in carbapenem-resistant *Klebsiella pneumoniae* strains by WZC sequencing

and implications for capsule depolymerase treatment. *Antimicrob. Agents Chemother.* **2015**, *59*, 1038–1047. [CrossRef] [PubMed]

27. Majkowska-Skrobek, G.; Latka, A.; Berisio, R.; Maciejewska, B.; Squeglia, F.; Romano, M.; Lavigne, R.; Struve, C.; Drulis-Kawa, Z. Capsule-targeting depolymerase, derived from Klebsiella KP36 phage, as a tool for the development of anti-virulent strategy. *Viruses* **2016**, *8*, 324. [CrossRef] [PubMed]
28. Achtman, M.; Mercer, A.; Kusecek, B.; Pohl, A.; Heuzenroeder, M.; Aaronson, W.; Sutton, A.; Silver, R.P. Six widespread bacterial clones among *Escherichia coli* K1 isolates. *Infect. Immun.* **1983**, *39*, 315–335. [PubMed]
29. Orskov, I.; Orskov, F.; Jann, B.; Jann, K. Serology, chemistry, and genetics of O and K antigens of *Escherichia coli*. *Bacteriol. Rev.* **1977**, *41*, 667–710. [PubMed]
30. Vimr, E.R.; Troy, F.A. Regulation of sialic acid metabolism in *Escherichia coli*: Role of N-acylneuraminate pyruvate-lyase. *J. Bacteriol.* **1985**, *164*, 854–860. [PubMed]
31. Smith, H.W.; Huggins, M.B. The association of the O18, K1 and H7 antigens and the ColV plasmid of a strain of *E. coli* with virulence and immunogenicity. *J. Gen. Microbiol.* **1980**, *121*, 387–400. [PubMed]
32. Bull, J.J.; Vimr, E.R.; Molineux, I.J. A tale of tails: Sialidase is key to success in a model of phage therapy against K1-capsulated *Escherichia coli*. *Virology* **2010**, *398*, 79–86. [CrossRef] [PubMed]
33. Scholl, D.; Kieleczawa, J.; Kemp, P.; Rush, J.; Richardson, C.C.; Merril, C.; Adhya, S.; Molineux, I.J. Genomic analysis of bacteriophages SP6 and K1-5, an estranged subgroup of the T7 supergroup. *J. Mol. Biol.* **2004**, *335*, 1151–1171. [CrossRef] [PubMed]
34. Whitfield, C.; Lam, M. Characterisation of coliphage K30, a bacteriophage specific for *Escherichia coli* capsular serotype K30. *FEMS Microbiol. Lett.* **1986**, *37*, 351–355. [CrossRef]
35. Leiman, P.G.; Battisti, A.J.; Bowman, V.D.; Stummeyer, K.; Muhlenhoff, M.; Gerardy-Schahn, R.; Scholl, D.; Molineux, I.J. The structures of bacteriophages K1E and K1-5 explain processive degradation of polysaccharide capsules and evolution of new host specificities. *J. Mol. Biol.* **2007**, *371*, 836–849. [CrossRef] [PubMed]
36. Bull, J.J.; Levin, B.R.; DeRouin, T.; Walker, N.; Bloch, C.A. Dynamics of success and failure in phage and antibiotic therapy in experimental infections. *BMC Microbiol.* **2002**, *2*, 35. [CrossRef]
37. Bull, J.J.; Otto, G.; Molineux, I.J. In vivo growth rates are poorly correlated with phage therapy success in a mouse infection model. *Antimicrob. Agents Chemother.* **2012**, *56*, 949–954. [CrossRef] [PubMed]
38. Rich, J.T.; Neely, J.G.; Paniello, R.C.; Voelker, C.C.; Nussenbaum, B.; Wang, E.W. A practical guide to understanding Kaplan-Meier curves. *Otolaryngol. Head Neck Surg.* **2010**, *143*, 331–336. [CrossRef] [PubMed]
39. Roach, D.R.; Leung, C.Y.; Henry, M.; Morello, E.; Singh, D.; Di Santo, J.P.; Weitz, J.S.; Debarbieux, L. Synergy between the host immune system and bacteriophage is essential for successful phage therapy against an acute respiratory pathogen. *Cell Host Microbe* **2017**, *22*, 38–47. [CrossRef] [PubMed]
40. Pelkonen, S.; Häyrinen, J.; Finne, J. Polyacrylamide gel electrophoresis of the capsular polysaccharides of *Escherichia coli* K1 and other bacteria. *J. Bacteriol.* **1988**, *170*, 2646–2653. [CrossRef] [PubMed]
41. Muhlenhoff, M.; Stummeyer, K.; Grove, M.; Sauerborn, M.; Gerardy-Schahn, R. Proteolytic processing and oligomerization of bacteriophage-derived endosialidases. *J. Biol. Chem.* **2003**, *278*, 12634–12644. [CrossRef] [PubMed]
42. Gerardy-Schahn, R.; Bethe, A.; Brennecke, T.; Mühlenhoff, M.; Eckhardt, M.; Ziesing, S.; Lottspeich, F.; Frosch, M. Molecular cloning and functional expression of bacteriophage PK1E-encoded endoneuraminidase Endo NE. *Mol. Microbiol.* **1995**, *16*, 441–450. [CrossRef] [PubMed]
43. Luke, D.R.; Brunner, L.J.; Vadiei, K. Bioavailability assessment of cyclosporine in the rat. Influence of route of administration. *Drug Metab. Dispos.* **1990**, *18*, 158–162. [PubMed]
44. Yamamura, Y.; Santa, T.; Kotaki, H.; Uchino, K.; Sawada, Y.; Iga, T. Administration-route dependency of absorption of glycyrrhizin in rats: Intraperitoneal administration dramatically enhanced bioavailability. *Biol. Pharm. Bull.* **1995**, *18*, 337–341. [CrossRef] [PubMed]
45. Kijanka, G.; Prokopowicz, M.; Schellekens, H.; Brinks, V. Influence of aggregation and route of injection on the biodistribution of mouse serum albumin. *PLoS ONE* **2014**, *9*, e85281. [CrossRef] [PubMed]
46. Torres-Barcelo, C. Phage Therapy Faces Evolutionary Challenges. *Viruses* **2018**, *10*, 323. [CrossRef] [PubMed]
47. Dennehy, J.J. What Can Phages Tell Us about Host-Pathogen Coevolution? *Int. J. Evol. Biol.* **2012**, *2012*, 396165. [CrossRef] [PubMed]
48. Nilsson, A.S. Phage therapy—Constraints and possibilities. *Ups J. Med. Sci.* **2014**, *119*, 192–198. [CrossRef] [PubMed]

49. Bull, J.J.; Vegge, C.S.; Schmerer, M.; Chaudhry, W.N.; Levin, B.R. Phenotypic resistance and the dynamics of bacterial escape from phage control. *PLoS ONE* **2014**, *9*, e94690. [CrossRef] [PubMed]
50. Levin, B.R.; Bull, J.J. Population and evolutionary dynamics of phage therapy. *Nat. Rev. Microbiol.* **2004**, *2*, 166–173. [CrossRef] [PubMed]
51. Smith, H.W.; Huggins, M.B. Successful treatment of experimental *Escherichia coli* infections in mice using phage: Its general superiority over antibiotics. *J. Gen. Microbiol.* **1982**, *128*, 307–318. [CrossRef] [PubMed]
52. Lourenco, M.; De Sordi, L.; Debarbieux, L. The Diversity of Bacterial Lifestyles Hampers Bacteriophage Tenacity. *Viruses* **2018**, *10*, 327. [CrossRef] [PubMed]
53. Cooper, C.J.; Khan Mirzaei, M.; Nilsson, A.S. Adapting Drug Approval Pathways for Bacteriophage-Based Therapeutics. *Front. Microbiol.* **2016**, *7*, 1209. [CrossRef] [PubMed]
54. Hagens, S.; Habel, A.; von Ahsen, U.; von Gabain, A.; Blasi, U. Therapy of experimental pseudomonas infections with a nonreplicating genetically modified phage. *Antimicrob. Agents Chemother.* **2004**, *48*, 3817–3822. [CrossRef] [PubMed]
55. Matsuda, T.; Freeman, T.A.; Hilbert, D.W.; Duff, M.; Fuortes, M.; Stapleton, P.P.; Daly, J.M. Lysis-deficient bacteriophage therapy decreases endotoxin and inflammatory mediator release and improves survival in a murine peritonitis model. *Surgery* **2005**, *137*, 639–646. [CrossRef] [PubMed]

5

Towards Inhaled Phage Therapy in Western Europe

Sandra-Maria Wienhold [1], Jasmin Lienau [1] and Martin Witzenrath [1,2,*]

1 Division of Pulmonary Inflammation, Charité–Universitätsmedizin Berlin, Freie Universität Berlin, Humboldt-Universität zu Berlin, and Berlin Institute of Health, 10117 Berlin, Germany; sandra.wienhold@charite.de (S.-M.W.); jasmin.lienau@charite.de (J.L.)

2 Department of Infectious Diseases and Respiratory Medicine, Charité–Universitätsmedizin Berlin, Freie Universität Berlin, Humboldt-Universität zu Berlin, and Berlin Institute of Health, 10117 Berlin, Germany

* Correspondence: martin.witzenrath@charite.de

Abstract: The emergence of multidrug-resistant bacteria constitutes a great challenge for modern medicine, recognized by leading medical experts and politicians worldwide. Rediscovery and implementation of bacteriophage therapy by Western medicine might be one solution to the problem of increasing antibiotic failure. In some Eastern European countries phage therapy is used for treating infectious diseases. However, while the European Medicines Agency (EMA) advised that the development of bacteriophage-based therapies should be expedited due to its significant potential, EMA emphasized that phages cannot be recommended for approval before efficacy and safety have been proven by appropriately designed preclinical and clinical trials. More evidence-based data is required, particularly in the areas of pharmacokinetics, repeat applications, immunological reactions to the application of phages as well as the interactions and effects on bacterial biofilms and organ-specific environments. In this brief review we summarize advantages and disadvantages of phage therapy and discuss challenges to the establishment of phage therapy as approved treatment for multidrug-resistant bacteria.

Keywords: bacteriophage; phage therapy; multidrug-resistant bacteria; antimicrobial resistance

1. Introduction

Antimicrobial drug resistance (AMR) is a growing challenge worldwide. The emergence of new resistance mechanisms and their broad distribution through vertical and horizontal gene transfer is alarming. Consequently, multidrug-resistant (MDR) bacteria are spreading globally [1]. Due to the lack of a global tracking system, the full impact of infections with MDR bacteria is still unknown. A recent study estimated that approximately 33,000 people died in 2015 in the European Union as consequence of an infection with a resistant pathogen [2]. In the U.S. about 23,000 people die each year due to infections with resistant bacteria and far more people are infected [3]. Besides the medical aspect the socio-economic burden for health care systems is enormous [3]. Previously, the focus was mainly on gram-positive bacteria such as methicillin-resistant *Staphylococcus aureus* (MRSA) or vancomycin-resistant enterococci (VRE) but in recent years gram-negative bacteria resistant against 3 or 4 classes of antimicrobial drugs or even pan-resistant bacteria are rapidly gaining importance. In this respect, particularly noteworthy are *Pseudomonas aeruginosa* and *Acinetobacter baumannii* [4]. Many advanced therapies for cancer or autoimmune diseases, as well as transplantations are no longer effective when patients suffer from untreatable nosocomial infections [5]. Even commensal and opportunistic bacteria could then become problematic and jeopardize medical progress [6]. Moreover, novel antibiotics are rare as the pharmaceutical industry has minimized research and development programs in infectious diseases for different reasons [7]. Meanwhile, as AMR poses a major public health concern, this issue has been discussed at the highest political levels (from the United Nations and the WHO to local authorities). The "Leaders´ Declaration G7 Summit, 7–8 June 2015" (held in Elmau, Germany) stated: "We will foster the prudent use of antibiotics and will engage in stimulating basic research, research on epidemiology, infection prevention and control, and the development of new antibiotics, alternative therapies, vaccines and rapid point-of-care diagnostics" [8].

Already 100 years ago, a decade before the discovery of penicillin, bacteriophages (phages) were considered for clinical use [9]. However, driven by the easy use and broader antibacterial spectrum of antibiotics, phage therapy was seldom used during the last few decades, especially in Western Countries [10]. Only in some countries of the former Soviet Union, such as Georgia and Russia but also in Poland, have physicians continued to use phages and generated valuable practical experience [11]. The recent rediscovery and reintroduction of bacteriophage therapy in the Western World may possibly provide an attractive solution to the increasing failure of antibiotics. Since then, phages have been shown to be effective in treating bacterial infections in several experimental animal studies, as well as in case reports and clinical trials in humans [12]. In *Staphylococcus aureus* induced sepsis in mice for example, intraperitoneal (i.p.) application of phages 6 h after infection resulted in survival rates of 67%, whereas only 10% of control mice survived [13]. Systemic phage lysin application increased survival of mice with severe pneumonia due to *S. pneumoniae* from 0 to 100% [14]. Furthermore, it was also shown that inhaled application of the bacteriophage endolysin Cpl-1 is a safe and efficient therapy in severe pneumococcal pneumonia in mice [15]. So far, lysins seem to be more effective for treating gram-positive bacteria and are currently being tested in clinical trials [16]. Improvement of the enzymes' penetrative abilities through the outer membranes is necessary for their efficient use in gram-negative bacteria [6,17].

In *P. aeruginosa* lung infection, intranasal application of phages, given 24 h prior or 2 h after infection, protected all mice from lethal infection [18]. In diabetic and nondiabetic mice with severe bacteraemia due to i.p. injection of MDR *P. aeruginosa*, a single i.p. injection of phages 20 min after bacterial injection increased survival [19]. The authors reported a survival rate of 90% in diabetic and 100% in nondiabetic mice even when treatment started 4 h after bacterial challenge. Treatment started 6 h after infection resulted in lower survival rates among diabetic mice. Further delay of treatment (12 h) also reduced the effectiveness of phage therapy in nondiabetic mice [19]. This suggests, phage therapy is effective in both immunocompetent and -incompetent mice. In the UK a clinical trial (double-blind placebo-controlled, randomized phase I/II) for treatment of chronic otitis media investigated the effect of a phage-cocktail of 6 phages against MDR *P. aeruginosa.* The study demonstrated physical improvement of the patients and distinctly lower *P. aeruginosa* counts compared to the placebo treated group after a single aural application. Notably, no side effects were reported [20]. These studies along with others indicate phage therapy could be a promising prospect for the treatment of MDR infectious diseases [21]. In laboratory animals, phages can generally be administered via different routes for example, i.p., subcutaneous (s.c.), intramuscular (i.m.), intravenous (i.v.), oral, inhaled or topical [22,23], with the success of phage therapy depending on both the application route and the target organ. After parenteral application, phages are quickly distributed in the systemic circulation [23,24]. McVay et al. [24] investigated different application routes for phage therapy in mice subjected to burn injury and subsequently infected with *P. aeruginosa.* Mice were treated i.m., s.c., i.p. or left untreated. In the untreated group only 6% of mice survived, whereas 28% and 22% of animals survived after i.m. or s.c. phage treatment, respectively. Intraperitoneal application yielded the highest effectiveness, resulting in 88% survival [24]. Oral application was shown to be effective in treating gastrointestinal infections [25,26], whereas topical application was successfully used to treat wound infections [27]. Nebulization of phages for inhaled application to treat lung infections has also been studied [28,29]. Huff et al. [30] reported that chickens, infected with *E. coli* into the thoracic air sac after pre-treatment with aerosolized phages showed significantly reduced mortality compared to untreated birds. However, Carmody et al. [31] demonstrated that intranasal inhalation of phages was less effective when compared to systemic application in a mouse model of lung infection caused by *Burkholderia cenocepacia*. Conversely, Semler et al. [32] observed that inhaled phage therapy was superior to i.p. injection in eliminating *Burkholderia cenocepacia* in murine lung infection.

Phages used for any medical application must be carefully selected and fully characterized [6]. Phages showing poor adsorption, replication and distribution should be excluded and exclusively obligate lytic phages should be applied [33]. Temperate phages may lead to the transfer of genes to the bacterial host, increasing its virulence by lysogenic conversion or transduction mechanisms or transferring virulence factors or antibiotic resistance genes from prophage genomes to the host bacteria [34,35]. The causative bacterial pathogen must be identified prior to phage selection, requiring fast and reliable pathogen detection and susceptibility screening [35]. Alternatively, bacteriophage cocktails including phages against the most common and typical pathogens in specific organs (e.g., "respiratory bacteria") could be employed [6]. In any case, phage therapy specific infrastructure, such as local, rapidly accessible phage libraries need to be established [6,36].

Whereas studies on effective phage therapy have been reported and extensively reviewed, there are hardly any reports on phage therapy failures in recent years. Reports of failures mainly date back to the early use of phage therapy [37]. In 2001, Sulakvelidze et al. [38] published a detailed overview of phage therapy in Eastern European countries starting in the 1920s. The authors stated that failures occur mostly due to poor phage preparations, limited knowledge regarding phage mode of action and inconsistencies between phages and host strains. Additionally, most studies were lacking placebo controls leading to controversial results [38]. Miedzybrodzki et al. [39] published a summary of 153 patients treated with phage therapy to different infections between 2008 and 2010 at the Hirszfeld Institute of Immunology and Experimental Therapy in Wrocław. 39.9% of all patients showed a good response to phage therapy and in 18.3% pathogen eradication and/or recovery was reported [39]. Moreover, there is one clinical trial from Bangladesh using phage cocktails targeting *Escherichia coli* (*E. coli*) in children with bacterial diarrhoea reporting no advantage of phage therapy [40]. Two different phage cocktails were tested and orally applied [40]. Phage therapy did not cause any side effects but also did not improve the clinical outcome compared to the control group receiving standard oral rehydration. The authors reported several limitations of the trial, including probable insensitivity of pathogenic *E. coli* strains to the applied phages and the possibility of low stomach pH affecting phage transport, as no antacid was given to the patients [40].

In this review we summarize the advantages and disadvantages of phage usage in terms of medical application and discuss challenges to the establishment of phage therapy as an approved treatment for MDR bacteria.

2. Advantages and Disadvantages of Phage Therapy

2.1. Phage Therapy Provides Several Advantages Over Conventional Antimicrobial Drugs Regarding Medical Application, Some of Which Are Addressed in the Following

2.1.1. Host Specificity and Potential to Spare Microbial Flora

Lytic bacteriophages are viruses that target and infect their specific host bacteria, replicate inside and destroy them [9]. Therefore, unlike indiscriminate antibiotics, bacteriophages are expected to spare the physiologically resident flora, thus avoiding the development of bacterial niches that typically result from antibiotic therapy and enable the settlement of antibiotic-resistant bacteria [41]. Moreover, an intact microbiome contributes to innate immunity vigilance [10,42,43]. Consequently, local gut immune response to bacterial challenge is dampened by preceding antimicrobial therapy, increasing susceptibility to intestinal colonization and infection with pathogenic microorganisms, including MDR bacteria [41]. Furthermore, disruption of the gut microbiome results in an impaired systemic immune response upon bacterial stimulation and ultimately insufficient bacterial elimination [44,45]. Thus, antibiotics [44] but not phage therapy may possibly compromise immunity through microbiome disruption, paving the way for subsequent MDR and non-MDR infections. However, this conjecture needs to be addressed in upcoming studies. Similarly interaction of resident phages (phageome) with commensals as well as function and dynamics of the phageome have not yet been completely unravelled [46].

2.1.2. Bacterial Phage Resistance

Phage infection and lysis occur independently of mechanisms used by antibiotics to kill bacteria. Therefore, antibiotic resistance does not imply phage resistance [47]. Resistance to phages, however, occurs naturally and to varying degrees in all bacterial cultures and communities. Different mechanisms of resistance development have been described, including phage adsorption to bacterial cell receptors, phage particle assembly in the bacterial cell or cell lysis processes [48,49]. Notably, resources in the environment to isolate new phages are abundant [50]. Thus, isolation of new phages for almost all bacterial species can be achieved quickly for example, by sampling the environment and phage screening overnight (so called phagogram) [6] for subsequent GMP production. Consequently, development of pan-phage resistant bacteria is very unlikely [51]. Interestingly, it has been reported that some bacteria evolving phage resistance might over time regain sensitivity to antibiotics [52,53] or lose their virulence [54,55].

2.1.3. Self-Replication, Self-Limitation and Anti-Biofilm Properties

Since bacteriophages can only target and infect their specific host bacteria, the lysis process is self-limiting [47]. Phages replicate as long as their host is accessible. Consequently, to initialize or continue the lytic cycle, phages need host bacterial cell contact, which is significantly impaired in the case of bacteria forming biofilms, remaining intracellularly or being less abundant. Phages encoding for depolymerases are able to degrade matrix exopolysaccharides of biofilms [56,57]. Consequently, phages and other antimicrobialsmight reach, infect and lyse bacteria inside the biofilm more easily [56,57], which is of particular interest in case of implants (e.g., vascular or joint devices) and airway infections [58–60]. Bedi et al. [61], showed a beneficial effect on the eradication of a biofilm formed by *Klebsiella pneumoniae* when antibiotic and phage were combined. Another study demonstrated that phage OMKO1 was able to reduce bacterial densities in a *P. aeruginosa in vitro* biofilm assay [62]. Moreover, this phage alone or in combination with an antibiotic was more effective in reducing the biofilm than antibiotics alone [62]. Nevertheless, the effectiveness depends on the phage and the host bacteria. Darch et al. [63] examined the ability of two phages to inhibit bacterial dissemination in a model of aggregate formation by *P. aeruginosa*. The two phages were able to kill *P. aeruginosa* and inhibit aggregate formation when applied simultaneously with the bacteria [63]. However, when applied after aggregate formation was already established, the authors did not observe complete elimination of aggregates, most likely due to exopolysaccharide production. Still phage application could prevent formation of new aggregates by proliferating bacteria [63]. Full elimination of a complex mature biofilm with one single phage seems unlikely but phage cocktails and combined therapy with antibiotics could be a potential strategy [56,57,64].

2.2. Some of the Disadvantages of Phage Therapy Are Addressed by the Following Aspects

2.2.1. Activity against Intracellular Pathogens

Phages are unlikely to be able to actively enter eukaryotic cells. Therefore, phages are less effective against intracellular bacteria for example, *Mycobacterium tuberculosis*, as well as against intracellularly-surviving and persistent clones of extracellular bacteria, for example, *A. baumannii* [38].

2.2.2. Liberation of Endotoxins

Although it seems unlikely that therapy with purified phages leads to relevant toxic side effects, major concerns encompass the potentially massive liberation of bacterial endotoxins after bacterial lysis. Similar observations have been made with the use of certain antibiotics [65], as well as immune reactions to bacterial components including endotoxin present in crude phage lysates [66].

Confrontation with large amounts of bacterial endotoxins could lead to clinical deterioration of septic patients [67,68]. However, Dufour et al [69] reported for two different *E. coli* phages fewer released endotoxins in vitro compared to β-lactams, while the phage-evoked endotoxin level was comparable to that evoked by amikacin [69].

2.2.3. Potential Risk of Anaphylaxis

Phages are members of microbial communities and are present in the environment as well as on and in the human body [70,71]. Despite this, therapy with phages requires a higher titre compared to their naturally occurring numbers. Moreover, the use of high phage titres in patients bears the theoretical risk of inducing extreme immune responses like anaphylaxis [38]. Although theoretically possible, anaphylaxis due to phage therapy has never been reported and does not seem to be a major concern in phage therapy [11,47].

2.2.4. Immune Response to Phages

Being composed of proteins and nucleic acids, phages in general are considered as innately non-toxic [47,72]. However, there is evidence for non-specific immunomodulatory characteristics of phages [73], as well as activation of phagocytosis and anti-inflammatory properties [74]. Roach et al. demonstrated that presence of neutrophils is necessary for phage therapy success against *P. aeruginosa* [75]. Moreover, a recent in vivo study revealed that an increased number of phages in the gut (applied via drinking water to mice) can aggravate colitis in a TLR9 and IFN-gamma dependent manner and that phages inside the gut could stimulate non-specific and phage-specific immunity [76].

It is also possible that the human immune system may recognize phages as foreign antigens and produce phage-neutralizing antibodies depending on the application route [77]. In order to minimize the risk of side-effects due to impurities, it is necessary in at least parenteral application routes to use highly purified phage preparations [78]. For a widespread use of human phage therapy according to Western European medical standards, more scientific evidence is needed. In particular further investigation is warranted in the areas of immunological reactions following single or repeated phage application, pharmacokinetics and -dynamics and interaction with bacterial biofilms and commensal flora.

3. Challenges in Clinical Use of Phage Therapy

3.1. Current State of Phage Therapy

Experience with human phage therapy dates back more than 100 years in Georgia, Russia and Poland. However, Jault et al [79] stated that these countries have not developed "evidence-based medical standards" so far and "if there are any, they are only available in Russian" [79]. Especially at the ELIAVA Institute of Bacteriophage in Tbilisi, significant effort has been put into the characterization and development of phage products. Phage cocktails are routinely used for treatment, including prescribed medicine and self-medication (over the counter products) [80,81]. In Poland, phage research is predominantly carried out at the Hirszfeld Institute of Immunology and Experimental Therapy in Wrocław [82]. The institute focuses on preparation of specific phage lysates for individual patients subsequent to identification of causative pathogens from patient's samples. After Poland's accession to the EU, the Phage Therapy Unit, an outpatient clinic working according to EU regulations, was established. In this unit phages are applied under terms of experimental treatment in accordance with the Declaration of Helsinki and Polish regulations [83,84]. Despite years of practical experience, numerous case reports [39,85–87] and data from clinical studies including investigations of immune response [20,88–93], the lack of peer-reviewed controlled clinical trials still renders an evidence-based evaluation of phage therapy by Western standards difficult [84]. Marketing authorization of phage therapy in Western Europe depends on several conditions, including production of phage preparations according to good manufacturing practice (GMP) conditions, the issue of patentability and official approval by European Authorities [35]. In the following section, we will discuss regulatory, production and clinical trial challenges to the establishment of phage therapy as a regulatory approved therapy.

3.2. Regulatory Challenges

The European Medicines Agency (EMA) held a workshop in 2015 together with relevant stakeholders including academia, industry, policy makers and patient organizations to identify possibilities for the development of bacteriophage-based therapies against bacterial infections [94]. Approximately 60 experts discussed practical and regulatory issues related to phage licensing pathways as opposed to conventional medicine, for example, whether or not the EU Directive 2001/83/EC (relating to medicinal products for human use) might be applicable for phages [84,94,95]. As EMA has not licensed any phage products so far, it is not clear which pathway to approval is most promising. Moreover, modification or updating of existing phage cocktails with new phages, necessities with regard to developing phage resistances or changing pathogens, are not yet covered by existing regulations [84]. Hence, currently new time and cost intensive re-production and re-approval under GMP conditions would be required [84]. As phage biology (and bacterial co-evolution) implies the necessity for fast turnover of specific phages in clinical use, the process of development and approval needs to be shortened, which could be achieved by approval of production processes rather than specific phage products. Additionally, it must be clarified whether each phage of a cocktail or the complete cocktail is considered a medicinal product and needs regulatory approval.

3.3. Production Challenges

For a broad medical application, phages have to be produced in large scale by pharmaceutically licensed facilities. Consequently, there will be a commercial interest in the optimization of processes and the reduction of costs, which is indeed not trivial as non-linear dynamics of phages and host bacteria have to be considered [96]. In order to scale up phage manufacturing Krysiak-Baltyn et al. [96] proposed a computational model appropriate for modelling phage production, including varying infection parameters. This model might be suitable to cut costs or to improve productivity [96]. With the increasing interest in phage therapy, the issue of intellectual property (IP) protection comes to the fore [97]. To date the options for IP protection of naturally occurring phages are limited because there are abundant resources to isolate phages from the environment [36]. Therefore, other possibilities should be considered. For example, there are several options to implement IP protection in the manufacturing process, for example, every new phage, new preparation (consisting of approved single phages) or the production method, in order to increase attractiveness of the field to economic stakeholders [39,98,99].

3.4. Clincial Trial Challenges and Ongoing Projects

Recently, results of the first European randomized, controlled phase 1/2 trial aimed at evaluating the efficacy and tolerability of a topical applied phage cocktail (PP1131) against *P. aeruginosa* in burn wounds (PhagoBurn, www.phagoburn.eu) have been published [79]. The authors reported that patients treated with the phage cocktail showed slower decrease of bacterial burden in the burn wounds compared to patients receiving standard therapy (1% sulfadiazine silver emulsion cream). This finding must be interpreted with caution, as the study had several limitations: The patient cohort was relatively small (standard therapy n = 13, PP1131 n = 12) and inhomogeneous, as patients treated with phages were older, were burned to a lesser extent and showed higher bacterial burden at therapy start compared to those treated with standard therapy [79]. Importantly, there have been some stability issues of the phage cocktail used, as the authors reported a decrease in plaque forming units (pfu) during the study, which was associated with the application of a lower than intended dose of active phages. Future studies should address stability and shelf-life of each phage product including phage cocktails. The relatively large cocktail of 12 phages resulted in double the expected production time and thus reduced time to recruit patients [79]. Although the study terminated prematurely due to insufficient efficacy, it was the first trial using a cocktail of phages purified according to GMP standards and approved by national health regulators [79].

The German Phage4Cure (http://phage4cure.de/) consortium aims to address the safety, tolerability and efficacy of a purified inhaled bacteriophage cocktail against chronic airway infection with *P. aeruginosa* [100]. The goal of the four project partners (Fraunhofer Institute for Toxicology and Experimental Medicine, ITEM; the Leibniz Institute DSMZ-German Collection of Microorganisms and Cell Cultures GmbH; Charité–Universitätsmedizin Berlin; and Charité Research Organisation GmbH, CRO) is to pave the way for clinical applications of bacteriophages in Germany and Western Europe by applying GMP standards in the entire production chain of the phage product and by getting approval for phage therapy from regulatory authorities [100]. The project gained governmental financial support (funded by the German Federal Ministry of Education and Research) and regulatory authorities, namely BfArM (Federal Institute for Drugs and Medical Devices), are closely involved [100]. The Phage4Cure team is focusing on bacteriophages targeting *P. aeruginosa*, which is characterized by high abundance, rapid growth, distinct ability to form biofilms and a highly flexible genome, aspects that contribute its wide distribution and difficulties in combatting this bacterium [101]. *P. aeruginosa* is intrinsically resistant to several classes of antibiotics and there is increasing evidence of strains resistant to antibiotics of last resort [101]. Immunocompromised patients and patients with pre-injured lungs, particularly those with cystic fibrosis (CF) are frequently colonized by bacteria with 80% of CF patients older than 18 years harbouring *P. aeruginosa* [102]. CF is a genetic disorder caused by a mutation in the cystic fibrosis transmembrane conductance regulator (CFTR) gene that affects the lungs, as well as the pancreas, liver, kidneys and intestine [103]. Non-cystic fibrosis (non-CF) bronchiectasis represents a chronic and heterogeneous airway disease with diverse aetiology. Like patients with CF, non-CF bronchiectasis patients are highly susceptible to pulmonary infections. Most patients with bronchiectasis are colonized with antibiotic resistant bacteria (e.g., *Acinetobacter, Pseudomonas, Burkholderia*), with *P. aeruginosa* infections being associated with poor prognosis [104–108]. As patients with bacterial colonization but not infection are clinically relatively stable, effectiveness and tolerability of inhaled phage therapy may well be tested. Consequently, *P. aeruginosa* colonization in CF and non-CF bronchiectasis patients was chosen by the consortium Phage4Cure as therapeutic target to pave the way to a clinical trial with phages produced under GMP conditions and, ultimately, to regulatory approval. On the basis of their expertise, each partner will work on different aspects of the project, ranging from phage selection and characterization (DSMZ; as discussed by Korf et al. in this issue of the journal) to drug production and stability testing (ITEM). Following phage production and thorough preclinical evaluation (Charité and ITEM), clinical phase 1 and 2 trials are planned to be performed at Charité. If successful, the project may lead to first-time establishment of phages as approved inhaled therapy for CF and non-CF bronchiectasis patients in Germany and may possibly provide a GMP-compliant phage purification platform process as a blueprint for phage therapy development with respect to other indications [6,100]. Further projects related to the implementation of phage therapy in Western Europe include PhagoMed and PhagoFlow. The biotech company PhagoMed Biopharma GmbH (https://www.phagomed.com/), based in Vienna, focuses on the development of phage-based therapies for bacterial infections [109]. Supported by grants and private investments, PhagoMed evaluates, inter alia, the treatment of infected prostheses with phages. PhagoFlow aims at testing a magistral prescription of phages in patients with wounds infected by MDR bacteria and is being carried out at the military hospital Berlin, together with DSMZ and Fraunhofer ITEM [110]. Magistral preparation in the EU is defined as "any medicinal product prepared in a pharmacy in accordance with a medical prescription for an individual patient" (Article 3 of Directive 2001/83 and Article 6 quarter, § 3 of the Law of 25 March 1964) [111] and is therefore a practical way to produce treatments adjusted to the special needs of an individual without being dependent on commercial manufacturing [111]. In Belgium, the magistral preparation is already used for phages [111] and could provide a solution for individual patients but cannot cover the requirements of a larger patient cohort. GMP and GCP guidelines also apply for magistral applications. To promote a European solution to conquer the regulatory challenges of personalized and phage based medicinal products, the idea of a "biological master file", a concept already existing for chemical drugs but not for biologically active substances, was suggested by Fauconnier [112]. In summary, the main prerequisites for the establishment of a bacteriophage-based therapy are specific regulations for phage-based pharmaceuticals, increased clinical trial evidence and an infrastructure for efficient and rapid phage provision [6,36,113].

After decades of sleeping like Rip van Winkle, phage therapy is currently awakening in Western Europe due to the noise made by antimicrobial resistance, causing relevant research activity in the field. New valuable data addressing current concerns regarding clinical use of phages can be expected. However, whether phages will be approved by regulatory authorities and get market access is currently unpredictable.

Author Contributions: S.M.W., J.L. and M.W. wrote the manuscript. All authors have approved the submitted version.

Acknowledgments: The authors thank all partners involved in the Phage4Cure consortium for fruitful discussion and Alexander Taylor for proofreading the manuscript. We acknowledge the support of the German Research Foundation (DFG) and the Open Access Publication Fund of Charité–Universitätsmedizin Berlin.

References

1. Alanis, A.J. Resistance to antibiotics: Are we in the post-antibiotic era? *Arch. Med. Res.* **2005**, *36*, 697–705. [CrossRef] [PubMed]
2. Cassini, A.; Högberg, L.D.; Plachouras, D.; Quattrocchi, A.; Hoxha, A.; Simonsen, G.S.; Colomb-Cotinat, M.; Kretzschmar, M.E.; Devleesschauwer, B.; Cecchini, M.; et al. Attributable deaths and disability-adjusted life-years caused by infections with antibiotic-resistant bacteria in the EU and the European Economic Area in 2015: A population-level modelling analysis. *Lancet Infect. Dis.* **2019**, *19*, 56–66. [CrossRef]
3. Antibiotic/Antimicrobial Resistance (AR/AMR). Available online: https://www.cdc.gov/drugresistance/ (accessed on 14 February 2019).
4. Souli, M.; Galani, I.; Giamarellou, H. Emergence of extensively drug-resistant and pandrug-resistant Gram-negative bacilli in Europe. *Euro Surveill* **2008**, *13*, 19045. [PubMed]
5. Reardon, S. WHO Warns Against 'Post-Antibiotic' Era. 2014. Available online: https://www.nature.com/news/who-warns-against-post-antibiotic-era-1.15135 (accessed on 10 March 2019).
6. Rohde, C.; Wittmann, J.; Kutter, E. Bacteriophages: A Therapy Concept against Multi-Drug-Resistant Bacteria. *Surg. Infect. (Larchmt)* **2018**, *19*, 737–744. [CrossRef] [PubMed]
7. Norrby, S.R.; Nord, C.E.; Finch, R. Lack of development of new antimicrobial drugs: A potential serious threat to public health. *Lancet Infect. Dis.* **2005**, *5*, 115–119. [CrossRef]
8. Leaders' Declaration G7 Summit, 7–8 June 2015. Available online: https://www.bundesregierung.de/breg-de/service/datenschutzhinweis/g7-abschlusserklaerung-und-weitere-dokumente-387344 (accessed on 14 February 2019).
9. D'Herelle, F.; Smith. *G.H. The Bacteriophage and Its Behavior*; by F. d'Herelle Translated by George H. Smith; The Williams & Wilkins Company: Baltimore, MD, USA, 1926.
10. Duckworth, D.H.; Gulig, P.A. Bacteriophages: Potential treatment for bacterial infections. *BioDrugs* **2002**, *16*, 57–62. [CrossRef]
11. Kutateladze, M.; Adamia, R. Bacteriophages as potential new therapeutics to replace or supplement antibiotics. *Trends Biotechnol.* **2010**, *28*, 591–595. [CrossRef] [PubMed]
12. Kortright, K.E.; Chan, B.K.; Koff, J.L.; Turner, P.E. Phage Therapy: A Renewed Approach to Combat Antibiotic-Resistant Bacteria. *Cell Host Microbe* **2019**, *25*, 219–232. [CrossRef]
13. Takemura-Uchiyama, I.; Uchiyama, J.; Osanai, M.; Morimoto, N.; Asagiri, T.; Ujihara, T.; Daibata, M.; Sugiura, T.; Matsuzaki, S. Experimental phage therapy against lethal lung-derived septicemia caused by Staphylococcus aureus in mice. *Microbes Infect.* **2014**, *16*, 512–517. [CrossRef] [PubMed]
14. Witzenrath, M.; Schmeck, B.; Doehn, J.M.; Tschernig, T.; Zahlten, J.; Loeffler, J.M.; Zemlin, M.; Müller, H.; Gutbier, B.; Schütte, H.; et al. Systemic use of the endolysin Cpl-1 rescues mice with fatal pneumococcal pneumonia. *Crit. Care Med.* **2009**, *37*, 642–649. [CrossRef]
15. Doehn, J.M.; Fischer, K.; Reppe, K.; Gutbier, B.; Tschernig, T.; Hocke, A.C.; Fischetti, V.A.; Löffler, J.;

Suttorp, N.; Hippenstiel, S.; et al. Delivery of the endolysin Cpl-1 by inhalation rescues mice with fatal pneumococcal pneumonia. *J. Antimicrob. Chemother.* **2013**, *68*, 2111–2117. [CrossRef]

16. Fischetti, V.A. Development of Phage Lysins as Novel Therapeutics: A Historical Perspective. *Viruses* **2018**, *10*, 310. [CrossRef] [PubMed]
17. Gerstmans, H.; Rodríguez-Rubio, L.; Lavigne, R.; Briers, Y. From endolysins to Artilysin®s: Novel enzyme-based approaches to kill drug-resistant bacteria. *Biochem. Soc. Trans.* **2016**, *44*, 123–128. [CrossRef] [PubMed]
18. Debarbieux, L.; Leduc, D.; Maura, D.; Morello, E.; Criscuolo, A.; Grossi, O.; Balloy, V.; Touqui, L. Bacteriophages can treat and prevent Pseudomonas aeruginosa lung infections. *J. Infect. Dis.* **2010**, *201*, 1096–1104. [CrossRef] [PubMed]
19. Shivshetty, N.; Hosamani, R.; Ahmed, L.; Oli, A.K.; Sannauallah, S.; Sharanbassappa, S.; Patil, S.A.; Kelmani, C.R. Experimental protection of diabetic mice against Lethal P. aeruginosa infection by bacteriophage. *Biomed. Res. Int.* **2014**, *2014*, 793242. [CrossRef] [PubMed]
20. Wright, A.; Hawkins, C.H.; Anggård, E.E.; Harper, D.R. A controlled clinical trial of a therapeutic bacteriophage preparation in chronic otitis due to antibiotic-resistant Pseudomonas aeruginosa; a preliminary report of efficacy. *Clin. Otolaryngol.* **2009**, *34*, 349–357. [CrossRef]
21. Parracho, H.M.; Burrowes, B.H.; Enright, M.C.; McConville, M.L.; Harper, D.R. The role of regulated clinical trials in the development of bacteriophage therapeutics. *J. Mol. Genet. Med.* **2012**, *6*, 279–286. [CrossRef]
22. Ryan, E.M.; Gorman, S.P.; Donnelly, R.F.; Gilmore, B.F. Recent advances in bacteriophage therapy: How delivery routes, formulation, concentration and timing influence the success of phage therapy. *J. Pharm. Pharmacol.* **2011**, *63*, 1253–1264. [CrossRef]
23. Qadir, M.I.; Mobeen, T.; Masood, A. Phage therapy: Progress in pharmacokinetics. *Braz. J. Pharm. Sci.* **2018**, *54*, 66. [CrossRef]
24. McVay, C.S.; Velásquez, M.; Fralick, J.A. Phage therapy of Pseudomonas aeruginosa infection in a mouse burn wound model. *Antimicrob. Agents Chemother.* **2007**, *51*, 1934–1938. [CrossRef]
25. Zhao, J.; Liu, Y.; Xiao, C.; He, S.; Yao, H.; Bao, G. Efficacy of Phage Therapy in Controlling Rabbit Colibacillosis and Changes in Cecal Microbiota. *Front. Microbiol.* **2017**, *8*, 957. [CrossRef] [PubMed]
26. Wagenaar, J.A.; van Bergen, M.A.P.; Mueller, M.A.; Wassenaar, T.M.; Carlton, R.M. Phage therapy reduces Campylobacter jejuni colonization in broilers. *Vet. Microbiol.* **2005**, *109*, 275–283. [CrossRef] [PubMed]
27. Kumari, S.; Harjai, K.; Chhibber, S. Topical treatment of Klebsiella pneumoniae B5055 induced burn wound infection in mice using natural products. *J. Infect. Dev. Ctries.* **2010**, *4*, 367–377.
28. Golshahi, L.; Seed, K.D.; Dennis, J.J.; Finlay, W.H. Toward modern inhalational bacteriophage therapy: Nebulization of bacteriophages of Burkholderia cepacia complex. *J. Aerosol Med. Pulm. Drug Deliv.* **2008**, *21*, 351–360. [CrossRef]
29. Turgeon, N.; Toulouse, M.-J.; Martel, B.; Moineau, S.; Duchaine, C. Comparison of five bacteriophages as models for viral aerosol studies. *Appl. Environ. Microbiol.* **2014**, *80*, 4242–4250. [CrossRef] [PubMed]
30. Huff, W.E.; Huff, G.R.; Rath, N.C.; Balog, J.M.; Donoghue, A.M. Prevention of Escherichia coli infection in broiler chickens with a bacteriophage aerosol spray. *Poult. Sci.* **2002**, *81*, 1486–1491. [CrossRef] [PubMed]
31. Carmody, L.A.; Gill, J.J.; Summer, E.J.; Sajjan, U.S.; Gonzalez, C.F.; Young, R.F.; LiPuma, J.J. Efficacy of bacteriophage therapy in a model of Burkholderia cenocepacia pulmonary infection. *J. Infect. Dis.* **2010**, *201*, 264–271. [CrossRef]
32. Semler, D.D.; Goudie, A.D.; Finlay, W.H.; Dennis, J.J. Aerosol phage therapy efficacy in Burkholderia cepacia complex respiratory infections. *Antimicrob. Agents Chemother.* **2014**, *58*, 4005–4013. [CrossRef] [PubMed]
33. Abedon, S.T.; Thomas-Abedon, C. Phage therapy pharmacology. *Curr. Pharm. Biotechnol.* **2010**, *11*, 28–47. [CrossRef]
34. Nobrega, F.L.; Costa, A.R.; Kluskens, L.D.; Azeredo, J. Revisiting phage therapy: New applications for old resources. *Trends Microbiol.* **2015**, *23*, 185–191. [CrossRef]
35. Pelfrene, E.; Willebrand, E.; Cavaleiro Sanches, A.; Sebris, Z.; Cavaleri, M. Bacteriophage therapy: A regulatory perspective. *J. Antimicrob. Chemother.* **2016**, *71*, 2071–2074. [CrossRef] [PubMed]
36. Sybesma, W.; Rohde, C.; Bardy, P.; Pirnay, J.-P.; Cooper, I.; Caplin, J.; Chanishvili, N.; Coffey, A.; de Vos, D.; Scholz, A.H.; et al. Silk Route to the Acceptance and Re-Implementation of Bacteriophage Therapy-Part II. *Antibiotics* **2018**, *7*, 35. [CrossRef]
37. Smith, J. The bacteriophage in the treatment of typhoid fever. *BMJ* **1924**, *2*, 47–49. [CrossRef] [PubMed]

38. Sulakvelidze, A.; Alavidze, Z.; Morris, J.G. Bacteriophage therapy. *Antimicrob. Agents Chemother.* **2001**, *45*, 649–659. [CrossRef] [PubMed]
39. Międzybrodzki, R.; Borysowski, J.; Weber-Dąbrowska, B.; Fortuna, W.; Letkiewicz, S.; Szufnarowski, K.; Pawełczyk, Z.; Rogóż, P.; Kłak, M.; Wojtasik, E.; et al. Clinical aspects of phage therapy. *Adv. Virus Res.* **2012**, *83*, 73–121. [PubMed]
40. Sarker, S.A.; Sultana, S.; Reuteler, G.; Moine, D.; Descombes, P.; Charton, F.; Bourdin, G.; McCallin, S.; Ngom-Bru, C.; Neville, T.; et al. Oral Phage Therapy of Acute Bacterial Diarrhea With Two Coliphage Preparations: A Randomized Trial in Children from Bangladesh. *EBioMedicine* **2016**, *4*, 124–137. [CrossRef]
41. Buffie, C.G.; Pamer, E.G. Microbiota-mediated colonization resistance against intestinal pathogens. *Nat. Rev. Immunol.* **2013**, *13*, 790–801. [CrossRef]
42. Maynard, C.L.; Elson, C.O.; Hatton, R.D.; Weaver, C.T. Reciprocal interactions of the intestinal microbiota and immune system. *Nature* **2012**, *489*, 231–241. [CrossRef] [PubMed]
43. Marsland, B.J.; Gollwitzer, E.S. Host-microorganism interactions in lung diseases. *Nat. Rev. Immunol.* **2014**, *14*, 827–835. [CrossRef]
44. Robak, O.H.; Heimesaat, M.M.; Kruglov, A.A.; Prepens, S.; Ninnemann, J.; Gutbier, B.; Reppe, K.; Hochrein, H.; Suter, M.; Kirschning, C.J.; et al. Antibiotic treatment-induced secondary IgA deficiency enhances susceptibility to Pseudomonas aeruginosa pneumonia. *J. Clin. Investig.* **2018**, *128*, 3535–3545. [CrossRef] [PubMed]
45. Belkaid, Y.; Hand, T.W. Role of the microbiota in immunity and inflammation. *Cell* **2014**, *157*, 121–141. [CrossRef]
46. Shkoporov, A.N.; Hill, C. Bacteriophages of the Human Gut: The "Known Unknown" of the Microbiome. *Cell Host Microbe* **2019**, *25*, 195–209. [CrossRef] [PubMed]
47. Loc-Carrillo, C.; Abedon, S.T. Pros and cons of phage therapy. *Bacteriophage* **2011**, *1*, 111–114. [CrossRef]
48. Labrie, S.J.; Samson, J.E.; Moineau, S. Bacteriophage resistance mechanisms. *Nat. Rev. Microbiol.* **2010**, *8*, 317–327. [CrossRef] [PubMed]
49. Rostøl, J.T.; Marraffini, L. (Ph)ighting Phages: How Bacteria Resist Their Parasites. *Cell Host Microbe* **2019**, *25*, 184–194. [CrossRef]
50. Haq, I.U.; Chaudhry, W.N.; Akhtar, M.N.; Andleeb, S.; Qadri, I. Bacteriophages and their implications on future biotechnology: A review. *Virol. J.* **2012**, *9*, 9. [CrossRef] [PubMed]
51. Ormälä, A.-M.; Jalasvuori, M. Phage therapy: Should bacterial resistance to phages be a concern, even in the long run? *Bacteriophage* **2013**, *3*, e24219. [CrossRef] [PubMed]
52. Rohde, C.; Resch, G.; Pirnay, J.-P.; Blasdel, B.G.; Debarbieux, L.; Gelman, D.; Górski, A.; Hazan, R.; Huys, I.; Kakabadze, E.; et al. Expert Opinion on Three Phage Therapy Related Topics: Bacterial Phage Resistance, Phage Training and Prophages in Bacterial Production Strains. *Viruses* **2018**, *10*, 178. [CrossRef] [PubMed]
53. Chan, B.K.; Sistrom, M.; Wertz, J.E.; Kortright, K.E.; Narayan, D.; Turner, P.E. Phage selection restores antibiotic sensitivity in MDR Pseudomonas aeruginosa. *Sci. Rep.* **2016**, *6*, 26717. [CrossRef]
54. Smith, H.W.; Huggins, M.B.; Shaw, K.M. The control of experimental Escherichia coli diarrhoea in calves by means of bacteriophages. *J. Gen. Microbiol.* **1987**, *133*, 1111–1126. [CrossRef]
55. Holst Sørensen, M.C.; van Alphen, L.B.; Fodor, C.; Crowley, S.M.; Christensen, B.B.; Szymanski, C.M.; Brøndsted, L. Phase variable expression of capsular polysaccharide modifications allows Campylobacter jejuni to avoid bacteriophage infection in chickens. *Front. Cell. Infect. Microbiol.* **2012**, *2*, 11. [PubMed]
56. Abedon, S.T. Ecology of Anti-Biofilm Agents I: Antibiotics versus Bacteriophages. *Pharmaceuticals* **2015**, *8*, 525–558. [CrossRef]
57. Abedon, S.T. Bacteriophage exploitation of bacterial biofilms: Phage preference for less mature targets? *FEMS Microbiol. Lett.* **2016**, *363*, fnv246. [CrossRef]
58. Curtin, J.J.; Donlan, R.M. Using bacteriophages to reduce formation of catheter-associated biofilms by Staphylococcus epidermidis. *Antimicrob. Agents Chemother.* **2006**, *50*, 1268–1275. [CrossRef] [PubMed]
59. Kwiatek, M.; Parasion, S.; Rutyna, P.; Mizak, L.; Gryko, R.; Niemcewicz, M.; Olender, A.; Łobocka, M. Isolation of bacteriophages and their application to control Pseudomonas aeruginosa in planktonic and biofilm models. *Res. Microbiol.* **2017**, *168*, 194–207. [CrossRef]
60. Fong, S.A.; Drilling, A.; Morales, S.; Cornet, M.E.; Woodworth, B.A.; Fokkens, W.J.; Psaltis, A.J.; Vreugde, S.; Wormald, P.-J. Activity of Bacteriophages in Removing Biofilms of Pseudomonas aeruginosa Isolates from Chronic Rhinosinusitis Patients. *Front. Cell. Infect. Microbiol.* **2017**, *7*, 418. [CrossRef] [PubMed]

61. Bedi, M.S.; Verma, V.; Chhibber, S. Amoxicillin and specific bacteriophage can be used together for eradication of biofilm of Klebsiella pneumoniae B5055. *World J. Microbiol. Biotechnol.* **2009**, *25*, 1145–1151. [CrossRef]
62. Chan, B.K.; Turner, P.E.; Kim, S.; Mojibian, H.R.; Elefteriades, J.A.; Narayan, D. Phage treatment of an aortic graft infected with Pseudomonas aeruginosa. *Evol. Med. Public Health* **2018**, *2018*, 60–66. [CrossRef] [PubMed]
63. Darch, S.E.; Kragh, K.N.; Abbott, E.A.; Bjarnsholt, T.; Bull, J.J.; Whiteley, M. Phage Inhibit Pathogen Dissemination by Targeting Bacterial Migrants in a Chronic Infection Model. *mBio* **2017**, *8*, e00240-17. [CrossRef]
64. Chaudhry, W.N.; Concepción-Acevedo, J.; Park, T.; Andleeb, S.; Bull, J.J.; Levin, B.R. Synergy and Order Effects of Antibiotics and Phages in Killing Pseudomonas aeruginosa Biofilms. *PLoS ONE* **2017**, *12*, e0168615. [CrossRef]
65. Holzheimer, R.G. Antibiotic induced endotoxin release and clinical sepsis: A review. *J. Chemother.* **2001**, *13* (Suppl. 4), 159–172. [CrossRef] [PubMed]
66. Skurnik, M.; Pajunen, M.; Kiljunen, S. Biotechnological challenges of phage therapy. *Biotechnol. Lett.* **2007**, *29*, 995–1003. [CrossRef] [PubMed]
67. Mignon, F.; Piagnerelli, M.; van Nuffelen, M.; Vincent, J.L. Effect of empiric antibiotic treatment on plasma endotoxin activity in septic patients. *Infection* **2014**, *42*, 521–528. [CrossRef]
68. Peng, Z.-Y.; Wang, H.-Z.; Srisawat, N.; Wen, X.; Rimmelé, T.; Bishop, J.; Singbartl, K.; Murugan, R.; Kellum, J.A. Bactericidal antibiotics temporarily increase inflammation and worsen acute kidney injury in experimental sepsis. *Crit. Care Med.* **2012**, *40*, 538–543. [CrossRef] [PubMed]
69. Dufour, N.; Delattre, R.; Ricard, J.-D.; Debarbieux, L. The Lysis of Pathogenic Escherichia coli by Bacteriophages Releases Less Endotoxin Than by β-Lactams. *Clin. Infect. Dis.* **2017**, *64*, 1582–1588. [CrossRef] [PubMed]
70. Breitbart, M.; Haynes, M.; Kelley, S.; Angly, F.; Edwards, R.A.; Felts, B.; Mahaffy, J.M.; Mueller, J.; Nulton, J.; Rayhawk, S.; et al. Viral diversity and dynamics in an infant gut. *Res. Microbiol.* **2008**, *159*, 367–373. [CrossRef]
71. Manrique, P.; Bolduc, B.; Walk, S.T.; van der Oost, J.; de Vos, W.M.; Young, M.J. Healthy human gut phageome. *Proc. Natl. Acad. Sci. USA* **2016**, *113*, 10400–10405. [CrossRef] [PubMed]
72. Kutter, E.; de Vos, D.; Gvasalia, G.; Alavidze, Z.; Gogokhia, L.; Kuhl, S.; Abedon, S.T. Phage therapy in clinical practice: Treatment of human infections. *Curr. Pharm. Biotechnol.* **2010**, *11*, 69–86. [CrossRef]
73. Górski, A.; Międzybrodzki, R.; Borysowski, J.; Dąbrowska, K.; Wierzbicki, P.; Ohams, M.; Korczak-Kowalska, G.; Olszowska-Zaremba, N.; Łusiak-Szelachowska, M.; Kłak, M.; et al. Phage as a modulator of immune responses: Practical implications for phage therapy. *Adv. Virus Res.* **2012**, *83*, 41–71. [PubMed]
74. Górski, A.; Jończyk-Matysiak, E.; Łusiak-Szelachowska, M.; Międzybrodzki, R.; Weber-Dąbrowska, B.; Borysowski, J. The Potential of Phage Therapy in Sepsis. *Front. Immunol.* **2017**, *8*, 1783. [CrossRef]
75. Roach, D.R.; Leung, C.Y.; Henry, M.; Morello, E.; Singh, D.; Di Santo, J.P.; Weitz, J.S.; Debarbieux, L. Synergy between the Host Immune System and Bacteriophage Is Essential for Successful Phage Therapy against an Acute Respiratory Pathogen. *Cell Host Microbe* **2017**, *22*, 38–47.e4. [CrossRef] [PubMed]
76. Gogokhia, L.; Buhrke, K.; Bell, R.; Hoffman, B.; Brown, D.G.; Hanke-Gogokhia, C.; Ajami, N.J.; Wong, M.C.; Ghazaryan, A.; Valentine, J.F.; et al. Expansion of Bacteriophages Is Linked to Aggravated Intestinal Inflammation and Colitis. *Cell Host Microbe* **2019**, *25*, 285–299.e8. [CrossRef] [PubMed]
77. Łusiak-Szelachowska, M.; Zaczek, M.; Weber-Dąbrowska, B.; Międzybrodzki, R.; Kłak, M.; Fortuna, W.; Letkiewicz, S.; Rogóż, P.; Szufnarowski, K.; Jończyk-Matysiak, E.; et al. Phage neutralization by sera of patients receiving phage therapy. *Viral Immunol.* **2014**, *27*, 295–304. [CrossRef]
78. Chan, B.K.; Abedon, S.T.; Loc-Carrillo, C. Phage cocktails and the future of phage therapy. *Future Microbiol.* **2013**, *8*, 769–783. [CrossRef]
79. Jault, P.; Leclerc, T.; Jennes, S.; Pirnay, J.P.; Que, Y.-A.; Resch, G.; Rousseau, A.F.; Ravat, F.; Carsin, H.; Le Floch, R.; et al. Efficacy and tolerability of a cocktail of bacteriophages to treat burn wounds infected by Pseudomonas aeruginosa (PhagoBurn): A randomised, controlled, double-blind phase 1/2 trial. *Lancet Infect. Dis.* **2019**, *19*, 35–45. [CrossRef]

80. Kutateladze, M.; Adamia, R. Phage therapy experience at the Eliava Institute. *Med. Mal. Infect.* **2008**, *38*, 426–430. [CrossRef] [PubMed]
81. Kutateladze, M. Experience of the Eliava Institute in bacteriophage therapy. *Virol. Sin.* **2015**, *30*, 80–81. [CrossRef]
82. Weber-Dąbrowska, B.; Jończyk-Matysiak, E.; Żaczek, M.; Łobocka, M.; Łusiak-Szelachowska, M.; Górski, A. Bacteriophage Procurement for Therapeutic Purposes. *Front. Microbiol.* **2016**, *7*, 1177. [CrossRef] [PubMed]
83. Phage Therapy Unit of the Medical Centre of the Institute of Immunology and Experimental Therapy PAS. Available online: https://www.iitd.pan.wroc.pl/en/OTF/ (accessed on 14 February 2019).
84. Hill, C.; Mills, S.; Ross, R.P. Phages & antibiotic resistance: Are the most abundant entities on earth ready for a comeback? *Future Microbiol.* **2018**, *13*, 711–726. [PubMed]
85. Chanishvili, N. *A Literature Review of the Practical Application of Bacteriophage Research*; Nova Biomedical Books: New York, NY, USA, 2012.
86. Hoyle, N.; Zhvaniya, P.; Balarjishvili, N.; Bolkvadze, D.; Nadareishvili, L.; Nizharadze, D.; Wittmann, J.; Rohde, C.; Kutateladze, M. Phage therapy against Achromobacter xylosoxidans lung infection in a patient with cystic fibrosis: A case report. *Res. Microbiol.* **2018**, *169*, 540–542. [CrossRef] [PubMed]
87. Zhvania, P.; Hoyle, N.S.; Nadareishvili, L.; Nizharadze, D.; Kutateladze, M. Phage Therapy in a 16-Year-Old Boy with Netherton Syndrome. *Front. Med. (Lausanne)* **2017**, *4*, 94. [CrossRef] [PubMed]
88. Rhoads, D.D.; Wolcott, R.D.; Kuskowski, M.A.; Wolcott, B.M.; Ward, L.S.; Sulakvelidze, A. Bacteriophage therapy of venous leg ulcers in humans: Results of a phase I safety trial. *J. Wound Care* **2009**, *18*, 237–243. [CrossRef] [PubMed]
89. Weber-Dabrowska, B.; Mulczyk, M.; Górski, A. Bacteriophages as an efficient therapy for antibiotic-resistant septicemia in man. *Transplant. Proc.* **2003**, *35*, 1385–1386. [CrossRef]
90. Markoishvili, K.; Tsitlanadze, G.; Katsarava, R.; Morris, J.G.; Sulakvelidze, A. A novel sustained-release matrix based on biodegradable poly(ester amide)s and impregnated with bacteriophages and an antibiotic shows promise in management of infected venous stasis ulcers and other poorly healing wounds. *Int. J. Dermatol.* **2002**, *41*, 453–458. [CrossRef]
91. Łusiak-Szelachowska, M.; Żaczek, M.; Weber-Dąbrowska, B.; Międzybrodzki, R.; Letkiewicz, S.; Fortuna, W.; Rogóż, P.; Szufnarowski, K.; Jończyk-Matysiak, E.; Olchawa, E.; et al. Antiphage activity of sera during phage therapy in relation to its outcome. *Future Microbiol.* **2017**, *12*, 109–117. [CrossRef]
92. Borysowski, J.; Międzybrodzki, R.; Wierzbicki, P.; Kłosowska, D.; Korczak-Kowalska, G.; Weber-Dąbrowska, B.; Górski, A. A3R Phage and Staphylococcus aureus Lysate Do Not Induce Neutrophil Degranulation. *Viruses* **2017**, *9*, 36. [CrossRef] [PubMed]
93. Międzybrodzki, R.; Borysowski, J.; Kłak, M.; Jończyk-Matysiak, E.; Obmińska-Mrukowicz, B.; Suszko-Pawłowska, A.; Bubak, B.; Weber-Dąbrowska, B.; Górski, A. In Vivo Studies on the Influence of Bacteriophage Preparations on the Autoimmune Inflammatory Process. *Biomed. Res. Int.* **2017**, *2017*, 3612015.
94. European Medicines Agency (EMA). Workshop on the Therapeutic Use of Bacteriophages. 2015. Available online: https://www.ema.europa.eu/documents/other/workshop-therapeutic-use-bacteriophages-summary_en.pdf (accessed on 14 February 2019).
95. European Commission. Directive 2001/83/EC of the European Parliament and of the Council of 6 November 2001 on the Community Code Relating to Medicinal Products for Human Use (consolidated version: 16/11/2012). In EudraLex—The Rules Governing Medicinal Products in the European Union (Volume 1), Pharmaceutical Legislation: Medicinal Products For Human Use. Available online: https://ec.europa.eu/health/sites/health/files/files/eudralex/vol-1/dir_2001_83_consol_2012/dir_2001_83_cons_2012_en.pdf (accessed on 14 February 2019).
96. Krysiak-Baltyn, K.; Martin, G.J.O.; Gras, S.L. Computational Modelling of Large Scale Phage Production Using a Two-Stage Batch Process. *Pharmaceuticals* **2018**, *11*, 31. [CrossRef]
97. Henein, A. What are the limitations on the wider therapeutic use of phage? *Bacteriophage* **2013**, *3*, e24872. [CrossRef] [PubMed]
98. Verbeken, G.; Pirnay, J.-P.; de Vos, D.; Jennes, S.; Zizi, M.; Lavigne, R.; Casteels, M.; Huys, I. Optimizing the European regulatory framework for sustainable bacteriophage therapy in human medicine. *Arch. Immunol. Ther. Exp. (Warsz)* **2012** *60*, 161–172. [CrossRef] [PubMed]

99. Pirnay, J.-P.; de Vos, D.; Verbeken, G.; Merabishvili, M.; Chanishvili, N.; Vaneechoutte, M.; Zizi, M.; Laire, G.; Lavigne, R.; Huys, I.; et al. The phage therapy paradigm: Prêt-à-porter or sur-mesure? *Pharm. Res.* **2011**, *28*, 934–937. [CrossRef]
100. Bacteriophages Join the Fight Again Infection, Research Alliance Launched, Aimed at Establishing Bacteriophages as an Approved Drug. Press Release 09.11.2017. Available online: https://www.charite.de/service/pressemitteilung/artikel/detail/bakteriophagen_als_arzneimittel_im_kampf_gegen_infektionen/ (accessed on 14 February 2019).
101. Poole, K. Pseudomonas aeruginosa: Resistance to the max. *Front. Microbiol.* **2011**, *2*, 65. [CrossRef] [PubMed]
102. Pressler, T.; Bohmova, C.; Conway, S.; Dumcius, S.; Hjelte, L.; Høiby, N.; Kollberg, H.; Tümmler, B.; Vavrova, V. Chronic Pseudomonas aeruginosa infection definition: EuroCareCF Working Group report. *J. Cyst. Fibros.* **2011**, *10* (Suppl. 2), S75–S78. [CrossRef]
103. O'Sullivan, B.P.; Freedman, S.D. Cystic fibrosis. *Lancet* **2009**, *373*, 1891–1904. [CrossRef]
104. Tunney, M.M.; Einarsson, G.G.; Wei, L.; Drain, M.; Klem, E.R.; Cardwell, C.; Ennis, M.; Boucher, R.C.; Wolfgang, M.C.; Elborn, J.S. Lung microbiota and bacterial abundance in patients with bronchiectasis when clinically stable and during exacerbation. *Am. J. Respir. Crit. Care Med.* **2013**, *187*, 1118–1126. [CrossRef] [PubMed]
105. Rogers, G.B.; van der Gast, C.J.; Cuthbertson, L.; Thomson, S.K.; Bruce, K.D.; Martin, M.L.; Serisier, D.J. Clinical measures of disease in adult non-CF bronchiectasis correlate with airway microbiota composition. *Thorax* **2013**, *68*, 731–737. [CrossRef] [PubMed]
106. King, P.T.; Holdsworth, S.R.; Freezer, N.J.; Villanueva, E.; Holmes, P.W. Microbiologic follow-up study in adult bronchiectasis. *Respir. Med.* **2007**, *101*, 1633–1638. [CrossRef] [PubMed]
107. Angrill, J.; Agustí, C.; de Celis, R.; Rañó, A.; Gonzalez, J.; Solé, T.; Xaubet, A.; Rodriguez-Roisin, R.; Torres, A. Bacterial colonisation in patients with bronchiectasis: Microbiological pattern and risk factors. *Thorax* **2002**, *57*, 15–19. [CrossRef]
108. McDonnell, M.J.; Jary, H.R.; Perry, A.; MacFarlane, J.G.; Hester, K.L.M.; Small, T.; Molyneux, C.; Perry, J.D.; Walton, K.E.; de Soyza, A. Non cystic fibrosis bronchiectasis: A longitudinal retrospective observational cohort study of Pseudomonas persistence and resistance. *Respir. Med.* **2015**, *109*, 716–726. [CrossRef] [PubMed]
109. PhagoMed. Available online: http://www.phagomed.com/2018/08/28/viruses-against-bacteria/ (accessed on 14 February 2019).
110. Geförderte Projekte des Innovationsausschusses zur Förderbekanntmachung Versorgungsforschung vom 20.Oktober 2017, PhagoFlow (page 25). Available online: https://innovationsfonds.g-ba.de/downloads/media/112/Liste-gefoerderter-Projekte-VSF-FBK_20-10-2017.pdf (accessed on 14 February 2019).
111. Pirnay, J.-P.; Verbeken, G.; Ceyssens, P.-J.; Huys, I.; de Vos, D.; Ameloot, C.; Fauconnier, A. The Magistral Phage. *Viruses* **2018**, *10*, 64. [CrossRef]
112. Fauconnier, A. Regulating phage therapy: The biological master file concept could help to overcome regulatory challenge of personalized medicines. *EMBO Rep.* **2017**, *18*, 198–200. [CrossRef] [PubMed]
113. Debarbieux, L.; Pirnay, J.-P.; Verbeken, G.; de Vos, D.; Merabishvili, M.; Huys, I.; Patey, O.; Schoonjans, D.; Vaneechoutte, M.; Zizi, M.; et al. A bacteriophage journey at the European Medicines Agency. *FEMS Microbiol. Lett.* **2016**, *363*, fnv225. [CrossRef] [PubMed]

6

Production of Bacteriophages by Listeria Cells Entrapped in Organic Polymers

Brigitte Roy [1,2,3], Cécile Philippe [1,3], Martin J. Loessner [4], Jacques Goulet [2] and Sylvain Moineau [1,3,*]

1 Département de Biochimie, de Microbiologie et de Bio-Informatique, Faculté des Sciences et de Génie, Université Laval, Québec, QC G1V OA6, Canada; brigitte.roy.12@ulaval.ca (B.R.); cecile.philippe.1@ulaval.ca (C.P.)

2 Département des Sciences des Aliments, Faculté des Sciences de L'agriculture et de L'alimentation, Université Laval, Québec, QC G1V OA6, Canada; Jacques.Goulet@fsaa.ulaval.ca

3 Félix d'Hérelle Reference Center for Bacterial Viruses and GREB, Faculté de Médecine Dentaire, Université Laval, Québec, QC G1V OA6, Canada

4 ETH Zurich, Institute of Food, Nutrition and Health, Schmelzbergstrasse, 7CH-8092 Zürich, Switzerland; martin.loessner@ethz.ch

* Correspondence: Sylvain.Moineau@bcm.ulaval.ca

Abstract: Applications for bacteriophages as antimicrobial agents are increasing. The industrial use of these bacterial viruses requires the production of large amounts of suitable strictly lytic phages, particularly for food and agricultural applications. This work describes a new approach for phage production. Phages H387 (*Siphoviridae*) and A511 (*Myoviridae*) were propagated separately using *Listeria ivanovii* host cells immobilised in alginate beads. The same batch of alginate beads could be used for four successive and efficient phage productions. This technique enables the production of large volumes of high-titer phage lysates in continuous or semi-continuous (fed-batch) cultures.

Keywords: *Listeria ivanovii*; bacteriophages; alginate; production; disinfection; phagodisinfection

---

1. Introduction

Listeria monocytogenes is responsible for fatal cases of listeriosis in humans via contaminated food products [1]. This bacterial species is ubiquitous in nature and can contaminate the food processing line at any critical point. The increasing resistance of these pathogens to disinfectants under certain conditions requires the use of higher concentrations of chemical products [2]. Furthermore, bacteria exposed to disinfectants may be more likely to develop antibiotic resistance [3,4]. Despite strict regulatory policies, the occurrence of *L. monocytogenes* still has detrimental consequences for the food industry.

The search for alternatives to overcome these challenges has rekindled interest for bacterial viruses (bacteriophages) in agriculture [5], aquaculture [6], food safety [7], and even in infectious diseases [8,9]. The use of strictly lytic (i.e., virulent) phages infecting *Listeria* as biosanitisers represents an ecological alternative that could reduce the use of chemical compounds and lower the concentrations of toxic residues in the environment [10]. Specific biodisinfectants consisting of suspensions of phages can provide a natural means to control pathogens in processed foods and on contact surfaces. For example, the virulent phage A511 has a very broad host range against several strains of *Listeria* spp. [11–13] and could be included in the formulation of this type of biodisinfectants.

Phage biocontrol of *L. monocytogenes* strains was first introduced in 2006 with the commercial product ListShield, which contained a cocktail of phages applicable to various foods. Another product is Phageguard Listex P100, which also aimed to reduce *L. monocytogenes* in a range of food products [14–18]. Moreover, it has been demonstrated that different virulent phages can reduce the *L. monocytogenes* population after adhesion to stainless steel or polypropylene surfaces, and a synergistic effect has been observed by combining phages with quaternary ammonium [19–21].

However, even if virulent phages have shown great potential for killing pathogenic or opportunistic food-borne bacteria [22], their production on a large scale often remains challenging. Phage production still involves traditional methods using tubes or Erlenmeyer flasks, or it is done in bioreactors as a batch process [23]. High phage titers can be obtained [24,25], but batch processes require significant manpower and non-operational periods of time that may be limiting [26].

Attempts have been made to overcome the disadvantages of the batch process with continuous phage production. Studies involving chemostats [25,27] have been conducted, as well as two-stage continuous processes or cellstat [25,28–30], which consists of culturing bacteria, separately, in the first stage to feed to a second stage when phages are produced. Although chemostat allows the cultivation of microorganisms at a physiological steady state [31], the bacterial culture may be less genetically stable, as mutations can occur [32]. Cellstat is recognised as a phage production system for strictly lytic phages [33] that avoids direct phage exposure and pressure but requires the use of two different bioreactors [34].

With the aim of reducing production time and costs, we investigated here a different phage production procedure that employs host bacteria entrapped in a porous gel matrix. Alginate gel was selected for the matrix because of its low cost and widespread use in a range of applications in medicine, pharmacy, biotechnology, and the food industry [35,36]. An alginate matrix with entrapped bacterial cells can be produced in a single-step process and has virtually no impact on the viability of the cells. Alginate can also form a gel in the presence of divalent cations, such as calcium, which are also often necessary as co-factors for phage multiplication [37,38].

Entrapped cells will still grow because nutrients diffuse through the gel matrix [39], and while microcolonies spread deeper in the beads, the bacterial density has been shown to be higher near to or at the surface of the beads [40–42]. Such a growth pattern leads to bacterial cell release in the medium by micro-fracture events in the matrix. Only bacterial cells released from the gel become infected and contribute to the propagation of virulent phages. Those cells remaining in the gel have been shown to be protected from the phages, as the bacterial viruses do not migrate into the beads because of their size [43–45]. Protein diffusion through the matrix is highly reduced when molecular weight is above 150 kDa [46].

Relevant advantages of using entrapped cells to produce strictly lytic phages are that the phage lysate can be easily recovered and the alginate beads can be reused for successive phage propagations. Multiple phage lytic cycles can also be favoured, because this protective system prevents the rapid decline of the phage-sensitive host population. This process also provides an opportunity to produce phages in continuous or semi-continuous (fed-batch) cultures. Taken together, the use of calcium alginate immobilised cells (in spheres or fibers) to produce phages is a bi-phasic technique that controls the bacterial population and preserves the integrity of the cells, as long as they remain entrapped in the matrix.

2. Materials and Methods

2.1. Bacteria, Phages, and Media

Listeria ivanovii WSLC 3009 and the broad-host-range virulent myovirus A511 [47] were obtained from the Institut für Mikrobiologie, ZIEL Institute for Food and Health, Technische Universität München (Germany). The siphovirus H387 [48,49] was obtained from the Félix d'Hérelle Reference Center for Bacterial Viruses (www.phage.ulaval.ca) of the Université Laval (Québec, Canada). Bacterial strains were grown in Trypticase soy broth (TSB) or plated on Trypticase soy agar (TSA) at 30 °C. Phage titration was done using the double-layer plating technique [50] on TSA. Phage stocks ($>1 \times 10^8$ Plaque Forming Unit (PFU) mL^{-1}) were stored at 4 °C prior to use.

2.2. *Alginate Gels and Cell Immobilisation by Entrapment*

A 2–4% (*w*/*v*) aqueous solution of sodium alginate was prepared by suspending the polymer in distilled water. Solutions were sterilised by autoclaving (121 °C, 15 min). *L. ivanovii* cells were harvested by centrifugation (8000 rpm, 10 min) and resuspended in sterile TSB (3 mL). The cell suspensions were then mixed with sterile alginate [51]. Beads were formed by the dropwise addition of the alginate-cell mixtures into sterile $CaCl_2$ (200 mM) using a syringe and a 20 Gauge (G) needle. The cell-containing beads, 2 to 3 mm in diameter, were allowed to solidify for 1 to 2 h before $CaCl_2$ was replaced by fresh TSB containing 0.5 mM $CaCl_2$ to maintain the integrity of the alginate beads.

2.3. *Morphology of Cells Immobilised in Beads*

Alginate beads were observed by scanning electron microscopy (SEM) to visualise entrapped *Listeria* cells. The alginate beads were cut in half, and the specimens were fixed by immersion in glutaraldehyde (2.5% *v*/*v*) in 0.1 M sterile cacodylate buffer (pH 7.0) for 4 h. The samples were washed twice in 0.1 M sterile cacodylate for 20 min. Post-fixation was done in osmium tetroxide (2% *v*/*v*) in sterile cacodylate buffer for 30 min at 30 °C, and dehydration was completed using CO_2 in a critical point dryer (Model 3000 CPD, Bio-Rad, Mississauga, ON, Canada). The samples were mounted on stubs and covered with 15 nm of gold using a sputter coater (Emscope, Bio-Rad). A Nanolab LE 2100 (Vickers Instruments, Bausch and Lomb, Nepean, ON, Canada) scanning electron microscope operating at 15 hV was used to examine the bead surfaces.

2.4. *Phage Adsorption*

A set of alginate beads was made as described above but omitting the bacterial cells. Ten grams of pure alginate beads was transferred into TSB. Aliquots of phage suspensions (0.1 and 1 mL) were added and incubated at 30 °C for 12 h. The adsorption of phages on alginate beads was monitored by determining phage titers every 4 h. Two independent experiments were performed.

2.5. *Biomass Concentration*

To estimate the population of immobilised bacteria, 1 mL of alginate beads was dissolved in 9.0 mL of Na^+ citrate (50 mM), a sequestrant for Ca^{++}. The number of viable cells in the dissolved alginate gel was determined by direct plating on TSA for two independent experiments.

2.6. *Phage Production*

2.6.1. Free Cells

TSB (100 mL) was inoculated (5%) with an overnight culture of *L. ivanovii* 3009 from the Weihenstephan *Listeria* collection (WSLC) and grown to an optical density at 600 nm (OD_{600}) of 0.5–0.8. Phages were added at multiplicities of infection (MOIs) of 0.1 (1:10) and 1 (1:1), and the mixture was incubated for 16 h at 30 °C. Phage titers were measured every 4 h for two independent experiments.

2.6.2. Immobilised Cells Used for Single and Successive Phage Propagations

Beads containing entrapped microorganisms were transferred at least 2–4 times into prewarmed (30 °C) fresh TSB before phage production. Ten grams of beads containing *L. ivanovii* cells was added to 100 mL of TSB (OD_{600} of 0.5–0.8), and phage suspensions (at MOIs of 0.1 and 1) were added to the cultures. The flasks were incubated at 30 °C for 16 h, and phage titers were also determined as described above for two independent experiments. Between each successive production, the beads were stored overnight at 4 °C in sterile 2% (*w*/*v*) $CaCl_2$. The beads were then washed twice with sterile 2% $CaCl_2$ and reactivated as described above before each production.

2.7. Statistical Analysis

Mean and standard deviation values were calculated using Microsoft Excel (Microsoft, Redmond, WA, USA).

3. Results and Discussion

3.1. Morphological Observations

For the efficient use of alginate microbeads, morphological characteristics such as size and shape are important [52]. The produced alginate beads had proper sphericality and were typically 2 to 3 mm in size (Figure 1). Scanning electron micrographs of entrapped *Listeria* revealed no major changes in cell morphology (Figure 1). The mechanical constraints of the polymer did not seem to interfere with cell growth.

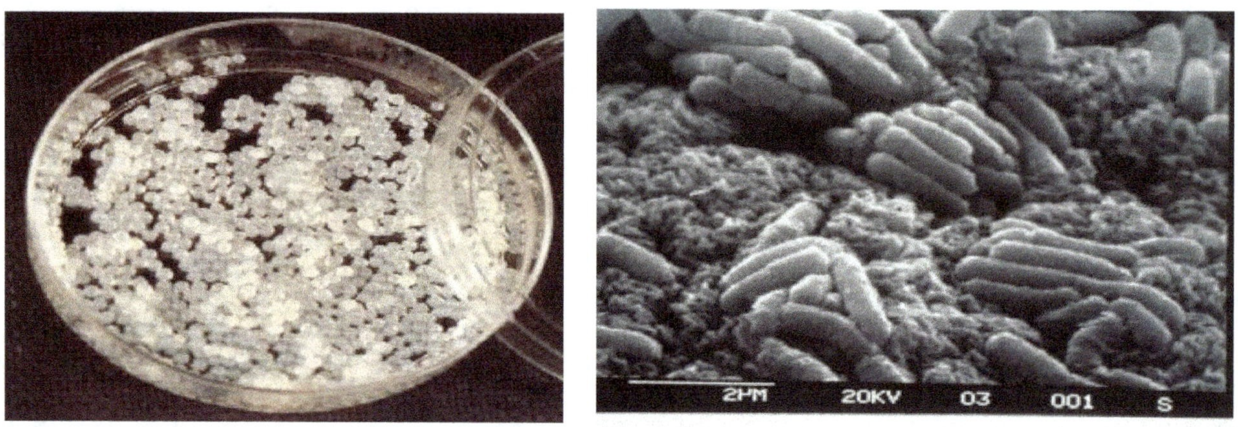

Figure 1. Observation of entrapped alginate bacteria. (**Left**) Visual appearance of alginate beads containing *Listeria ivanovii* WSLC 3009 (10^8 Colony Forming Unit (CFU) mL^{-1}) in a Petri dish. (**Right**) Scanning electron micrograph of *L. ivanovii* WSLC 3009 immobilised in alginate beads ($\times$10,000).

3.2. Phage Adsorption

Phage adsorption onto the gel matrix is a parameter that may impact the overall performance of the production system. The electrostatic adsorption of phages onto polymer beads could decrease the number and infectivity of phage particles in the medium. For this reason, the organic material selected for phage production should be tested for ionic attraction of viral particles. No decreases in the titers of phages A511 and H387 were observed in the medium after contact with the alginate beads. These results suggest that no major ionic interactions exist between the organic polymer and the phages.

3.3. Biomass Concentration

The concentration of entrapped cells in alginate beads has been studied for several types of bacteria [39,51,53,54]. Alginate is non-toxic to most living cells [55] and provides protection against external stresses such as temperature, pH, and toxic molecules. Figure 2 shows that three successive transfers (reactivations) of entrapped *L. ivanovii* cells in fresh TSB could raise the bacterial cell concentration inside the gel to almost 1×10^9 cells mL^{-1}, while five transfers increased the bacterial counts to almost 10^{10} cells mL^{-1}. Because the number of bacteria released into a medium is related to, among other parameters, the saturation level of the cells in the alginate structure, the yield of phage production will likely be influenced by the concentration of bacteria in the beads and at the bead surface.

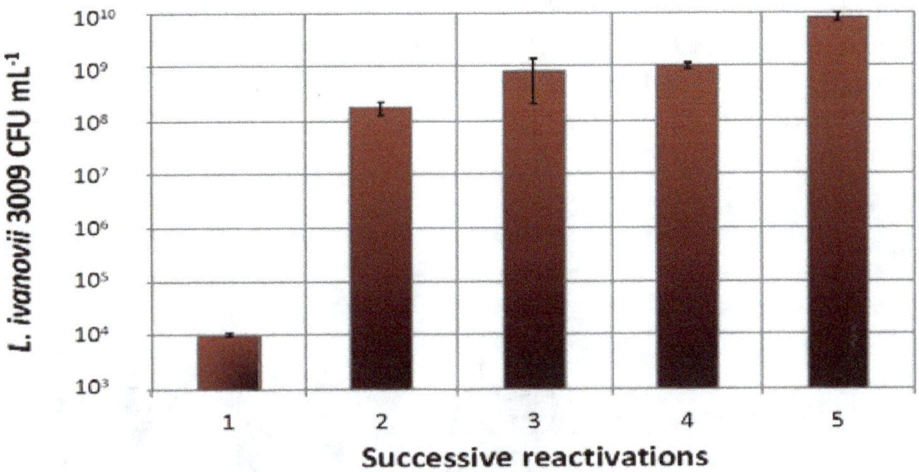

Figure 2. Transfers of *Listeria ivanovii* WSLC 3009 immobilised cells in fresh Trypticase soy broth (TSB) medium. Each reactivation was followed by an interval of 12 h. Bacterial concentrations were measured after 12 h of growth at 30 °C. Mean values were calculated from two independent experiments, and error bars correspond to standard deviations.

3.4. Phage Production

3.4.1. Free Cells

Phage productions in liquid medium were performed with both phages individually (Figure 3). All phage productions were characterized by a lag phase for the first 4 h, followed by a sharp increase in phage titers at 8 h. Maximal phage titers were close to 10^{10} PFU mL^{-1} of medium after 12 h. Very small variations in phage titers were observed at different MOIs. After 16 h, the titer of phage H387 decreased when using a 1:10 ratio. It is unclear at this time what caused this decrease in the phage titer, but it could have been due to phage adsorption to cell debris.

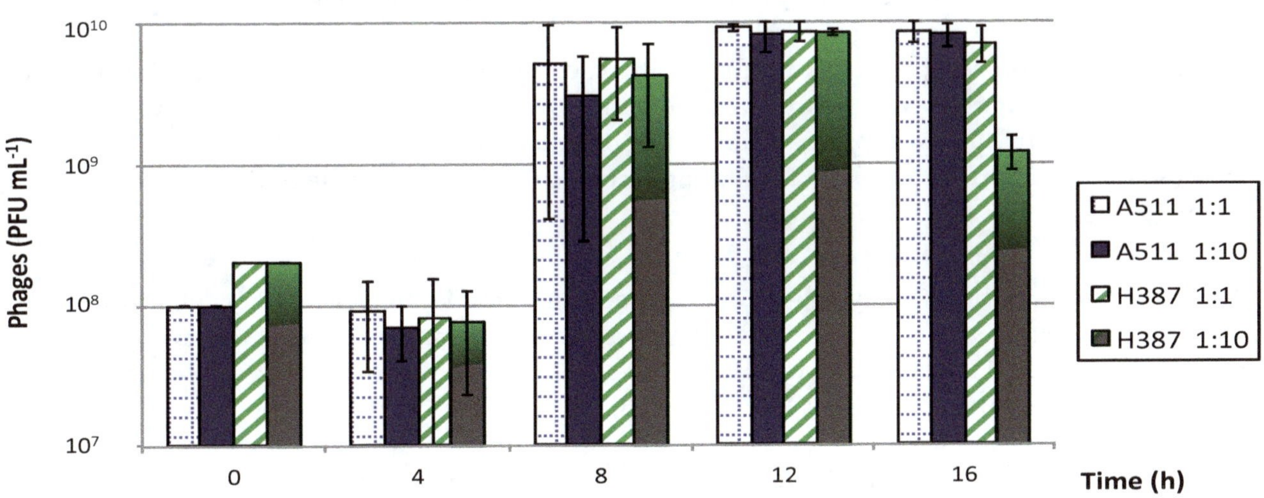

Figure 3. Production of phages A511 and H387 on *Listeria ivanovii* WSLC 3009 in liquid medium, using multiplicities of infection (MOIs) of 1 and 0.1. Phage counts were measured every 4 h. Mean values were calculated from two independent experiments, and error bars correspond to standard deviations.

3.4.2. Immobilised Cells Used for Single and Successive Phage Propagations

Microorganisms immobilised in polymers produce concentrated host bacteria that can be more easily and rapidly manipulated than free cells. Phage production using gel-entrapped host cells was compared to that of free cells in the same culture medium and under the same growing conditions. The highest production of virulent *Listeria* phages A511 and H387 was obtained after 12 h using a MOI of 1 (Figure 4). The maximum phage titers achieved using entrapped cells were slightly lower than for free cells. Some phage productions reached their maximum titer after 8 h of incubation, which was faster than for the free cells.

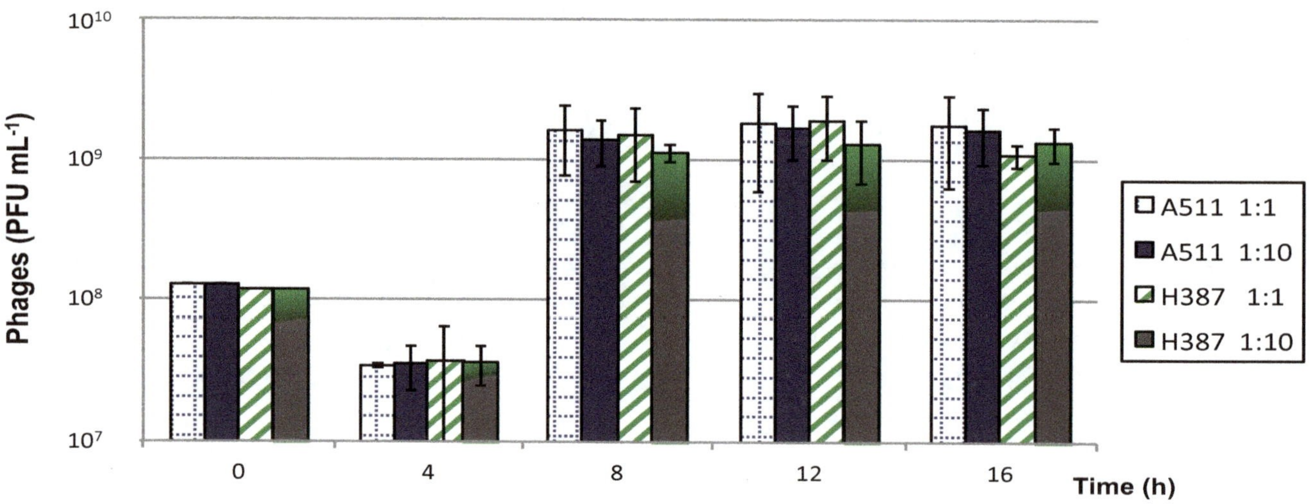

Figure 4. Production of phages A511 and H387 on *Listeria ivanovii* WSLC 3009 immobilised in alginate beads, using 1 and 0.1 multiplicities of infection (MOIs). Phage titers were measured every 4 h. Mean values were calculated from two independent experiments, and error bars correspond to standard deviations.

Two advantages of using gel-entrapped cells to produce virulent phages are that phage particles can be easily recovered by draining the culture medium (followed by centrifugation and filtration) and that phage propagation can be immediately resumed or pursued after a short or prolonged storage period. The same alginate beads with immobilised *L. ivanovii* cells were used for four successive phage productions. In all cases, phage titers were maintained at over 10^9 PFU mL^{-1} after the four productions (Figure 5). In general, the final phage titers of the virulent phage A511 were higher than for phage H387.

It has been shown previously that phages infecting some lactic acid bacteria cannot penetrate calcium alginate gels [43,44]. Because *Listeria* phages are the same size as dairy phages and even larger in the case of A511 [56,57], bacterial cells are well protected from phage infection as long as they remain entrapped in the gel. It is likely that this physical constraint, protecting the integrity of the bacterial population, allows the gel beads to be reused for successive phage production in new media. This advantage cannot be provided by free-cell amplification. Only small molecules can diffuse through the alginate matrix [43]. *L. ivanovii* cells entrapped in alginate beads are, therefore, protected against phages as well as against contamination by other bacteria. The production of phages after infection of the host bacteria likely only takes place on the beads' surface and in the medium after the cells have been released from the matrix. In fact, we noticed that the structure of the alginate gel was rather loose and easily broken up at the periphery of the beads, where cells usually most actively grow. These cells were likely released into the medium and infected by phages.

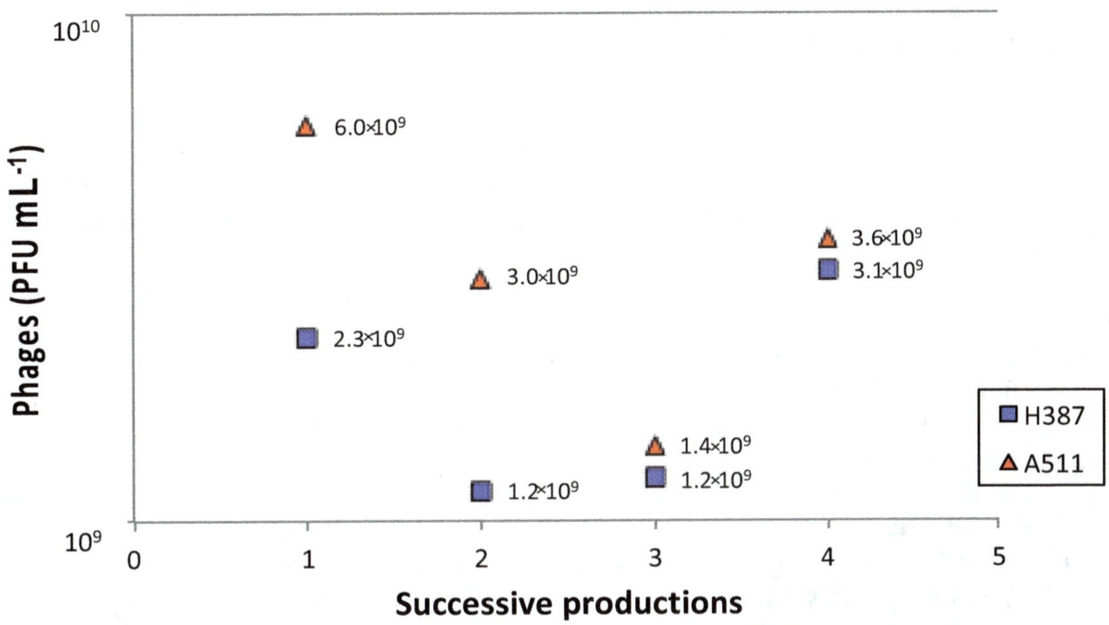

Figure 5. Successive productions of the two phages, A511 and H387, on *Listeria ivanovii* WSLC 3009 using a multiplicity of infection (MOI) of 1. Aliquots were withdrawn after 10 h of incubation. Mean values were calculated from two independent experiments.

While the process described here still requires optimisation, the gel entrapment of cells to produce specific phages offers the potential for the large-scale and rapid production of phages. Successive phage productions have shown that entrapped cells can be reused for at least four propagation cycles. Although the viral titer of lysate produced with entrapped cells was nearly 10-fold reduced compared to that of free-cell production, successive productions with the same beads should be globally seen as an interesting advantage. Continuous phage production using entrapped cells could be enhanced and applied to a large variety of phages.

Author Contributions: B.R. and J.G. conceived and designed the experiments; B.R. performed the experiments; B.R., M.J.L., J.G., and S.M. analysed the data; B.R., C.P., and S.M. wrote the paper.

Acknowledgments: We thank Alpha-Biotech Inc. and DAAD (Deutscher Akademischer Austauschdienst) for providing financial assistance for this study. We also thank Claude Champagne for discussion. S.M. holds the Canada Research Chair in Bacteriophages.

References

1. Radoshevich, L.; Cossart, P. *Listeria monocytogenes*: Towards a complete picture of its physiology and pathogenesis. *Nat. Rev. Microbiol.* **2018**, *16*, 32–46. [CrossRef] [PubMed]
2. Frank, F.J.; Koffe, A.R. Surface-adherent growth of *Listeria monocytogenes* is associated with increased resistance to surfactant sanitizers and heat. *J. Food Protect.* **1989**, *53*, 550–554. [CrossRef]
3. Directorate-General for Health and Consumers. *Assessment of the Antibiotic Resistance Effects of Biocides, 28th Plenary*; Commission Européenne, Scientific Committee on Emerging and Newly Identified Health Risks: Bruxelles, Belgium, 2009.
4. Pearce, H.; Messager, S.; Maillard, J.-Y. Effect of biocides commonly used in the hospital environment on the transfer of antibiotic-resistance genes in *Staphylococcus aureus*. *J. Hosp. Infect.* **1999**, *43*, 101–108. [CrossRef] [PubMed]
5. Buttimer, C.; McAuliffe, O.; Ross, R.P.; Hill, C.; O'Mahony, J.; Coffey, A. Bacteriophages and bacterial plant diseases. *Front. Microbiol.* **2017**, *8*, 34. [CrossRef] [PubMed]

6. Stalin, N.; Srinivasan, P. Efficacy of potential phage cocktails against *Vibrio harveyi* and closely related *Vibrio* species isolated from shrimp aquaculture environment in the south east coast of India. *Vet. Microbiol.* **2017**, *207*, 83–96. [CrossRef] [PubMed]
7. Bai, J.; Kim, Y.-T.; Ryu, S.; Lee, J.-H. Biocontrol and rapid detection of food-borne pathogens using bacteriophages and endolysins. *Front. Microbiol.* **2016**, *7*, 474. [CrossRef] [PubMed]
8. Abedon, S.T. Phage therapy of pulmonary infections. *Bacteriophage* **2015**, *5*, e1020260. [CrossRef] [PubMed]
9. Hagens, S.; Loessner, M.J. Phages of *Listeria* offer novel tools for diagnostics and biocontrol. *Front. Microbiol.* **2014**, *5*, 159. [CrossRef] [PubMed]
10. Lin, D.M.; Koskella, B.; Lin, H.C. Phage therapy: An alternative to antibiotics in the age of multi-drug resistance. *World J. Gastrointest. Pharmacol. Ther.* **2017**, *8*, 162–173. [CrossRef] [PubMed]
11. Loessner, M.J.; Busse, M. Bacteriophage typing of *Listeria* species. *Appl. Environ. Microbiol.* **1990**, *56*, 1912–1918. [PubMed]
12. Guenther, S.; Huwyler, D.; Richard, S.; Loessner, M.J. Virulent bacteriophages for biocontrol of *Listeria monocytogenes* in ready-to-eat foods. *Appl. Environ. Microbiol.* **2009**, *75*, 93–100. [CrossRef] [PubMed]
13. Klumpp, J.; Dorscht, J.; Lurz, R.; Bielmann, R.; Wieland, M.; Zimmer, M.; Calendar, R.; Loessner, M.J. The terminally redundant, non-permuted genome of *Listeria* bacteriophage A511: A model for the SPO1-like myoviruses of Gram-positive bacteria. *J. Bacteriol.* **2008**, *190*, 5753–5765. [CrossRef] [PubMed]
14. Silva, E.N.G.; Figueiredo, A.C.L.; Miranda, F.A.; de Castro Almeida, R.C. Control of *Listeria monocytogenes* growth in soft cheeses by bacteriophage P100. *Braz. J. Microbiol.* **2014**, *45*, 11–16. [CrossRef] [PubMed]
15. Chaitiemwong, N.; Hazeleger, W.C.; Beumer, R.R. Inactivation of *Listeria monocytogenes* by disinfectants and bacteriophages in suspension and stainless-steel carrier tests. *J. Food Protect.* **2014**, *77*, 2012–2020. [CrossRef] [PubMed]
16. Chibeu, A.; Agius, L.; Gao, A.; Sabour, P.M.; Kropinski, A.M.; Balamurugan, S. Efficacy of bacteriophage LISTEX™P100 combined with chemical antimicrobials in reducing *Listeria monocytogenes* in cooked turkey and roast beef. *Int. J. Food Microbiol.* **2013**, *167*, 208–214. [CrossRef] [PubMed]
17. Miguéis, S.; Saraiva, C.; Esteves, A. Efficacy of LISTEX P100 at different concentrations for reduction of *Listeria monocytogenes* inoculated in sashimi. *J. Food Protect.* **2017**, *12*, 2094–2098. [CrossRef] [PubMed]
18. Greer, G.G. Homologous bacteriophage control of *Pseudomonas* growth on beef spoilage. *J. Food Protect.* **1986**, *49*, 104–109. [CrossRef]
19. Ganegama Arachchi, G.J.; Cridge, A.G.; Dias-Wanigasekera, B.M.; Cruz, C.D.; McIntyre, L.; Liu, R.; Flint, S.H.; Mutukumira, A.N. Effectiveness of phages in the decontamination of *Listeria monocytogenes* adhered to clean stainless steel, stainless steel coated with fish protein, and as a biofilm. *J. Ind. Microbiol. Biotechnol.* **2013**, *10*, 1105–1116. [CrossRef] [PubMed]
20. Gray, J.A.; Chandry, P.S.; Kaur, M.; Kocharunchitt, C.; Bowman, J.P.; Fox, E.M. Novel biocontrol methods for *Listeria monocytogenes* biofilms in food production facilities. *Front. Microbiol.* **2018**, *9*, 605. [CrossRef] [PubMed]
21. Roy, B.; Ackermann, H.-W.; Pandian, S.; Picard, G.; Goulet, J. Biological inactivation of adhering *Listeria monocytogenes* by listeriaphages and a quaternary ammonium compound. *Appl. Environ. Microbiol.* **1993**, *59*, 2914–2917. [PubMed]
22. Lee, S.; Kim, M.G.; Lee, H.S.; Heo, S.; Kwon, M.; Kim, G. Isolation and characterization of *Listeria* phages for control of growth of *Listeria monocytogenes* in milk. *Korean J. Food Sci. Anim. Resour.* **2017**, *37*, 320–328. [CrossRef] [PubMed]
23. Agboluaje, M.; Sauvageau, D. Bacteriophage production in bioreactors. *Methods Mol. Biol.* **2018**, *1692*, 173–193.
24. Sargeant, K.; Yeo, K.G.; Lethbridge, J.H.; Shooter, K.V. Production of bacteriophage T7. *Appl. Microbiol.* **1968**, *16*, 1483–1488. [PubMed]
25. Chen, B.Y.; Lim, H.C. Bioreactor studies on temperature induction of the Qmutant of bacteriophage λ in *Escherichia coli*. *J. Biotechnol.* **1996**, *51*, 1–20. [CrossRef]
26. Sauvageau, D.; Cooper, D.G. Two-stage, self-cycling process for the production of bacteriophages. *Microb. Cell Fact.* **2010**, *9*, 81. [CrossRef] [PubMed]
27. Los, M.; Wegrzyn, G.; Neubauer, P. A role for bacteriophage T4 rI gene function in the control of phage development during pseudolysogeny and in slow growing host cells. *Res. Microbiol.* **2003**, *154*, 547–552. [CrossRef]

28. Park, S.H.; Park, T.H. Analysis of two-stage continuous operation of *Escherichia coli* containing bacteriophage λ vector. *Bioprocess Eng.* **2000**, *23*, 187–190. [CrossRef]
29. Chen, X.A.; Cen, P.L. A novel three-stage process for continuous production of penicillin G acylase by a temperature-sensitive expression system of *Bacillus subtilis* phage phi105. *Chem. Biochem. Q.* **2005**, *19*, 367–372.
30. Oh, J.S.; Cho, D.; Park, T.H. Two-stage continuous operation of recombinant *Escherichia coli* using the bacteriophage λ Q-vector. *Bioprocess Biosyst. Eng.* **2005**, *28*, 1–7. [CrossRef] [PubMed]
31. Ziv, N.; Brandt, N.J.; Gresham, D. The use of chemostats in microbial systems biology. *J. Vis. Exp.* **2013**, *80*, 50168. [CrossRef] [PubMed]
32. Chao, L.; Levin, B.R.; Stewart, F.M. A complex community in a simple habitat: An experimental study with bacteria and phage. *Ecology* **1977**, *58*, 369–378. [CrossRef]
33. Schwienhorst, A.; Lindemann, B.F.; Eigen, M. Growth kinetics of a bacteriophage in continuous culture. *Biotechnol. Bioeng.* **1996**, *50*, 217–221. [CrossRef]
34. Nabergoj, D.; Kuzmić, N.; Drakslar, B.; Podgornik, A. Effect of dilution rate on productivity of continuous bacteriophage production in cellstat. *Appl. Microbiol. Biotechnol.* **2018**, *102*, 3649–3661. [CrossRef] [PubMed]
35. Diviès, C.; Prévost, H.; Cavin, J.F. Les bactéries immobilisées dans l'industrie laitière. *Process. Mag.* **1989**, *1041*, 28–33.
36. Gacesa, P. Alginates. *Carbohydr. Polym.* **1988**, *53*, 161–182. [CrossRef]
37. Ackermann, H.-W.; Dubow, M.S. Phage multiplication. In *Viruses of Prokaryotes*; CRC Press, Inc.: Boca Raton, FL, USA, 1987; Volume 1, pp. 49–85.
38. Mahony, J.; Tremblay, D.M.; Labrie, S.J.; Moineau, S.; van Sinderen, D. Investigating the requirement for calcium during lactococcal phage infection. *Int. J. Food Microbiol.* **2015**, *201*, 47–51. [CrossRef] [PubMed]
39. Gosmann, B.; Rehm, H.J. Influence of growth behaviour and physiology of alginate-entrapped microorganisms on the oxygen consumption. *Appl. Microbiol. Biotechnol.* **1988**, *29*, 554–559. [CrossRef]
40. Cachon, R.; Catté, M.; Nommé, R.; Prévost, H.; Diviès, C. Kinetic behaviour of *Lactococcus lactis* ssp. *lactis* bv. *diacetylactis* immobilized in calcium alginate gel beads. *Process Biochem.* **1995**, *6*, 503–510.
41. Prévost, H.; Diviès, C.; Rousseau, E. Continuous yoghurt production with *Lactobacillus bulgaricus* and *Streptococcus thermophilus* entrapped in Ca-alginate. *Biotechnol. Lett.* **1985**, *4*, 247–252. [CrossRef]
42. Audet, P.; Paquin, C.; Lacroix, C. Immobilized growing lactic acid bacteria with κ-carrageenan—Locust bean gum gel. *Appl. Microbiol. Biotechnol.* **1988**, *1*, 11–18. [CrossRef]
43. Steenson, L.R.; Klaenhammer, T.R.; Swaisgood, H.E. Calcium alginate-immobilized cultures of lactic streptococci are protected from bacteriophages. *J. Dairy Sci.* **1987**, *70*, 1121–1127. [CrossRef]
44. Champagne, C.P.; Morin, N.; Couture, R.; Gagnon, C.; Jelen, P.; Lacroix, C. The potential of immobilized cell technology to produce freeze-dried, phage-protected cultures of *Lactococcus lactis*. *Food Res. Intern.* **1992**, *25*, 419–427. [CrossRef]
45. Champagne, C.P.; Moineau, S.; Lafleur, S.; Savard, T. The effect of bacteriophages on the acidification of a vegetable juice medium by microencapsulated *Lactobacillus plantarum*. *Food Microbiol.* **2017**, *63*, 28–34. [CrossRef] [PubMed]
46. Tanaka, H.; Matsumura, M.; Veliky, I.A. Diffusion characteristics of substrates in Ca alginate gel beads. *Biotechnol. Bioeng.* **1984**, *1*, 53–58. [CrossRef] [PubMed]
47. Zink, R.; Loessner, M.J. Classification of virulent and temperate bacteriophages of *Listeria* spp. on the basis of morphology and protein analysis. *Appl. Environ. Microbiol.* **1992**, *58*, 296–302. [PubMed]
48. Ackermann, H.-W.; Dubow, M.S. Description and identification of new phages. In *Viruses of Prokaryotes*; CRC Press, Inc.: Boca Raton, FL, USA, 1987; Volume 1, pp. 103–142.
49. Ortel, S.; Ackermann, H.-A. Morphologie von Neuen Listeriaphagen. *Zentralbl. Bakteriol. Mikrobiol. Hyg. Ser. A Med. Microbiol. Infect. Dis. Virol. Parasitol.* **1985**, *260*, 423–427.
50. Adams, M.H. Methods of study of bacterial viruses. In *Bacteriophages*; Interscience Publishers, Inc.: New York, NY, USA, 1959; pp. 443–457.
51. Boyaval, P.; Lebrun, A.; Goulet, J. Étude de l'immobilisation de *Lactobacillus helveticus* dans des billes d'alginate de calcium. *Le Lait* **1985**, *65*, 185–199. [CrossRef]
52. Börner, R.A.; Aliaga, M.T.A.; Mattiasson, B. Microcultivation of anaerobic bacteria single cells entrapped in alginate microbeads. *Biotechnol. Lett.* **2013**, *35*, 397–405. [CrossRef] [PubMed]

53. Kurosawa, H.; Matsumura, M.; Tanaka, H. Oxygen diffusivity in gel beads containing viable cells. *Biotechnol. Bioeng.* **1989**, *34*, 926–932. [CrossRef] [PubMed]
54. Chen, K.-C.; Huang, C.-T. Effects of the growth of *Trichosporon cutaneum* in calcium alginate gel beads upon bead structure and oxygen transfer characteristics. *Enzym. Microb. Technol.* **1988**, *10*, 284–292. [CrossRef]
55. Ogbonna, J.C.; Amano, Y.; Nakamura, K. Elucidation of optimum conditions for immobilization of viable cells by using calcium alginate. *J. Ferment. Bioeng.* **1989**, *67*, 92–96. [CrossRef]
56. Klumpp, J.; Loessner, M.J. *Listeria* phages: Genomes, evolution, and application. *Bacteriophage* **2013**, *3*, e26861. [CrossRef] [PubMed]
57. Ackermann, H.-W. Bacteriophage taxonomy. *Microbiol. Aust.* **2011**, *32*, 90–94.

7

Protection of Phage Applications in Crop Production: A Patent Landscape

Dominique Holtappels [1], Rob Lavigne [1], Isabelle Huys [2,*] and Jeroen Wagemans [1,*]

1 Laboratory of Gene Technology, KU Leuven, 3001 Heverlee, Belgium; dominique.holtappels@kuleuven.be (D.H.); rob.lavigne@kuleuven.be (R.L.)
2 Clinical Pharmacology and Pharmacotherapy, KU Leuven, 3000 Leuven, Belgium
* Correspondence: Isabelle.huys@kuleuven.be (I.H.); Jeroen.wagemans@kuleuven.be (J.W.)

Abstract: In agriculture, the prevention and treatment of bacterial infections represents an increasing challenge. Traditional (chemical) methods have been restricted to ensure public health and to limit the occurrence of resistant strains. Bacteriophages could be a sustainable alternative. A major hurdle towards the commercial implementation of phage-based biocontrol strategies concerns aspects of regulation and intellectual property protection. Within this study, two datasets have been composed to analyze both scientific publications and patent documents and to get an idea on the focus of research and development (R&D) by means of an abstract and claim analysis. A total of 137 papers and 49 patent families were found from searching public databases, with their numbers increasing over time. Within this dataset, the majority of the patent documents were filed by non-profit organizations in Asia. There seems to be a good correlation between the papers and patent documents in terms of targeted bacterial genera. Furthermore, granted patents seem to claim rather broad and cover methods of treatment. This review shows that there is indeed growing publishing and patenting activity concerning phage biocontrol. Targeted research is needed to further stimulate the exploration of phages within integrated pest management strategies and to deal with bacterial infections in crop production.

Keywords: phage biocontrol; patent landscape; crop production

---

1. Introduction

Soon after the discovery of bacteriophages by d'Herelle and Twort at the beginning of the 20th century [1,2], the potential to use these bacterial viruses as a therapeutic was recognized. Although the first applications of phages focused on human medicine [3], other fields including agriculture soon began to explore the potential of bacteriophages as biocontrol agents [4]. The first isolation of phages infecting plant pathogenic bacteria (PPB) dates back to 1924, when it was shown that *Xanthomonas campestris* pv. *campestris*, causing black rot in *Brassicaceae*, could be lysed by the filtrate of diseased cabbages [4,5]. In the following years, interest in phages as biocontrol agents remained relatively high [4]. However, the discovery of broad-spectrum antibiotics and other bactericidal chemicals resulted in a dwindling interest in phage therapy research in general [6].

Within the agricultural sector, the prevention and treatment of bacterial infections represents an increasing challenge. For farmers, devastating losses by bacterial pathogens are generally estimated to reach 10% of the total production [7] and for some bacterial species like *Xanthomonas campestris* pv. *campestris*, crop yield can be reduced by 25% [8]. Other major threats include *Ralstonia solanacearum*, *Xylella fastidiosa*, and *Pseudomonas syringae* pathovars [9]. In recent years, general antibiotics like streptomycin, as well as copper-based chemicals, have been restricted in crop production to ensure public health and to limit the occurrence of resistant strains [10–13]. Because of these restrictions, the search for sustainable, natural biocontrol of PPBs has reached a critical stage, especially considering the increased food production needs [14]. Governments have decided to implement integrated pest management strategies (IPMs) as the standard for crop protection (e.g., the European Parliament and the Council of the European Union (2009) Directive 2009/128/EC of the European Parliament and of the Council of 21 October 2009) [15]. These strategies are based on the implementation of sustainable pest control strategies with the emphasis on biological control not to eradicate pests, but to maintain their populations to avoid economical losses [15]. As phages are the natural predators of bacteria, and thus fit into this framework of IPM, research on phage-based biocontrol is coming back into the picture. Some critical proofs of concept on the efficacy of phages as biocontrol agents have been demonstrated in recent years, as reviewed elsewhere [4].

A major hurdle towards the commercial implementation of these phage-based biocontrol strategies in crop protection concerns aspects of regulation and intellectual property protection. The cost to develop new crop protectants can reach $286 million and may take eleven years [16,17]. Therefore, patents can act as a tool to stimulate innovations in the field. They provide the applicant(s) the right to prohibit others to use their invention for a time-span of twenty years in a specific geographical area in which the patent has been filed. As a consequence, when an applicant wants to have an exclusive right for the invention in different countries, the patent application should be filed for each country individually (full application procedure available [18]). This exclusive right could assure a return-on-investment to the patent holder and hence serve as an incentivizing tool for research and innovation [19,20]. However, patenting biological substances like bacteriophages has been shown to be difficult [21,22]. Nevertheless, the question remains as to whether phages and phage-containing products are protectable by patents and what the scope is of these patents. Here, we present a patent landscape on the existing patents within the field of phage biocontrol using natural phages in agriculture and correlate this with a systematic survey of the scientific literature. A database containing the relevant patent documents within this research area has been set up and analyzed. The number, geographical distribution, and legal status were examined and the scope of the patents was investigated by means of a claim analysis. In parallel, a database of scientific publications within the same research topic was analyzed to enable comparisons with the patent information. This analysis allows us to draw conclusions on the amount and scope of protection of phage-based biocontrol applications in crop production.

2. Materials and Methods

2.1. Dataset Scientific Publications

A dataset consisting of scientific publications on the topic of phage biocontrol in crop production was created by searching Web of Science and PubMed using Boolean search operators combined with a set of keywords relevant for this topic (((“phage”[Title/Abstract] OR “phage therapy” [Title/Abstract] OR “bacteriophage” [Title/Abstract] OR “phage biocontrol” [Title/Abstract] OR “bacteriophage therapy” [Title/Abstract])) AND ((“plant”[Title/Abstract] OR “crop”[Title/Abstract])). The database was manually curated by eliminating non-relevant papers (papers discussing human phage therapy or phage biocontrol in food). Therefore, all abstracts of the scientific publications were manually curated to verify the relevance to the topic. The last update of the dataset was on 17 February 2019 (Supplementary Table S1) and can be considered as an up-to-date snapshot of the situation.

2.2. Patent Search, Legal Status, and Geographical Distribution

An algorithm based on Verbeure et al. (2006) [23] was used to set up a dataset of relevant patent applications and granted patents. In short, a classification search was performed using the International Patent Classification system (IPC) (A01N63—C12N7) combined with a set of keywords relevant for phage applications in the agricultural sector (bacteriophage, phage, phage biocontrol, phage therapy, bacteriophage therapy, plant, crop) in public databases (EspaceNet, Patent Scope, Google Patents). The dataset was manually evaluated and was last updated 17 February 2019 (Supplementary Table S2).

The patent landscape was performed according to Huys et al. (2009) [24]. Three different categories of the legal status were used as retrieved from EspaceNet by evaluating the "Global dossier" in the case of non-European patents or the "INPADOC legal status" and "EP register" for European patents: pending (patent application in consideration), granted (patent that is active in a specific territory), dead (meaning that the application or patent is abandoned) (e.g., WO2014177996 (A1)), refused (e.g., JP2005073562 (A)), withdrawn or deemed to be withdrawn (e.g., CN103430973 (A)), or lapsed (e.g., US19840662065). A patent and/or application is considered "active" when the application is still pending or when the patent is granted. On the contrary, if the patent and/or application is dead, it is considered "non-active".

The applicants and the geographical span of the patents were evaluated by looking at the patent document and its attributed number. The documents were categorized according to continent to have a better overview (Africa (ZA), Asia (CN, IN, JP, KR), Oceania (AU, NZ), Europe (DE, EA, EP, ES, GB, HU, IT), North America (CA, US), South America (AR, BR, CL, CR, GT, MX, PE)).

2.3. Categorization of Patent Documents and Scientific Publications

To have an understanding of the core focus of patent documents and scientific publications in terms of genera of bacteria being addressed, both were categorized among the most prominent bacterial genera causing plant bacterial diseases, as determined by Mansfield et al. 2012: *Agrobacterium, Dickeya, Erwinia, Pectobacterium, Pseudomonas, Ralstonia, Xanthomonas, Xylella*, and Other [9]. Here, "Other" was defined as any other bacterial genus or if the document did not specify the bacterium addressed. The categorization was based on a claim analysis (both dependent and independent claims) of the patent documents and an abstract analysis of the scientific publications.

A detailed independent claim analysis was performed for the granted, active patents to determine the scope of the patent. Independent claims were analyzed as these generally define the broadest scope. Claims were categorized into four categories: (i) the phage itself ("phage"), (ii) the composition of the phage cocktail and the final product ("composition"), (iii) methods for producing and/or obtaining phages ("production"), and (iv) the use of phages to treat (non-human) bacterial diseases ("treatment"). One limitation of this research is that the authors had to rely on automatic translations of the claims in Asian patents in order to understand their scope. The same categories were applied on the scientific publications by interpreting the abstracts of the papers, enabling a comparison between the scope of patents and scientific papers.

Moreover, the impact of the independent claims was evaluated based on Huys et al. 2009 [24] according to Art. 69, Art. 83, and the Protocol of the European Patent Convention (EPC) ("fair protection for the patentee with a reasonable degree of certainty for third parties"). In the case of U.S. patents, the claim interpretation was based on U.S. Utility Patent Act §112, demanding a "clear written description" and "best mode for carrying out the invention". Non-European and non-U.S. patents were interpreted by the authors in a similar way. Using this methodology, three impact levels could be defined: narrow, intermediate, and broadly-defined claims. The circumvention of the claims was estimated according to the author's appraisal. Narrow defined claims (green) cover specific details of the invention and can easily be circumvented, for example, changes in the genomic sequence of the phage, adaptations to the product composition, different protocols, and methods of treatment not covered by the claims. Intermediate claims (orange) cover the invention as such without describing details (e.g., a specific phage for a specific bacterium, a composition of a product or production process). These claims can be circumvented, though this would require substantial inventiveness. The authors categorized production and treatment claims as intermediate when these claims cover broad methods of production of treatment, but only for a particular phage. On the other hand, broadly defined claims (red) cover every aspect of the invention, but are vaguely described and hence claim outside the invention. However, no full freedom-to-operate analysis for each individual invention was conducted, as this is beyond the scope of this study.

3. Results

3.1. Patent Search, Scientific Papers, and Legal Status

Searching the different databases resulted in the identification of 49 different patent families within the field of phage biocontrol in crop production. A patent family is defined as a group of patents and/or patent applications that have been filed in different countries, but protect one and the same invention and have the same inventor(s). To highlight specific patent families, the first attributed application number was chosen to represent the family. Within the database, the families comprise in total 97 patents and applications (both active and non-active). Figure 1 shows the different patent families organized per year (priority year—dark blue area chart). It shows that the number of patent families slightly increases in time (peak at 2013) and decreases again as less patents were filed in 2016. The information on patent applications from 2017, 2018, and 2019 is not complete as these applications may not have been published yet.

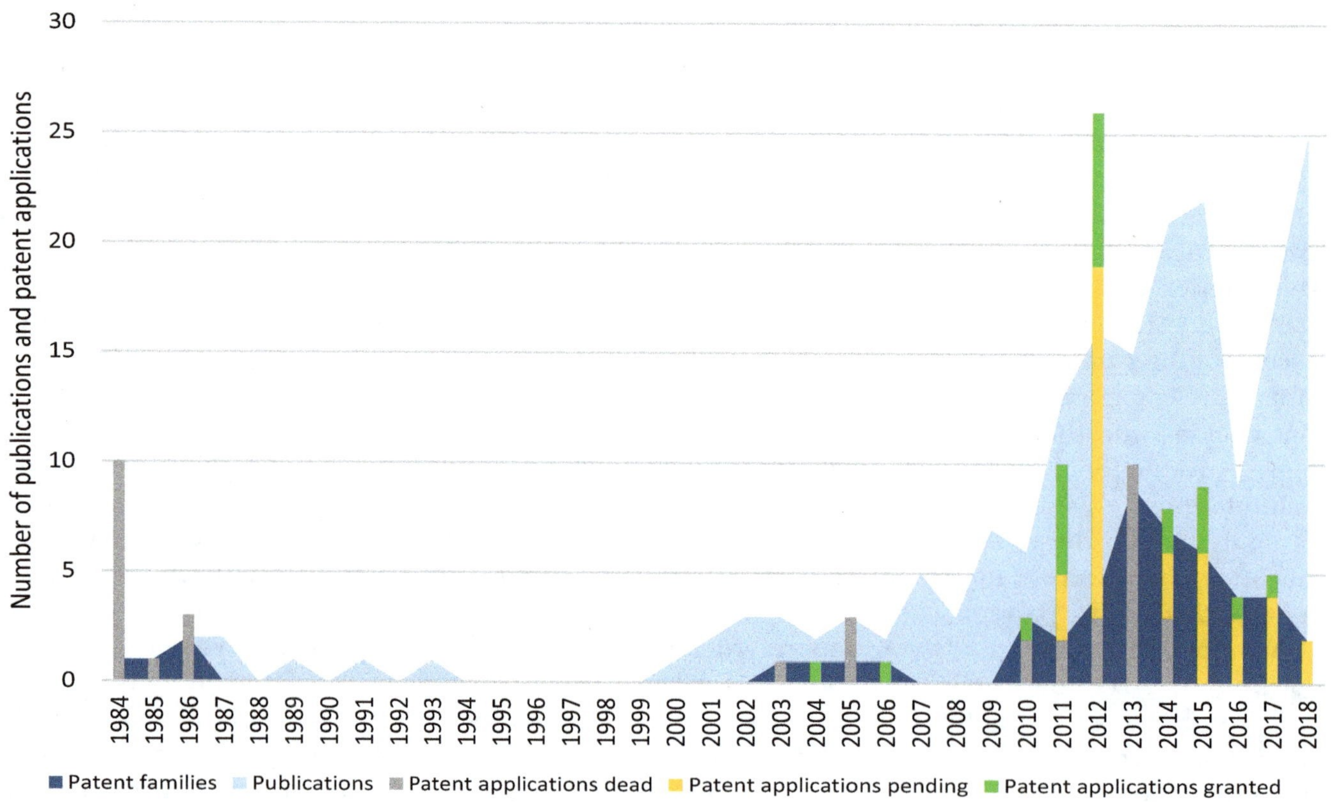

Figure 1. An overview of the number of scientific publications, patent families, patents, and patent applications in the field of phage biocontrol in crop production organized by year. The light blue area chart represents the number of scientific publications and the dark blue area chart the number of patent families per priority year. The bars represent the number of patent applications per priority year: green ("Granted patents") corresponds to the number of granted patents, yellow ("Pending applications") to pending applications, and grey ("Dead applications and patents") to dead patents and applications. This last group consists of patents and applications that are abandoned, refused, withdrawn, deemed to be withdrawn, or lapsed.

In sharp contrast, 137 scientific publications (1984–2019) were found within Web of Science and PubMed (Figure 1—light blue area chart). Publications on phage biocontrol were scarce in the eighties and nineties of the 20th century. However, from the year 2000 onwards, this number has increased steadily (25 peer reviewed publications in 2018). In other words, there is an increasing trend in the number of publications over the past decade, demonstrating a discrepancy between scientific publishing and patent filing. However, not all patent applications from 2017, 2018, and 2019 are publically available, as the 18-month period before publishing has not passed yet.

When looking at the patent documents in more detail (Figure 1—bar charts), a distinction should be made between "Granted", "Pending", and "Dead", based on their legal status as derived from Espacenet. In total, 59 patents and patent applications (61%) are active, 22 patents (23%) have been granted, 37 applications (38%) are pending, and 38 patent documents (39%) can be considered dead. From the latter, 39% are applications that were deemed to be withdrawn, 16% are rejected applications, and 16% are lapsed patents. Figure 1 shows an overview of the percentages of granted, pending, and dead documents with the same priority year. The first active patent from the dataset dates from 2004 (JP4532959 (B2)). In 2011, there were two families filed, represented by GB20110010647 and JP20110102153, containing in total six patents and four applications, respectively. All the applications and patents within the first family remain active—50% is granted and 50% is pending—whereas two out of four patent applications from the latter family have been rejected. The year 2012 has the most patents—26 in total, divided among four different families represented by GB20120017097, KR101584214, MX2012011440, and US201261716245. This last family contains four granted patents and sixteen applications. The family represented by GB20120017097 consists of one pending and two dead applications and one granted patent (US9278141 (B2)). In 2013, there was a peak in the amount of patent families filed as the number reached nine families. These families consist in total of ten applications, all of which are dead. The majority of these applications were deemed to be withdrawn (80%), meaning that the designation fee was not paid.

3.2. *Applicants and Geographical Distribution*

Analyzing the applicants of the different patent documents, it shows that 56% (54) of the 97 patent documents have been filed by academia, whereas 37% (36) are linked to industry (without joint applicants), and 7% (7) are joint applicants. This means that the family, or patent documents belonging to a family, have more than one applicant and thus the rights of the patent are distributed among the different partners. The most prominent academic applicants based on the amount of patent families filed by these applicants are the University of Hiroshima (JP) (21% of patent families –6/28) and the Rural Development Administration (KR) (14%, 4/28). The most prolific company in terms of patent filing is Qingdao Biological Technology Corporation LTD (CN), accounting for 50% (8/16). However, it is worthwhile to mention that all patents within the database from the Qingdao Biological Technology Corporation LTD have been withdrawn. Remarkably, only 4 out of 21 granted patents are filed by applicants from the private sector and all of these patents belong to the same family (represented by GB20110010647—Fixed Phage).

Figure 2 provides an overview of the relative contributions by countries in terms of filed and granted patent applications. One percent of all patent documents were filed in Africa (ZA), 3% in Oceania (AU, NZ), 13% in Europe (DE, EA, EP, ES, GB, HU, IT), and 13% worldwide. The majority of the patent documents have been filed in North America and Asia—16% in the USA and Canada and 43% in Asia. These Asian documents consist of 45% (19/42) Chinese, 31% (13/42) Japanese, 21% (9/42) Korean, and 2% (1/42) Indian applications and patents. When analyzing the legal status of the different patents organized per continent, 33% (14/42) of the Asian patents have been granted, 26% (11/42) of the applications are pending, and 40% (17/42) are dead. The large portion of dead patents and applications is also visible among the European (54%, 7/13) and North American (44%, 7/16) documents. Only 8% (1/13) of European patents have been granted, while this figure is 25% (4/16) for North American patents. The amount of pending applications is similar at 38% (5/13) and 31% (5/16) of the European and North American applications, respectively. On the other hand, in the case of the South American patent applications, 89% (8/9) are pending and 11% are dead. Notably, 7/9 of these South American patents are part of the same patent family (US2016309723).

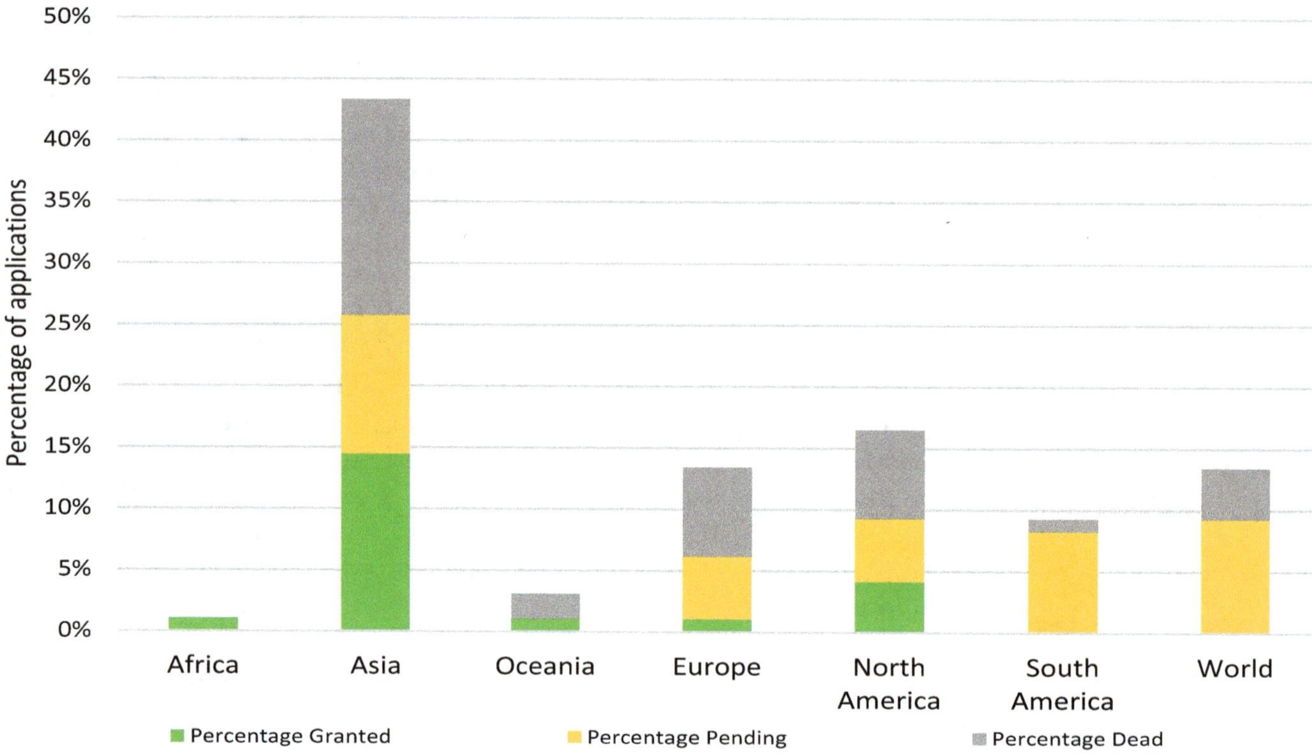

Figure 2. Percentage of patents and applications organized per continent. The total height of the bars indicate the percentage of patents and applications per continent. Africa (ZA), Asia (CN, IN, JP, KR), Oceania (AU, NZ), Europe (DE, EA, EP, ES, GB, IT), North America (CA, US), South America (AR, BR, CL, CR, GT, MX, PE), and world applications. In green, the percentage of granted patents; in yellow, the percentage of pending applications; and in grey, the percentage of dead applications and dead patents.

Furthermore, China has the highest percentage of dead patents, with 63% (12/19). The majority of these patent were deemed to be withdrawn after the admission fee was not paid (92%). On the contrary, Japan and Korea have the highest amount of granted patents, 38% (5/13) and 67% (6/9) of the patents filed, respectively, are granted and still active.

3.3. Categorization of Patents and Scientific Publications

As the most prominent bacterial species belong to the genera of *Agrobacterium, Dickeya, Erwinia, Pectobacterium, Pseudomonas, Ralstonia, Xanthomonas*, and *Xylella* [9], patent families and scientific publications were categorized and quantified among these groups according to (in)dependent claims (patent applications) and abstracts (scientific publications) (Figure 3). Combinations of genera were created when phages against certain pathogens were combined in a single cocktail (*Dickeya/Pectobacterium* and *Xanthomonas/Xylella*). A patent family or publication was classified as "Other" if it concerns a phage infecting bacteria of other genera (e.g., *Streptomyces*—"McKenna, F., et al. 2001. Novel In vivo use of a polyvalent Streptomyces phage to disinfest Streptomyces scabies-infected seed potatoes. Plant Pathol. 50:666–675." [25]) or if the paper/publication has no specification of the type of phage neither in the independent nor in the dependent claims (e.g., WO2016154602—"A method of preparing a phage composition for killing or degrading fitness of a pest").

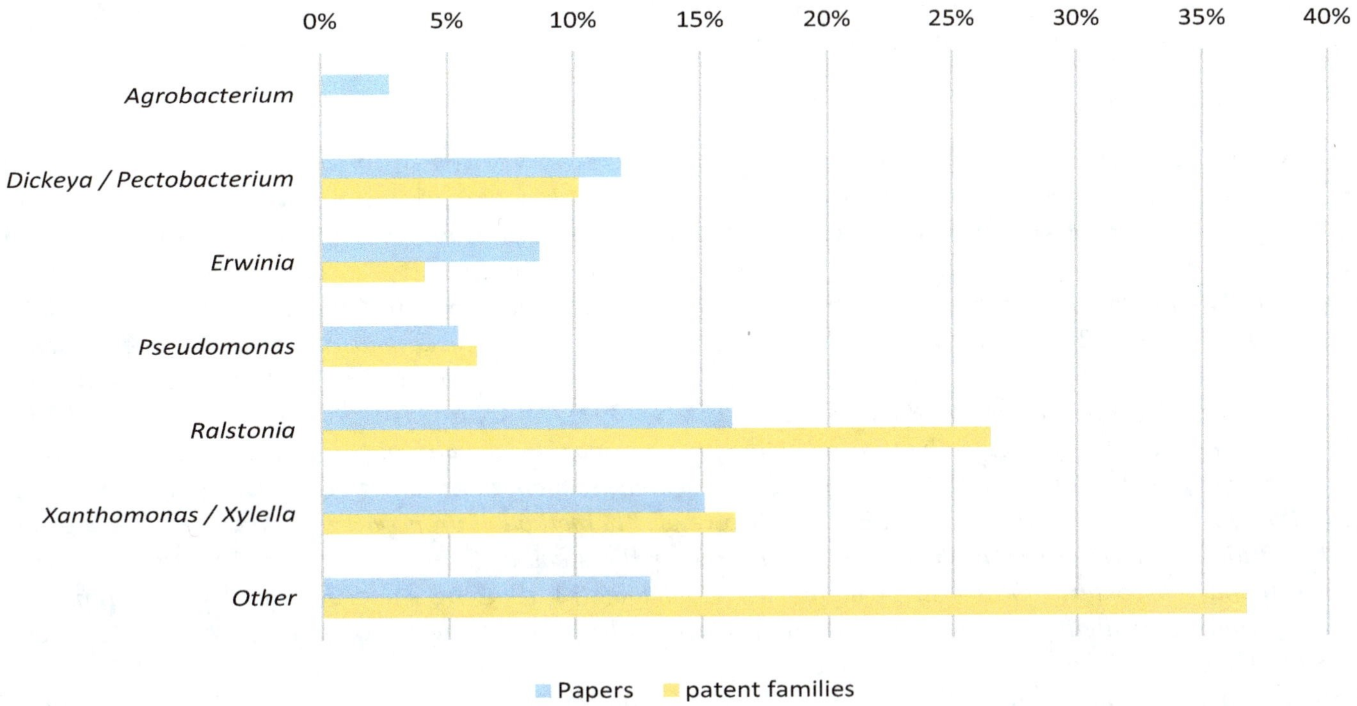

Figure 3. Distribution of patent families and scientific publications classified according to the bacterial genera that is tackled by the phage product. On the basis of Mansfield et al., 2012, seven categories (*Agrobacterium, Dickeya/Pectobacterium, Erwinia, Pseudomonas, Ralstonia, Xanthomonas/Xylella,* and Other) were made to classify patent families and publications. Groupings of bacterial genera (*Dickeya/Pectobacterium* and *Xanthomonas/Xylella*) were created as phage cocktails were created to tackle both bacterial genera. The last category "Other" consists of patent families and publications that do not specify the bacterial pathogen that is being targeted or that tackle an alternative bacterial genera.

The least researched bacterial genera within both databases are *Agrobacterium* (0% patent families, 3% publications), *Pseudomonas* (6% patent families, 5% publications), and *Erwinia* (4% patent families, 9% publications). The most represented bacterial genera within the datasets as suggested by Figure 3 are *Ralstonia, Xanthomonas/Xylella,* and *Dickeya/Pectobacterium*. Sixteen percent of the scientific publications discuss phages infecting *Ralstonia*; 15% *Xanthomonas, Xylella,* or a combination of *Xanthomonas and Xylella*; and 12% *Dickeya, Pectobacterium,* or a combination of *Dickeya* and *Pectobacterium*. In the case of the patent applications, a similar trend can be observed—27% *Ralstonia*, 16% *Xanthomonas / Xylella,* and 10% *Dickeya / Pectobacterium*.

A closer inspection of the different categories reveals that three patent families within the category of *Ralstonia* have included a private company as co-applicant (23%, 3/13). On the other hand, inventions from all patent families filed by public institutes have also been published in scientific papers (Supplementary Table S3). In the case of the category of *Xanthomonas / Xylella*, a similar trend can be observed, as there are three families filed by industrial applicants represented by WO2015200519 by Auxergen (US), US2017142976 by Fairhaven Vineyards (US), and HU1700178 Enviroinvest Koernyezetvedelmi es biotechnologiai (HU).

The other families are filed by the University of Hiroshima (JP), Texas A&M University (US), University Huazhong (CN), and the National institute for Agro-Environmental Sciences (JP), all situated in the public sector. This is also the case for *Dickeya* and *Pectobacterium*, as no patents were filed by private institutes. The applicants here include the Rural Development Administration (KR) and the national university of Seoul (KR). The majority of the families filed by private institutes are classified as "Other" (37%), indicating that the patents are not discussing the major genera of bacteria, but rather do not specify the phages nor their host. Hence, the claims are defined broadly.

Within this group, the majority of the families are filed by industrial applicants (88%): Fixed phage (GB), Epibiome (US), Qingdao Biological Technology Corporation LTD (CN), and Internalle (US).

3.4. Claim and Abstract Analysis

A claim analysis was performed to determine the scope of the individual patents along with an analysis of the scientific publications. Among the dataset of 91 patent documents analyzed, 21 were active, granted patents. In total, 79 independent claims were systematically analyzed and classified into four different categories (Figure 4): (1) Phage (e.g., *"A bacteriophage able to lyse cells of Ralstonia solanacearum selected from the group of the following: (a) vRsoP-WF2 (DSM 32039), vRsoP-WM2 (DSM32040), vRsoP-WR2 (DSM32041); or (b) a podovirus whose genome has the sequence of SEQ ID NO: 1 (corresponding to vRsoP-WF2), SEQ ID NO: 2 (corresponding to vRsoP- WM2), or SEQ ID NO: 3 (corresponding to vRsoP-WR2)"*—ES2592352), (2) Composition (e.g., *"A composition for inhibiting or preventing the growth of Pectobacterium carotovorum, which comprises as an active ingredient bacteriophage PM-2 (KACC97022P) having an entire genome sequence consisting of the nucleotide sequence of SEQ ID NO: 1."*—KR101797463), (3) Production (e.g., *"A method of propagating a virulent bacteriophage that includes X fastidiosa in its host range, comprising the steps of the following: (a) infecting a culture of Xanthomonas bacteria with said virulent bacteriophage; (b) allowing said bacteriophage to propagate; and (c) isolating virulent bacteriophage particles from the culture."*—"Production claim": AU2013331060), and (4) Treatment (e.g., *"A method of preventing or reducing symptoms or disease associated with Xylella fastidiosa or Xanthomonas in a plant, comprising contacting said plant with particles of at least one virulent bacteriophage, wherein Xylella fastidiosa and/or Xanthomonas axonopodis are hosts of the bacteriophage, wherein the bacteriophage is a Xfas 300-type bacteriophage and displays the following characteristics: (a) the bacteriophage is capable of lysing said Xylella fastidiosa and/or Xanthomonas bacteria; (b) the bacteriophage infects a cell by binding to a Type IV pilus; (c) the bacteriophage comprises a non-contractile tail with a capsid size ranging from 58–68 nm in diameter and belongs to the Podoviridae family; (d) the genomic size of the bacteriophage is about 43,300 bp to 44,600 bp; and (e) the bacteriophage prevents or reduces symptoms associated with Pierce's disease in a plant or plants."*—US9357785). The same categories were used to classify the scientific publications based on the abstract of the publication. Both scientific papers and patents can fall in different categories as they may discuss one or more phages and their basic characterization, the composition of a cocktail, and the testing of this cocktail in bioassays and/or field trials. As Figure 4 shows, there are differences between the relative contributions of scientific papers and patents that address a specific topic. The majority of the scientific papers focus on the isolation and basic characterization of one or more phages (84%). Thirty-six percent of the manuscripts discuss the composition of a phage cocktail and 39% use this cocktail in bioassays and/or field trials. The least represented topic discusses production methods of phage (4%). In contrast, the majority of the patents (90%) protect the use of phages to treat a plant in one way or another. Seventy-six percent of the patents claim the composition of a product containing phage, 62% protect the phage itself, and 24% contain claims protecting the production of the phage product. On the other hand, no patents within the database contain claims to protect methods of detection nor of the phage nor of the host.

When evaluating the 77 independent claims of all active, granted patents, the majority of the claims are process claims protecting different methods to use phages as a treatment for bacterial infection (40%—Supplementary Figure S1). Furthermore, this data shows that 30% of the claims protect the composition of the phage product. This means that a combination of phages is protected and/or the formulation of the final product. Nineteen percent can be considered as compound claims as the claim is protecting the phage(s) as an active ingredient and only 10% of the claims are production claims.

The 77 independent claims were also categorized within three classes: narrow, intermediate, and broadly-defined. This gives an indication of whether a specific claim can be easily circumvented (narrowly-defined) or not (broadly-defined). Table 1 gives an overview of all the granted patents and the independent claims that belong to these patents. Twenty-six percent of the claims are narrow claims (e.g., "*The invention relates to a method for applying a bacteriophage of R. solanacearum, characterized in that the bacteriophage liquid of R. solanacearum is placed in a sterile syringe needle obliquely inserted into the stem of the tobacco plant, and then the bacterial phage liquid is covered with sterile mineral oil to prevent evaporation. And pollution, so that the R. solanaceans phage directly enters the stem of the tobacco through a sterile syringe needle; the sterile mineral oil is prepared by pouring 300 mL of mineral oil into a 500 mL screw bottle and sterilizing at 121 °C 30 min, then stored and reserved after cooling; the sterile syringe needle is prepared by using a sterile blister needle overnight, rinsing twice with sterile water, drying at 50 °C after autoclaving, and after cooling to room temperature, Packed and stored for use; each tobacco stem is injected with 50–100 µL of R. solanacearum phage solution; in the sterile syringe needle inserted into the stem of the tobacco plant, the amount of sterile mineral oil is 50–100 µL*"—"Treatment claim": CN104542717). Thirty percent of the claims are intermediate as they do not cover specific details on the invention (e.g., "*A method for controlling bacterial wilt disease bacteria, which comprises spraying the bacteriophage strain according to any one of claims 1 to 3 to a plant or soil.*"—"Treatment claim": JP4532959). Finally, 44% can be defined as broad claims (e.g., "*An isolated bacteriophage which is toxic to X. fastidiosa and Xanthomonas species, wherein said bacteriophage is at least one member selected from the group consisting of Xfas 100 phage type bacteriophage and Xfas 300 phage type bacteriophage Of the bacteriophage, wherein the Xfas 100 phage type is selected from the group consisting of SEQ ID NO: 11, SEQ ID NO: 12, SEQ ID NO: 13, SEQ ID NO: 14, SEQ ID NO: 15, SEQ ID NO: 16, SEQ ID NO: 17, and SEQ ID NO: 18 Wherein the Xfas 300 phage type comprises a genome having a DNA sequence that is 99% or more identical to the sequence of SEQ ID NO: 19, SEQ ID NO: 20, SEQ ID NO: 21, SEQ ID NO: 22, SEQ ID NO: 23 and SEQ ID NO: 24 Select from It comprises a sequence a genome having the same DNA sequence 99% or more that is, the bacteriophage.*"—"Phage claim": JP6391579).

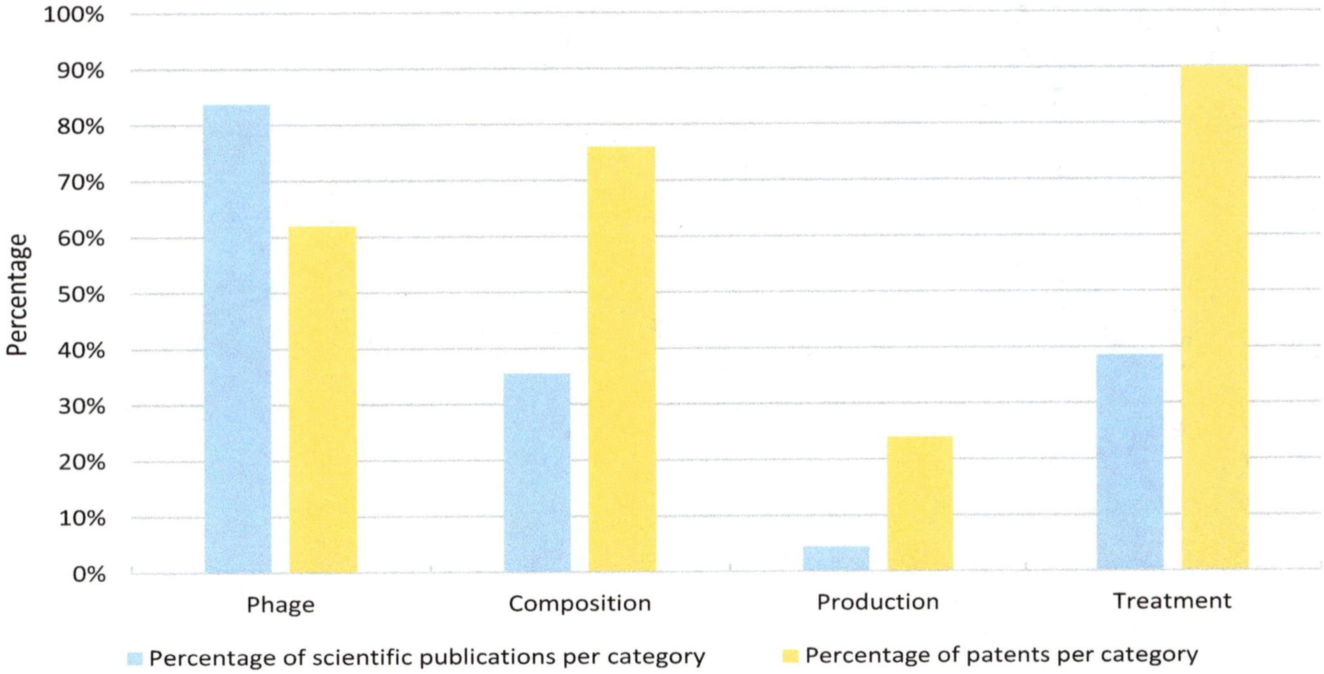

Figure 4. Claim and abstract analysis of the active, granted patents and scientific publications. In total, 79 independent claims from 21 patents and 137 abstracts from scientific papers were categorized among four different categories: (1) Phage—here the phage was described as the active ingredient or the isolation of a phage was described, (2) Cocktail—this category contains claims that protect the combination of phages and publications that describe a phage cocktail, (3) Production—ways of how the phage is produced, and (4) Treatment—claims that protect the use of phages to fight a specific bacterial infection or methods and application strategies for using the phage (e.g., bioassays, field trials). In blue, the percentages of publications are shown; in yellow, the percentage of claims are shown. Note: one publication and patent can be categorized in multiple categories.

Table 1. Claim analysis of the granted patents. Within this table, all granted patents have been organized according to the bacterial genera they describe, their patent number, the applicant (private sector in blue and public sector in yellow) and the nationality of the applicant (CN China, ES Spain, GB United Kingdom, JP Japan, KR Korea, and US United States), and the filing year. Moreover, the claims were categorized according the four different categories: (1) Phage: claims protecting one or multiple phages and their genome sequence, (2) Composition: claims discussing the composition of a phage product, (3) Production: methods to produce phages, and (4) Treatment: methods to use phages as a treatment for plant diseases. If a patent contains claims that belong to a specific category, it is quantified. The colors indicate the scope of a claim or set of claims: very narrow, intermediate, or broadly-defined (green, orange, and red, respectively).

Bacterial Genera	Patent Number	Applicant	Filing Year	Type of Claim			
				Phage	Composition	Production	Treatment
Other	US9539343	Fixed Phage (GB)	2012		1		1
	CN103747792	Fixed Phage (GB)	2012		1		1
	JP6230994	Fixed Phage (GB)	2012		1		1
	US9278141	Fixed Phage (GB)	2013		5		
	CN104630154	University of Zhejiang (CN)	2015	1	1	1	2
	KR101887987	Pukyong National University (KR)	2016	1	1		1
Dickeya/ Pectobacterium	KR101368328	Rural development Administration (KR)	2010	1	1		
	KR101790019	Rural development administration (KR)	2014	1	1		1
	KR101797463	Rural development Administration (KR)	2014	1	1		1
	KR101891298	Seoul National University (KR)	2016	1	2		1
Pseudomonas	KR101584214	Chungbuk National University (KR)	2012		1		1
Ralstonia	JP4532959	Sanin Kensetsu Kogyo (JP)	2004	3	2		2
	JP4862154	University of Hiroshima (JP)	2006	1	1		3
	US9380786	University of Hiroshima (JP)	2012				1
	JP5812466	University of Hiroshima (JP)	2011	1			3
	CN104542717	Guizhou Tobacco science research institute (CN)	2015			1	1
	ES2592352	University of Valencia (ES)	2015	1	1		2
Xanthomonas/ Xylella	AU2013331060	Texas A&M University (US)	2013	1	1	2	4
	JP6391579	Texas A&M University (US)	2013	1	1	2	2
	US9357785	Texas A&M University (US)	2013				1
	ZA201502230	Texas A&M University (US)	2013	1	1	2	2

The claims categorized as "Phage claims" are generally narrowly-defined (41%), as the claims protect the phage and its genomic sequence. However, highly similar phages with differences in their genomic sequence fall outside the scope of these claims. Thus, the claims can be circumvented. A judge, however, may interpret by the claim as equivalent by the doctrine of equivalence. The isolation of a different phage that targets the same bacterium also circumvents the claim. On the other hand, the majority of the "Composition claims" and "Production claims" are difficult to circumvent as they are broadly defined (56% and 75%, respectively).

As mentioned above, 4 out of 21 granted patents have been filed by a private organization (Fixed Phage) and these patents belong to the same patent family. When looking at the claims for these patents, one notices that all the claims are broadly-defined. As the invention discusses the use of phages in a composition to fight bacterial infections without defining the phage itself, the majority of the claims protect the composition of the product rather than the phage or the production of the product.

4. Discussion

Within this study, we analyzed publishing and patenting activities in phage biocontrol as a crop protectant using the number of scientific papers and patent documents as a measuring tool for assessing interest in this area. Furthermore, we looked into the applicants, geographical distribution, legal status, and scope of the patent documents by categorizing both the patents and scientific manuscripts by claims and abstracts. This allowed us to make a general comparison between the focus of patents and scientific literature and the willingness of R&D to look into the potential of phages as a part of IPM.

4.1. Despite a Growing Interest in Phage Biocontrol, Patenting Activities Remain Limited

The increasing number of scientific publications (Figure 1) shows that there is indeed a growing interest in using phages as an alternative to existing plant protecting products. The number of patent filings seems to fall behind in 2016, but increases slightly in 2017. However, it is premature to determine a trend because not all the applications filed in 2017 and 2018 have passed the 18-month period before publication and thus are not made publicly available [26]. Fifty-six percent of the patent documents were filed by non-profit organizations like the University of Hiroshima (JP), the Rural Development Administration of South-Korea (KR), and Texas A&M University (US). This confirms the slightly stronger interest from non-profit organizations in protecting phage biocontrol inventions compared with industry. It might also suggest that private companies are still dangling in the start-up phase or have not picked up the topic yet (apart from a few early adopters). This could also indicate that the expertise still remains in non-profit and needs to be transferred to the private sector.

The assessment of the legal status of the documents shows a high fraction of dead documents (39%). Within this group of dead applications, 16% of the applications were rejected as the invention was not considered novel (US2009053179) and/or did not include an inventive step (JP2005073562). The majority of the dead documents are applications that were deemed to be withdrawn (39%) and patents that are lapsed (16%—no oppositions were filed, e.g., EP0182106). In both cases, the applicants did not pay the fees needed to maintain the rights of the patent. For some patent applications, this is because of a negative search report (GB2519913 and WO2007044428), in which the invention was not found novel nor inventive. On the other hand, not paying the fees may also imply internal shifts of interest for commercial or other reasons. Hurdles in the regulation of biopesticides may influence such decisions as well. In Europe, for instance, the registration exists for two phases: registration of the active ingredient at European level by the European Food Safety Authority (EFSA), and the authorization of the formulated product at member state level leading to bureaucratic difficulties and high cost [17]. In the United States, a similar procedure should be taken as the product needs to be registered by the Environmental Protection Agency (EPA) [27]. Other countries including China and South Korea have similar agencies [28,29]. As phages are highly specific and can only infect a few strains of one bacterial species, they are often combined in a cocktail [30]. In terms of registrations, this means that every phage in the cocktail should be registered as an active ingredient (Regulation (EC) No

1107/2009) and reformulations of the product require re-registrations [4]. The cost of such registrations may be high, for example, the registration costs of products corresponding to a "New Active Ingredient, Non-food use; outdoor; reduced risk" can reach $436,004 in the United States [31] and in Europe, the total R&D costs (including registration fees) are estimated to reach $286 million [16]. Moreover, phage genomes are variable as a result of evolutionary fluxes [32], thus phages cannot be considered as stable, fixed products that could impede registration [33]. Luckily, this can partially be addressed by recent insights on genome-based taxonomy that phages sharing 95% nucleotide similarity are considered as isolates the same species [34]. Changes in the regulation including fast track registration, priority registration, and zonal authorization (i.e., authorization for all of the EU instead of registration per country) could function as an incentive to further develop innovations and promote patenting in biocontrol [35]. These reasons could also explain the low number of filed applications in Europe and North America, as observed in Figure 2. Nevertheless, a first phage product line, AgriPhage™, was registered in the United States (2005) by Omnilytics (part of Phagelux). AgriPhage™ is approved by the Environmental Protection Agency (EPA) and contains products with phages against *Xanthomonas campestris* pv. *vesicatoria* and *Pseudomonas syringae* pv. *tomato*. Currently, Omnilytics has added cocktails against *Erwinia amylovora* and *Clavibacter michiganensis* subsp. *michiganensis* to their product line [36]. Notably, none of these products or phages were found by the authors in the public assessed databases. This may imply that the patents could be licensed (e.g., from an academic partner); the applications are not publicly available yet; or the product is not patented, opening the discussion of whether patenting is indeed crucial for commercial activities of phage applications in agriculture. Also, in Europe, a few phage-containing products are on the market. In Hungary, Enviroinvest has a product (available since March 2018) on the Hungarian market called Erwiphage PLUS, containing bacteriophages targeting *Erwinia amylovora* [37]. Moreover, the Scottish company APS Biocontrol distributes a product line Biolyse®, a food-packaging aid that contains phages that prevent soft rot disease in stored potatoes [38].

4.2. Efforts in Asia to Protect Phage Biocontrol Preparations

The geographical distribution of the patent documents (Figure 2) shows that the majority were filed in Asia (43%). This observation might be explained by local governmental stimuli to promote patenting to cause rapid economic growth [39,40]. China, for instance, has implemented so-called patent promotion policies. These policies stimulate patenting as tax incentives and subsidies are linked to patent ownership, and have caused a booming growth in the number of Chinese patent applications and patents [40]. Furthermore, Asia, in general, is taking measures to reduce the amount of chemical pesticides and fertilizers. China, for instance, has launched a "national research program on reduction in chemical pesticides and fertilizers in China" ($340 million) [35]. Within the study presented here, 19% of all documents were filed in China. In contrast, 63% of these documents are dead, from which 92% are applications that were deemed to be withdrawn as fees were not paid. This might implicate that the applicants lost their confidence in the invention. The number of granted, active patents is high in Japan and South Korea, further illustrating Asian efforts to develop new biocontrol strategies. A study from the Food and Agriculture Organization from the United Nations (FAO) and the Asia and Pacific Plant Protection Commission (APPPC) has shown that both Japan and South Korea are promoting integrated pest management strategies by setting pesticide reduction targets (KR) and appointing IPM expert groups (JP) [41].

4.3. Scientific Publications and Patent Documents Show a Correlation in Terms of Targeted Pathogens

To get a more profound idea about the focus of the patent and scientific literature, both datasets were classified according to the most prominent bacterial genera causing plant diseases [9] (Figure 3). In general, the percentages of scientific publications and patent families discussing a specific bacterial genus correspond quite well. Within the datasets presented here, the most studied bacterial genus is *Ralstonia*; not surprisingly, as these bacteria cause disease in a wide range of cash crops like tomato, potato, tobacco, eggplant, and banana [42]. In the dataset, tomato is the most researched crop.

The majority of the documents categorized within this group were filed by non-profit organizations rather than industrial applicants. This suggests that the actual interest from industry is still rather limited compared with that of academia. The second most prominent group is the combination of *Xanthomonas* and *Xylella*. Both pathogens can have a significant impact in crop production and hence, it is not remarkable that these bacteria are largely represented in phage biocontrol research [43,44]. Furthermore, the majority of the applications were filed by the public sector. The *Pseudomonas* genus, including that of *Pseudomonas syringae* and its pathovars, is less represented within both databases. This is striking as *P. syringae* pathovars are considered as one of the most important PPBs causing disease in different crops (tomato, bean, kiwi, leek, and others) [45]. As Figure 3 shows, there is a discrepancy within the *"Other"* group. This category combines documents that talk about other bacterial genera or do not specify the bacterium that is being addressed. The majority of the patents and patent applications were classified in this category because these do not specify a particular bacterial genus. From these patent documents, we observe that all the granted patents filed by industrial applicants have chosen this option (Table 1). This might suggest that industry defines claims containing bacteriophages as broad as possible to get patent exclusive rights to any phage product that falls under the protection of the patent. By applying this strategy, companies are taking risks in their patenting strategy because these broad claims are more susceptible in terms of novelty anticipation, which may invalidate them [46].

4.4. Granted Patents Include Broad Claims

The main focus of the scientific publications and the granted patents indicate a difference in emphasis (Figure 4). While the majority of the manuscripts discuss the isolation of one or more bacteriophages and their basic characterization, the majority of the patents claim a method of treating a bacterial infection by means of a phage product. Only 39% of scientific papers address the latter, although this could be considered as the ultimate goal of phage biocontrol. This illustrates that first efforts are made in the field, but that there are still opportunities for further innovations.

Limited efforts have been made towards patenting detection strategies for and by phages in the field of phage biocontrol in crop production. As phages are highly specific to a specific bacterium and can locate their host in a complex matrix of bacteria, they can easily be used as a detection tool [47]. However, this study suggests that little published evidence is available in this area by both the scientific community and the industrial early adopters, as there are no claims protecting possible methods of detection and only a small minority (8%) of scientific papers discuss this matter.

The claims that belong to the "Phage" category consist of claims that protect a natural occurring phage. According to Art. 3 of the Biotechnology Directive 98/44/EC (European Commission), natural phages can be patented because the phage is isolated from the environment [22]. The techniques to isolate phages, however, are similar to those used in 1920, which makes the patentability of natural phages fragile [21]. Nevertheless, claims for isolated phages can be of great value as patents covering such claims may give the right to prevent others from using that particular phage. On the contrary, as phages are abundantly present in the environment, the chances of finding a similar, yet different phage, which may circumvent the claim, exists. However, as the literature on phages applicable for phage biocontrol increases, anticipation of novelty as a patentability requirement of a particular phage may become an issue. In the United States, the requirement of novelty is more complicated, as the phage will be excluded for patentability if on the one side it is known or used within the United States, or on the other side, published or patented wherever in the world [22].

Figure 4 also shows that there is limited evidence on the optimization of the production of phage cocktails based on both scientific and patent literature. One could argue that the production of phages is phage-dependent (specific bacterial strains, media, temperature) and thus keeping the production of phages secret could be a valid strategy to maintain a competitive edge [19].

On the other hand, many patents claim the combination of phages or phages as part of a formulation. This is illustrated by Supplementary Figure S1. Claiming a combination of phages can act as a buffer to reduce the risk of resistance development of the target bacterium. Phages are known to have different infection strategies and highly diverse genomes, leading to the chance that a certain bacterium develops resistance (by altering receptors, CRISPRs, restriction enzymes) against two or even three phages in one cocktail are theoretically small [4,48,49]. The strength of these claims can be questioned as minor changes to the cocktail could already be sufficient to circumvent claims.

Table 1 depicts in which categories the individual patents can be classified. Here, it is clear that the different patents combine different types of claims. Combined with the scope of the claims, this might support the previous statement that companies employ a "throw everything at the wall to see what sticks" patenting strategy because of the uncertainty and the ignorance in how to achieve a strong protection for the invention [19].

4.5. Phages and Other Viruses as Part of an Integrated Pest Management Strategy

To safeguard public health and minimize impact on the environment, traditional pesticides used in crop production are currently being stigmatized. This triggers the research community to evaluate new, alternative methods to deal with different kinds of pests like fungi, bacteria, and insects. The use of relatively high concentrations of natural predators to eradicate a certain pest, also known as augmentative biocontrol, is gaining in popularity [35]. In this regard, bacteriophages and other viruses, like insect viruses and mycoviruses, are ideal candidates as biocontrol agents because they are sustainable, specific, and do not leave residues on the crop. Moreover, they fit into the framework of integrated pest management, where the use of biocontrol agents is heavily promoted [35]. Viruses as biocontrol agents are, however, sometimes overlooked in IPM [15], which indicates that more efforts need to be taken to integrate these viral strategies. This review shows that there is indeed a basis within the scientific community to investigate the potential of phages to be used as biocontrol agents. In 2018, a Horizon 2020 consortium was established to investigate viruses and their potential to serve as a possible solution against pests as both a probiotic and viral treatment strategy (https://viroplant.eu/). Initiatives like these, together with more in-depth research, are needed to provide fundamental insights to close the gap between academia and industry in this matter and to stimulate the industry to invest in phage biocontrol.

Author Contributions: Conceptualization, D.H., R.L., I.H., and J.W.; methodology, D.H. and I.H.; writing—original draft preparation, D.H.; writing—review and editing, R.L., I.H., and J.W.

References

1. Twort, F.W. An Investigation On The Nature Of Ultra-Microscopic Viruses. *Lancet* **1915**, *186*, 1241–1243. [CrossRef]
2. D'Herelle, F. Roux On an invisible microbe antagonistic toward dysenteric bacilli: Brief note by Mr. F. D'Herelle, presented by Mr. Roux. *Res. Microbiol.* **2007**, *158*, 553–554. [PubMed]
3. Pirnay, J.P.; De Vos, D.; Verbeken, G.; Merabishvili, M.; Chanishvili, N.; Vaneechoutte, M.; Zizi, M.; Laire, G.; Lavigne, R.; Huys, I.; et al. The phage therapy paradigm: Prêt-à-porter or sur-mesure? *Pharm. Res.* **2011**, *28*, 934–937. [CrossRef]
4. Buttimer, C.; McAuliffe, O.; Ross, R.P.; Hill, C.; O'Mahony, J.; Coffey, A. Bacteriophages and bacterial plant diseases. *Front. Microbiol.* **2017**, *8*, 34. [CrossRef]
5. Mallmann, W.; Hemstreet, C. Isolation ofan inhibitory substance from plants. *Agric. Res.* **1924**, *28*, 599–602.
6. Okabe, N.; Goto, M. Bacteriophages of Plant Pathogens. *Annu. Rev. Phytopathol.* **1963**, *1*, 397–418. [CrossRef]
7. Strange, R.; Scott, P.R. Plant disease: A threat to global food security. *Annu. Rev. Phytopathol.* **2005**, *43*, 83–116. [CrossRef] [PubMed]
8. Inagro IWT—Beheersing bacteriële pathogeen opkweek kolen-prei. Available online: http://leden.inagro.be/Wie-is-Inagro/Projecten/project/13960 (accessed on 27 December 2018).

9. Mansfield, J.; Genin, S.; Magori, S.; Citovsky, V.; Sriariyanum, M.; Ronald, P.; Dow, M.; Verdier, V.; Beer, S.V.; Machado, M.A.; et al. Top 10 plant pathogenic bacteria in molecular plant pathology. *Mol. Plant Pathol.* **2012**, *13*, 614–629. [CrossRef] [PubMed]
10. Cooksey, D.A. Genetics of Bactericide. *Annu. Rev. Phytopathol.* **1990**, *28*, 201–219. [CrossRef]
11. Frampton, R.A.; Pitman, A.R.; Fineran, P.C. Advances in bacteriophage-mediated control of plant pathogens. *Int. J. Microbiol.* **2012**, *2012*, 326452. [CrossRef]
12. Pietrzak, U.; McPhail, D.C. Copper accumulation, distribution and fractionation in vineyard soils of Victoria, Australia. *Geoderma* **2004**, *122*, 151–166. [CrossRef]
13. Copping, L.G.; Duke, S.O. Natural products that have been used commercially as crop protection agents. *Pest Manag. Sci.* **2007**, *63*, 524–554. [CrossRef] [PubMed]
14. Ray, D.K.; Mueller, N.D.; West, P.C.; Foley, J.A. Yield Trends Are Insufficient to Double Global Crop Production by 2050. *PLoS ONE* **2013**, *8*, e66428. [CrossRef] [PubMed]
15. Stenberg, J.A. A Conceptual Framework for Integrated Pest Management. *Trends Plant Sci.* **2017**, *22*, 759–769. [CrossRef] [PubMed]
16. Phillips, M.D. *The Cost of New Agrochemical Product Discovery, Development and Resgistration in 1995, 2000, 2005–8 and 2010 to 2014. R&D Expenditure in 2014 and Expectations for 2019. A Consultancy Study for CropLife International, CropLife America and the European Crop*; Pathhead: Midlothian, UK, 2016.
17. European Crop Protection Registering Plant Protection Products in the EU. Available online: https://www.ecpa.eu/sites/default/files/7450_Registrationbrochure_3.pdf%0Ahttp://www.ecpa.eu/files/attachments/20110125_PPPBrochure_ECPA.pdf (accessed on 5 February 2019).
18. WIPO—Protecting Your Inventions Abroad: Frequently Asked Questions About the Patent Cooperation Treaty (PCT). Available online: https://www.wipo.int/pct/en/faqs/faqs.html (accessed on 12 March 2019).
19. Todd, K. The Promising Viral Threat To Bacterial Resistance: The Uncertain Patentability of Phage Therapeutics and the Necessity of Alternative Incentives. *J. D. Expect.* **2019**, *68*, 767–805.
20. Williams, H.L. How do patents affect research investments? *Annu. Rev. Econ.* **2017**, *9*, 441–469. [CrossRef]
21. Pirnay, J.-P.; Verbeken, G.; Rose, T.; Jennes, S.; Zizi, M.; Huys, I.; Lavigne, R.; Merabishvili, M.; Vaneechoutte, M.; Buckling, A.; et al. Introducing yesterday's phage therapy in today's medicine. *Future Virol.* **2012**, *7*, 379–390. [CrossRef]
22. Verbeken, G. *Towards An Adequate Regulatory Framework For Bacteriophage Therapy*; KU Leuven and Royal Military Academy: Leuven, Belgium, 2015.
23. Verbeure, B.; Matthijs, G.; Van Overwalle, G. Analysing DNA patents in relation with diagnostic genetic testing. *Eur. J. Hum. Genet.* **2006**, *14*, 26–33. [CrossRef]
24. Huys, I.; Berthels, N.; Matthijs, G.; Van Overwalle, G. Legal uncertainty in the area of genetic diagnostic testing. *Nat. Biotechnol.* **2009**, *27*, 903–909. [CrossRef]
25. McKenna, F.; El-Tarabily, K.A.; Hardy, G.S.J.; Dell, B. Novel in vivo use of a polyvalent Streptomyces phage to disinfest Streptomyces scabies-infected seed potatoes. *Plant Pathol.* **2001**, *50*, 666–675. [CrossRef]
26. EPO—Basic Definitions. Available online: https://www.epo.org/searching-for-patents/helpful-resources/first-time-here/definitions.html (accessed on 14 February 2019).
27. Braverman, M. United States. In *Use and Regulation of Microbial Pesticides in Representative Jurisdictions Worldwide*; 2015; Available online: https://www.IOBC-Global.org (accessed on 14 February 2019).
28. Wang, B.; Li, Z. Use and Regulation of Biopesticides in China. In *Use And Regulation Of Microbial Pesticides In Representative Jurisdictions Worldwide*; 2015; Available online: https://www.IOBC-Global.org (accessed on 14 February 2019).
29. Kim, J.J.; Lee, S.G.; Lee, S.; Jee, H.-J. South Korea. In *Use and Regulation of Microbial Pesticides in Representative Jurisdictions Worldwide*; 2015; Available online: https://www.IOBC-Global.org (accessed on 14 February 2019).
30. Rombouts, S.; Volckaert, A.; Venneman, S.; Declercq, B.; Vandenheuvel, D.; Allonsius, C.N.; Van Malderghem, C.; Jang, H.B.; Briers, Y.; Noben, J.P.; et al. Characterization of novel bacteriophages for biocontrol of bacterial blight in leek caused by Pseudomonas syringae pv. porri. *Front. Microbiol.* **2016**, *7*, 1–15. [CrossRef]
31. EPA PRIA Fee Category Table—Registration Division—New Active Ingredients. Available online: https://www.epa.gov/pria-fees/pria-fee-category-table-registration-division-new-active-ingredients (accessed on 15 February 2019).

32. Barbosa, C.; Venail, P.; Holguin, A.V.; Vives, M.J. Co-Evolutionary Dynamics of the Bacteria Vibrio sp. CV1 and Phages V1G, V1P1, and V1P2: Implications for Phage Therapy. *Microb. Ecol.* **2013**, *66*, 897–905. [CrossRef]
33. European Commission. *Guidance Document For The Assessment Of The Equivalence Of Technical Grade Active Ingredients For Identical Microbial Strains Or Isolates Approved Under Regulation (EC) No 1107/2009*; European Commission Health and Food safety: Brussels, Belgium, 2014.
34. Adriaenssens, E.M.; Rodney Brister, J. How to name and classify your phage: An informal guide. *Viruses* **2017**, *9*, 70. [CrossRef]
35. Van Lenteren, J.C.; Bolckmans, K.; Köhl, J.; Ravensberg, W.J.; Urbaneja, A. Biological control using invertebrates and microorganisms: Plenty of new opportunities. *BioControl* **2018**, *63*, 39–59. [CrossRef]
36. AgriPhageTM Product Info AgriPhage. Available online: https://www.agriphage.com/product-info/ (accessed on 9 February 2019).
37. Enviroinvest Zrt. Erwiphage PLUS. Available online: http://www.erwiphage.com/ (accessed on 12 March 2019).
38. APS Biocontrol Ltd. Biolyse Products. Available online: https://www.apsbiocontrol.com/products (accessed on 12 March 2019).
39. Erstling, J.; Strom, R. Korea's Patent Policy and Its Impact on Economic Development: A Model for Emerging Countries. *San Diego Int. Law J.* **2009**, *11*, 441–481.
40. Long, C.X.; Wang, J. China's patent promotion policies and its quality implications. *Sci. Pub. Policy* **2018**, *46*, 91–104. [CrossRef]
41. APPPC; FAO. Plant Protion Profiles from Asia-Pacific countries—Chapter 3 Intergrated Pest Management. Available online: http://www.fao.org/docrep/010/ag123e/AG123E22.htm (accessed on 13 February 2019).
42. Álvarez, B.; Biosca, E.G. Bacteriophage-Based Bacterial Wilt Biocontrol for an Environmentally Sustainable Agriculture. *Front. Plant Sci.* **2017**, *8*, 1–7. [CrossRef]
43. Ryan, R.P.; Vorhölter, F.J.; Potnis, N.; Jones, J.B.; Van Sluys, M.A.; Bogdanove, A.J.; Dow, J.M. Pathogenomics of Xanthomonas: Understanding bacterium-plant interactions. *Nat. Rev. Microbiol.* **2011**, *9*, 344–355. [CrossRef]
44. Janse, J.D.; Obradovic, A. Xylella Fastidiosa: Its Biology, Diagnosis, Control And Risks. *J. Plant Pathol.* **2010**, *92*, S1.35–S1.48.
45. Xin, X.F.; Kvitko, B.; He, S.Y. Pseudomonas syringae: What it takes to be a pathogen. *Nat. Rev. Microbiol.* **2018**, *16*, 316–328. [CrossRef]
46. WIPO. IP and Business: Quality Patents: Claiming what Counts. Available online: https://www.wipo.int/wipo_magazine/en/2006/01/article_0007.html (accessed on 14 February 2019).
47. Schofield, D.A.; Bull, C.T.; Rubio, I.; Wechter, W.P.; Westwater, C.; Molineux, I.J. Development of an engineered bioluminescent reporter phage for detection of bacterial blight of crucifers. *Appl. Environ. Microbiol.* **2012**, *78*, 3592–3598. [CrossRef] [PubMed]
48. Labrie, S.J.; Samson, J.E.; Moineau, S. Bacteriophage resistance mechanisms. *Nat. Rev. Microbiol.* **2010**, *8*, 317–327. [CrossRef] [PubMed]
49. Chan, B.K.; Abedon, S.T.; Loc-Carrillo, C. Phage cocktails and the future of phage therapy. *Future Microbiol.* **2013**, *8*, 769–783. [CrossRef] [PubMed]

8

Criteria for Selecting Suitable Infectious Diseases for Phage Therapy

David R. Harper

Evolution Biotechnologies, Colworth Science Park, Sharnbrook, Bedfordshire MK44 1LZ, UK; drh@evolutionbiotech.com

Abstract: One of the main issues with phage therapy from its earliest days has been the selection of appropriate disease targets. In early work, when the nature of bacteriophages was unknown, many inappropriate targets were selected, including some now known to have no bacterial involvement whatsoever. More recently, with greatly increased understanding of the highly specific nature of bacteriophages and of their mechanisms of action, it has been possible to select indications with an increased chance of a successful therapeutic outcome. The factors to be considered include the characteristics of the infection to be treated, the characteristics of the bacteria involved, and the characteristics of the bacteriophages themselves. At a later stage all of this information then informs trial design and regulatory considerations. Where the work is undertaken towards the development of a commercial product it is also necessary to consider the planned market, protection of intellectual property, and the sourcing of funding to support the work. It is clear that bacteriophages are not a "magic bullet". However, with careful and appropriate selection of a limited set of initial targets, it should be possible to obtain proof of concept for the many elements required for the success of phage therapy. In time, success with these initial targets could then support more widespread use.

Keywords: bacteriophage; therapy; phage therapy; bacterial disease; infection; target selection

---

1. Introduction

When bacteriophages were first used as therapeutic agents from 1919 onwards [1] this was done in the context of an extremely limited knowledge of bacteriophage biology. Given the toxicity of antibacterial agents at the time, which included both mercury and arsenic, there was a clear need for new approaches. Unfortunately, many early uses of phage therapy were driven more by commercial pressures than by science. As a result, bacteriophages were used for a wide variety of indications, many of which had no bacterial component (Figure 1).

Unsurprisingly, with such indications as urticaria and herpes, there was unlikely to be therapeutic benefit due to the effects of bacteriophages. In addition, early bacteriophage preparations contained a large amount of bacterial debris which had a range of immunomodulatory effects, which were considered likely to be responsible for many of the observed clinical effects [2,3]. When data from 100 papers published in the early years of phage therapy was analysed for the American Medical Association, it was concluded that only a very few indications showed good evidence of beneficial effects, with convincing data only for *Staphylococcal* skin disease and some instances of cystitis [2]. With a very limited understanding of the nature of the agent, controversy over its effects, and complications arising from the crude nature of the early therapeutic preparations, it is perhaps unsurprising that phage therapy fell into disuse once chemical antibiotics became widely available. However, as antibiotic resistance changed from an abstract concern to a full-blown crisis [4], interest in phage therapy has been revived [5,6]. This drew on the much greater understanding of bacteriophages resulting from their use during that intervening period in experimental studies, notably in the area of molecular biology.

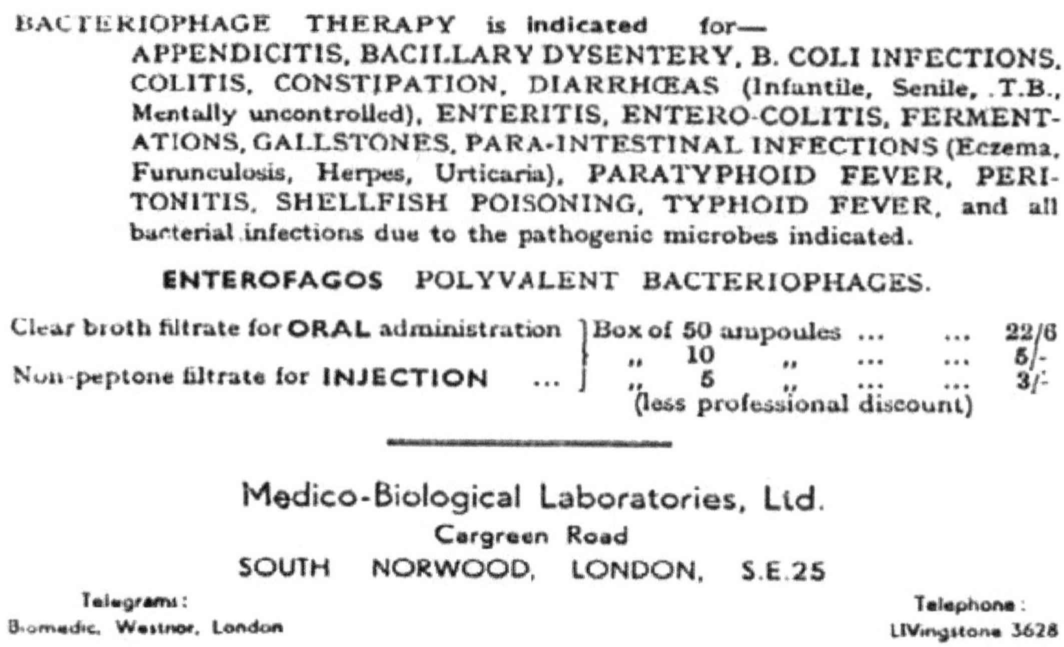

Figure 1. An advertisement for therapeutic bacteriophages from the 1920s (reprinted with the kind permission of Dr. J. Soothill).

With this increased understanding of bacteriophage biology came the opportunity for far more precision in their use [5]. Key properties of bacteriophages that had been clarified by this point included many aspects of their biology, such as their nature as bacterial viruses, their highly specific host requirements, and the molecular processes of infection. Technical advances also allowed the purification of bacteriophages away from bacterial contaminants, including the removal of highly active host cell components such as endotoxins. While we are still a long way from a full understanding of the biology of these complex viruses, we can now build on what we do know to use these unique agents far more effectively.

2. Selection of Therapeutic Approaches

2.1. Clinical Need

When a serious disease cannot be controlled by current therapies there is a need for new approaches. Much of the current interest in phage therapy is driven by concerns over antimicrobial drug resistance, and a working group evaluating a broad range of alternative approaches has concluded that phage therapy is a promising way to counter this issue [7]. There is also some evidence of both natural and engineered bacteriophages driving bacteria towards the loss of existing antibiotic resistance [8–10], suggesting a possible role for combinations of bacteriophages with conventional antibiotics.

The initial motivation for the selection of a therapeutic target is typically that there is an unmet need for control of a bacterial infection—that is, a lack of effective antibacterial approaches for a disease with serious medical or economic consequences. If effective controls exist there is rarely a driver for the development of novel therapies, except perhaps to provide an alternative due to commercial drivers. A therapy can be targeted at infections of humans, animals, or plants; conditions addressed by the use of bacteriophages range from ear infections in humans [11] to rot in harvested potatoes [12]. However, the focus of this article is on therapeutic uses and, thus, on unmet clinical need in humans (and, to an extent, animals). Lack of an effective therapy can arise from multiple factors, including evolved antimicrobial resistance or inherent resistance determinants, such as growth in biofilms [13,14].

Thus, unmet need underpins the development of new therapies and generates funding (whether as grants or commercial investment) that is necessary to undertake such work.

No phage therapy has yet been approved for market by the European Medicines Agency (EMA) in the EU or the Food and Drugs Administration (FDA) in the USA. Until this is achieved, phage therapy remains an experimental approach in these jurisdictions, however accepted it is in some other areas such as Eastern Europe. Thus, it is of critical importance to maximise the risk of success in development efforts, since failures can delay, or even destroy, the prospects for developing such approaches. An example of this is gene therapy, which is only now recovering from some early high-profile setbacks [15].

2.2. Key Elements of the Disease Target

Sufficient unmet need: While individual patients might be in dire need of a particular therapy, there generally need to be enough potential users to justify the costs of development and commercialisation. As an example, many early gene therapy treatments were directed at indications where there were only very small numbers of affected individuals. These "ultra-orphan" targets can help with approval, but the first gene therapy to be approved in Europe, Glybera, targeted a disease which occurs in less than one in a million people and had a consequently high price. The drug was withdrawn five years after launch, having been used just once [16].

Antimicrobial resistance: The driver for much of the interest in phage therapy is antimicrobial resistance, where infections may be largely or even completely resistant to conventional antibiotics. Bacteriophages, with their entirely different modes of action, are unaffected by such resistance. Bacteriophages can and will evolve to counter the evolution of bacteriophage resistance by the target bacteria [17]. Another major cause of resistance to conventional antibiotics is bacterial growth in biofilms, which can decrease bacterial sensitivity to antibiotics by over a thousand-fold [13,14]. Bacteriophages have unique capabilities in attacking bacteria in such a setting by targeting both the biofilm matrix and specialized cells growing within it [14]. Efficacy against biofilms has been demonstrated both in vitro and in vivo [11,14] and has the potential to be a significant driver for the adoption of phage therapy.

Disease results from bacterial infection: It (nowadays) goes without saying that the target for phage therapy should be bacterial in nature. Bacteriophages are highly specific, with only a relatively small number even crossing species boundaries. They are almost completely inert towards other cells. The days when herpes or urticaria could be regarded as a viable target are, fortunately, long gone.

Infection is caused by one type of bacteria or a small number of types: Bacteriophages are often referred to as "exquisitely specific" since most are able to infect and replicate in only a subset of strains within a single bacterial species, meaning that a mixture of bacteriophages (usually referred to as a "cocktail") is usually needed to target even a single bacterial species, though there are exceptions [5,18]. Thus, a polymicrobial infection is poorly suited to phage therapy. This is a very important difference to the historical use of broad spectrum chemical antibiotics. Although some broad spectrum bacteriophage treatments have been used in Eastern Europe, these contain extremely high numbers of relatively undefined bacteriophages, which would make approval by EMA or FDA complex. An early polymicrobial infection may change during treatment with conventional antibiotics, with a much more limited range of bacteria in the later stages of infection [11]. Such infections offer both unmet need (having failed to resolve with conventional treatments) and a limited range of bacterial targets. They are, thus, well suited to phage therapy approaches.

Bacteria causing the infection are identified: Unlike chemical antibiotics, it is unlikely that there will be broad spectrum phage therapeutic cocktails without an extremely complex regulatory process and prohibitive production costs. This is likely to limit first-line use, unless such a treatment is paired with a rapid point-of-care diagnostic test. A simpler approach, at least initially, is to focus on cases where the bacterial target has been identified but is resistant to clearance by existing methods. This was the approach taken in the only phase 2 trial to date to report positive results [11] by targeting late stage ear infections where one bacterial species (*Pseudomonas aeruginosa*) predominates. Additionally, testing must be able to identify and quantify the target bacteria in the intended recipients, both prior to and as part of the trial process.

Bacteria targeted are responsible for the clinical pathology: Given the specificity of bacteriophages, simply removing one component of a polymicrobial infection may not result in a positive clinical outcome. While regulators may accept microbiological endpoints (reduction of target bacterial numbers) in initial trials, in later work, improvement in clinical symptoms is likely to be required for trial success. This has been an issue with some work where positive outcomes were not observed [19].

Potential for useful preclinical work: While in vitro data is useful, good preclinical data derived from in vivo work is extremely useful in making the case for progression into human trials. This can either be from model systems [20,21] or from analogous infections in animals [11,22,23]. Where no suitable system is available, data collection to permit trials is likely to be more complex.

Suitability for clinical trials: Patients must be both available and accessible, in line with current ethical practices. If the patient group requires simultaneous treatment with other antibacterial agents (as is often the case with seriously ill patients, for example, under "expanded access" single patient uses) this can greatly complicate the interpretation of results, reducing the value of the data generated. There are, of course, also many issues relating to the design and conduct of clinical trials, from liaison with regulators to selection of endpoints. However, these fall outside the scope of this article. Nevertheless, it should be noted that even the most promising approach will not succeed with a poorly designed trial.

Site of infection is accessible: Bacteriophages are large nucleoprotein structures in the megadalton to gigadalton range. Chemical antibiotics are far smaller. This can lead to misunderstandings over how best to administer bacteriophages among those more used to existing approaches. Given the simplicity of delivery, attention has been focused on topical administration where it is possible to deliver bacteriophages directly to the infected site [11,22–26]. Unlike conventional antibiotics, bacteriophages are unlikely to be able to cross many barriers within the body with useful levels of efficiency, at least when these barriers are intact. These can be normal elements of the body, such as the gut wall or the blood-brain barrier, or part of the pathology of the infection, such as lung tubercles in tuberculosis [27] or closed comedones in acne [28]. However, the ability of bacteriophages to amplify exponentially from very small initial doses [23] can allow even limited bacteriophage numbers to produce a strong localized therapeutic effect.

Bacterial numbers are sufficient to support amplification: Localised amplification where their target is present is a unique feature of bacteriophages and underlies their proposed use as therapeutics in most cases. However, in order to support such amplification, there needs to be a sufficient supply of susceptible bacteria [29]. While this is more complex in vivo, it is clear that in some applications, particularly those with cleaned or disinfected sites of infection, bacterial densities may be insufficient to rely on in situ phage amplification [26]. Any therapeutic effect would thus be reduced. In contrast, even very low levels of bacteriophage can produce rapid and dramatic effects when bacterial numbers are high [23]. Thus, phage therapy is better suited to high density bacterial infections, which is, again, counterintuitive for those used to conventional antibiotics.

Limitations of oral dosing: Oral dosing is considered highly desirable for conventional antibiotics but is inherently limited for bacteriophages. One issue is the degradation of bacteriophages in the acid environment of the stomach, leading to limited oral bioavailability unless the administered bacteriophages are encapsulated [30] or the stomach acid is neutralized [19]. There is also evidence that bacteria that have established infection within the gut may be poorly accessible to bacteriophages, probably because they are located within the coating of the intestinal walls [31], leaving administered bacteriophages to simply pass by them on their way through.

Issues with systemic delivery: Although there is considerable evidence of efficacy in model systems [20,21], bacteriophages delivered via the circulation are challenged by a number of issues [32].

Both innate and adaptive immunity are major concerns. Bacteriophages are prime candidates for those elements of the innate response intended to provide a first response to invading viruses, notably phagocytosis [33]. In addition, the adaptive immune response will, in time, respond to bacteriophages, particularly after repeated administration. However, the ablative effect of such responses on bacteriophage efficacy appears to be limited [34]. Another major issue is delivery to the site of infection. Although bacteriophages have the unique ability to amplify locally even from a very small initial dose [11,23], they nevertheless have to reach and infect their target bacteria in order to be able to do so. Barriers that can be crossed by conventional antibiotics may be impervious to bacteriophages, favouring topical uses or use in body activities. However, a recent in-depth review of the subject noted bacteriophages as one of the most promising approaches to combating antimicrobial resistance even in systemic applications [7].

3. Bacteriophages

Intellectual property issues: It has long been argued that the patenting of phage therapy approaches is challenging. It is undeniable that the basic approach of phage therapy is firmly in the public domain. However, this is also true for monoclonal antibodies, and these have led to drugs with current market values in the tens of billions of dollars. It is also true that novel bacteriophages can be identified for almost any bacterial target, potentially bypassing patent protection. Again, this is also true for monoclonal antibodies. From a commercial point of view a patent is useful, but not actually essential since the progress of a drug or phage mix through the regulatory process underpins much of its value. However, patent protection is highly desirable, particularly in the early stages of development. There is considerable confusion over the patenting of naturally occurring biological materials [35], but it is clear that bacteriophage mixtures exhibiting activities different from those seen in nature can form the basis for patent awards.

Bacteriophages are available: It should go without saying that the bacteriophages used must be able to target the infecting bacteria, whether as part of a broadly effective cocktail [11] or by selection for the bacterial strain(s) present [36]. While it is thought that bacteriophages exist for all bacteria, they are sometimes hard to find, as with certain members of the *Streptococci* [37]. Alternatively, properties of the host bacteria can make isolation of bacteriophages difficult, as with slow-growing members of the *Mycobacteria*. However, for many bacterial species, isolation can be both rapid and simple.

Bacteriophages are effective in killing the target bacteria: While some bacteriophages cause rapid killing of their host, others do not. Selection of those which produce rapid lysis and liberate large numbers of progeny bacteriophage (high burst size) is usually assessed in vitro. The normal method for this initially is to monitor the formation of plaques, selecting those bacteriophages that form large, clear plaques [38]. Growth in liquid culture, often using plate-based optical density systems, is also used for this purpose.

Bacteriophages must target the bacteria responsible for the infection: Most bacteriophages kill only a subset of strains within a single bacterial species. In order to kill sufficient members of a representative panel of strains of that species (a diversity panel), the activity of individual bacteriophages is tested against that panel and a mixture selected which provides broad coverage. This may be a mixture of broadly effective bacteriophages along with those selected to cover specific strains from a diversity panel, for example those with concerning levels of resistance to conventional antibiotics. While 100% coverage of a large diversity panel is not usually required (for antibiotics or for bacteriophages), there are minimum levels (analogous to those defined for antibiotic development) which need to be attained for a generally applicable therapy. It is also advantageous to ensure that as many strains as possible are targeted by multiple bacteriophages, minimising the potential for resistance.

Cross-resistance: Generation of resistance in vitro may be used to confirm that cross-resistance to candidate therapeutic bacteriophages in a cocktail (implying similar biology of infection) is minimized. This involves the selection of bacteria which do not show similar resistance profiles against bacteriophage-resistant mutants of the target bacteria, and (as with antibiotics) minimizes the potential for the development of resistance in vivo.

Coverage: Isolates from different pathologies and geographic locations must be covered by the bacteriophages selected if a standardized cocktail is to be used [11,19,22,24–26], and this can be difficult to attain with some highly variable bacterial species. An alternative approach, of having a panel of bacteriophages with defined activities, from which personalized cocktails are prepared for individual patients [36,39] faces a number of currently unresolved regulatory challenges, as well as significant resourcing issues.

Bacteriophages are obligately lytic, not temperate: Obligately lytic bacteriophages that infect a permissive host produce rapid killing. The bacterial life cycle is simply "kill or be killed". However, in many cases bacteriophages are temperate. That is, they are capable of entering a latent state within the host bacteria (lysogeny) in which they are usually integrated into the bacterial genome. In such a state, host bacteria are often rendered resistant to superinfection with the same, or even closely related, bacteriophages [40,41]. As and when a lysogenic bacteriophage reactivates, it may carry bacterial genes with it to a new host, a process known as specialized transduction. In addition, it is now becoming clear that lysogenic bacteriophages may modulate genetic activity and actually benefit their bacterial host [40]. Thus, while lysogenic bacteriophages may reduce bacterial numbers both in vitro and in vivo [42], they are generally considered unsuitable for therapeutic use. Traditional tests for lysogeny include the formation of turbid plaques, where the clearance zone is clouded by surviving bacteria. More recently, genetic analysis can identify markers of lysogeny such as the presence in the bacteriophage genome of a functional integrase gene or known repressors linked to the establishment and maintenance of a lysogenic infection state. This then allows exclusion from the development pathway. For some bacteria, such as *Clostridium difficle*, all bacteriophages identified to date appear to be temperate [43], limiting the options for phage therapy in these settings.

Transduction and toxins: As well as the specialized transduction seen in lysogenic infections, bacteriophages can pick up a wide range of segments of bacterial DNA essentially at random and transfer them to a new host. This is considered undesirable in candidate therapeutic bacteriophages since virulence genes could be transferred by this route. In addition, some bacteriophages actually carry such genes, including both antibiotic resistance genes [44] and clinically significant bacterial toxins [45], while others have adapted forms that transfer virulence-associated genes [46]. It is necessary to exclude such bacteriophages from therapeutic development, usually by genetic analysis.

Stability: The most promising therapeutic bacteriophage is of no value if it loses activity too fast before it can be used to treat patients. Assessment of stability in suitable forms for therapeutic use is, thus, a vital part of development [47].

Quality of product: In order to be used as therapeutics, bacteriophages must be able to grow to sufficiently high titres in a suitable bacterial host. Such hosts are often selected for their non-pathogenic nature, including absence of toxins and even of lysogenic bacteriophage genomes. It is however necessary to ensure that the bacteriophages produced by such compliant hosts retain their virulence against target bacteria. Unlike early therapeutic products, it is also necessary to purify bacteriophages away from host bacterial components, in particular the endotoxins produced by Gram-negative bacteria for which strict limits are applied [48,49]. The whole issue of producing bacteriophages to the required standards (as a drug substance) then combining them to make a therapeutic cocktail (i.e., a drug product) while complying with necessary quality control standards (cGMP, except for all but the earliest trials) is both demanding and expensive. However, if such standards cannot be attained, perhaps because of a persistent contaminant, then all of the preceding work has been in vain.

Bacteriophages as biological control agents: Bacteriophages are not chemical antibiotics. Although this statement seems obvious, it has not stopped some groups from assuming that the same processes used in the development of chemical antibiotics must of necessity be applied a priori to therapeutic bacteriophages. While bacteriophages do need to conform with existing rules, the regulators show a significant degree of flexibility, and indeed enthusiasm, in working with these new paradigms [50–53]. This is an area which is likely to see significant changes. However, these will rely on good science and, in particular, on data from fully regulated clinical trials, which are still sparse in this area. One important difference to conventional antibiotics is that bacteriophages are unlikely to produce sterilising effects in vivo since, when bacterial numbers fall below the replication threshold [29], they will lose much of their effect. However, in such situations, lowering bacterial numbers far enough can inhibit their replication [52] and reduce toxin production, thus allowing the immune system of an infected patient to aid in resolving the infection [11,22].

4. Stages of target selection

The following stages need to be considered (see Figure 2):

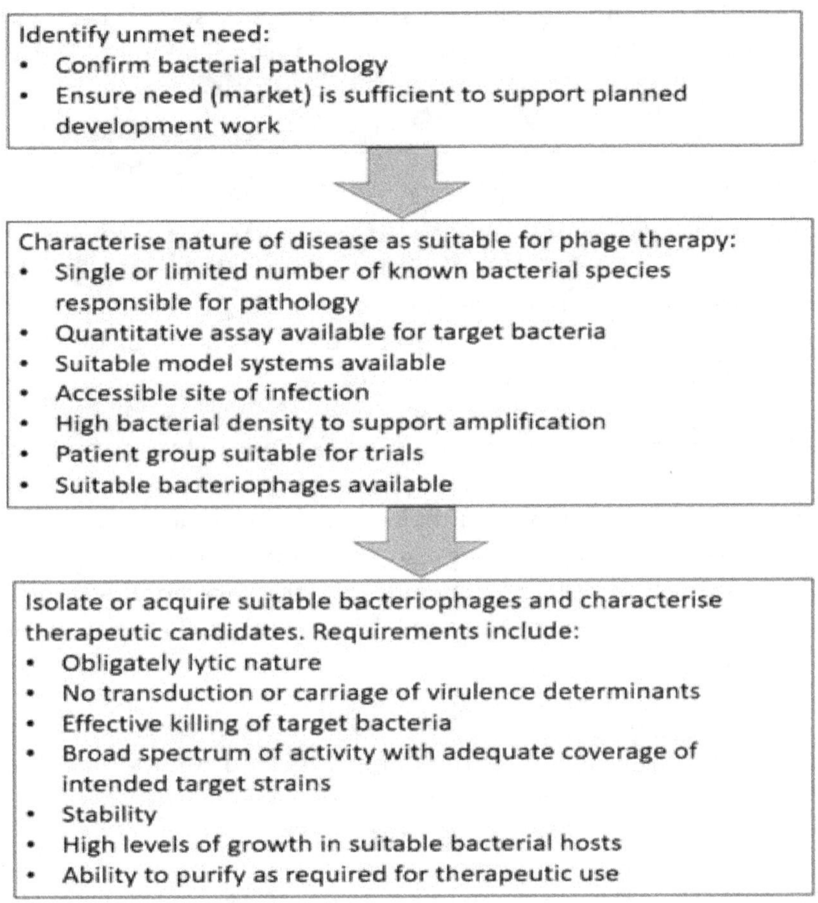

Figure 2. Steps in the selection of an initial target disease for phage therapy.

5. A Worked Example

As an example of the practical application of such considerations, *P. aeruginosa* appears to highly suitable as a phage therapy target, as outlined below and elsewhere [54]. As a result, it is proving a popular target for such intervention [11,22–26]. Indeed, the only successful phase 2 trial reported to date targeted late stage ear infections caused by *P. aeruginosa* [11].

In this study [11] the bacterial pathology had been confirmed both generally and in the specific cases by repeated microbiological assessment. The individual clinical need was severe (aiding patient recruitment and ethical review) and the market need was assessed as sufficient to support development, with the potential for expansion into other types of topical infection thereafter. While ear infections are initially polymicrobial, use of existing therapies that fail to clear the infection typically results in a "late-stage" infection dominated by *P. aeruginosa*, which was assessed prior to trial entry. A suitable trial centre was identified with strong clinical expertise, at which patients were accessible and willing to participate. *P. aeruginosa* is relatively simple to culture and to enumerate, and a previous veterinary field trial [22,55] had provided useful preclinical data. The ear is accessible, allowing direct application of bacteriophage onto the infected site, and had a high density of *P. aeruginosa* (2.3×10^6 to 4.5×10^{10} CFU/gram at the start of the trial, averaging well over 10^9 CFU/gram) [11]. Bacteriophages specific for *P. aeruginosa* are relatively widespread and simple to isolate from available sources [54]. Obligately lytic forms are common, showing rapid bacterial killing and releasing high numbers of progeny bacteriophages. Levels of transduction or toxin carriage are low, and broad activity of bacteriophages against *P. aeruginosa* is obtainable. The bacteriophages could be grown in culture to the required level and purified from such cultures. Though the presence of endotoxins in lysate of Gram-negative bacteria such as *P. aeruginosa* does require careful consideration of levels remaining in a candidate therapy, the low dosing levels used in the study (a single input dose of 2.4 ng) aided in this. With due consideration given to the above elements, the phase 1/2 clinical trial was conducted (albeit at a small scale) [11] and, uniquely to date, produced promising and positive results.

6. Summary

Phage therapy remains experimental in both human and veterinary medicine. With antibiotic resistance now acknowledged as a worldwide crisis [4], the need for new approaches to antibacterial therapy makes the development of this powerful approach a priority. Despite this, there is a real shortage of high quality clinical work on which to base progression of phage therapy through the regulatory approvals required to permit widespread use.

The selection of appropriate disease targets is an essential step in progressing this important technology. Trial failures are expensive in both time and resources and benefit nobody. Such failures carry the risk of causing serious damage to confidence in the field as a whole [15]. In order to maximise the chances of success, the selection of disease targets must be informed by sound knowledge of the disease to be treated, of the infecting bacteria, and of the nature and interactions of the bacteriophages to be used. Success against carefully selected initial targets is required to build the confidence to allow later work in more challenging applications

Based on the work to date, while it seems likely that bacteriophages will be used systemically and even orally in time, topical treatments where the bacteriophage can be placed onto an infection site with a high bacterial density offer the best chance of success. Such success is vital to moving phage therapy into clinical use, to save lives, and to improve lives.

Acknowledgments: The author would like to thank Ben Burrowes for his helpful comments on the manuscript.

References

1. D'Herelle, F. Sur le role du microbe bacteriophage dans la typhose aviare. *Comptes Rendus de l'Académie des Sciences Paris* **1919**, *169*, 932–934.
2. Eaton, M.D.; Bayne-Jones, S. Bacteriophage therapy: Review of the principles and results of the use of bacteriophage in the treatment of infections. *JAMA* **1934**, *103*, 1769–1776, 1847–1853, 1934–1939. [CrossRef]
3. Krueger, A.P.; Scribner, E.J. The bacteriophage: Its nature and its therapeutic use. *JAMA* **1941**, *116*, 2160–2167. [CrossRef]
4. Chan, M. WHO Director-General briefs UN on Antimicrobial Resistance. 2016. Available online: http://www.who.int/dg/speeches/2016/antimicrobial-resistance-un/en/ (accessed on 9 March 2018).
5. Harper, D.R.; Burrowes, B.H.; Kutter, E.M. Bacteriophage: Therapeutic Uses. In *Encyclopedia of Life Sciences*; John Wiley and Sons: Chichester, UK, 2014.

6. Harper, D.; Abedon, S.; Burrowes, B.; McConville, M. (Eds.) *Bacteriophgages: Biology, Technology, Therapy*; Springer: Cham, Switzerland, 2018; ISBN 978-3-319-40598-8. Available online: https://link.springer.com/referencework/10.1007/978-3-319-40598-8#about (accessed on 9 March 2018).
7. Czaplewski, L.; Bax, R.; Clokie, M.; Dawson, M.; Fairhead, H.; Fischetti, V.A.; Foster, S.; Gilmore, B.F.; Hancock, R.E.; Harper, D.; et al. Alternatives to antibiotics—A pipeline portfolio review. *Lancet Infect. Dis.* **2016**, *16*, 239–251. [CrossRef]
8. Hagens, S.; Habel, A.; Bläsi, U. Augmentation of the Antimicrobial Efficacy of Antibiotics by Filamentous Phage. *Microb. Drug Resist.* **2006**, *12*, 164–168. [CrossRef] [PubMed]
9. Chan, B.K.; Sistrom, M.; Wertz, J.E.; Kortright, K.E.; Narayan, D.; Turner, P.E. Phage selection restores antibiotic sensitivity in MDR Pseudomonas aeruginosa. *Sci. Rep.* **2016**, *6*, 26717. [CrossRef] [PubMed]
10. Lu, T.K.; Collins, J.J. Engineered bacteriophage targeting gene networks as adjuvants for antibiotic therapy. *PNAS* **2009**, *106*, 4629–4634. [CrossRef] [PubMed]
11. Wright, A.; Hawkins, C.; Änggård, E.; Harper, D.A. Controlled clinical trial of a therapeutic bacteriophage in chronic otitis due to antibiotic-resistant *Pseudomonas aeruginosa;* A preliminary report of efficacy. *Clin. Otolaryngol.* **2009**, *34*, 349–357. [CrossRef] [PubMed]
12. Blackwell, A. The Potential for Bacteriophage to Control Soft Rot Development in Store. Available online: https://potatoes.ahdb.org.uk/sites/default/files/publication_upload/APS%20Biocontrol%20Ltd.pdfDevelopmentDevelopment (accessed on 9 March 2018).
13. Ceri, H.; Olson, M.E.; Stremick, C.; Read, R.R.; Morck, D.; Buret, A. The Calgary biofilm device: New technology for rapid determination of antibiotic susceptibilities of bacterial biofilms. *J. Clin. Microbiol.* **1999**, *37*, 1771–1776. [PubMed]
14. Harper, D.R.; Parracho, H.M.; Walker, J.; Sharp, R.; Hughes, G.; Werthén, M.; Lehman, S.; Morales, S. Bacteriophages and biofilms. *Antibiotics* **2014**, *3*, 270–284. [CrossRef]
15. Kumar, S.R.; Markusic, D.M.; Biswas, M.; High, K.A.; Herzog, R.W. Clinical development of gene therapy: Results and lessons from recent successes. *Mol. Ther. Methods Clin. Dev.* **2016**, *3*, 16034. [CrossRef] [PubMed]
16. FiercePharma. With Its Launch Fizzling Out, UniQure Gives Up on $1M+ Gene Therapy Glybera. Available online: https://www.fiercepharma.com/pharma/uniqure-gives-up-1m-gene-therapy-glybera (accessed on 9 March 2018).
17. Brockhurst, M.A.; Koskella, B.; Zhang, Q.G. Bacteria-Phage Antagonistic Coevolution and the Implications for Phage Therapy. In *Bacteriophages: Biology, Technology, Therapy*; Harper, D., Abedon, S., Burrowes, B., McConville, M., Eds.; Springer Nature: Cham, Switzerland, 2017.
18. Sillankorva, S.M.; Oliveira, H.; Azeredo, J. Bacteriophages and Their Role in Food Safety. *Int. J. Microbiol.*, **2012**, *2012*, 863945. [CrossRef] [PubMed]
19. Sarker, S.A.; Sultana, S.; Reuteler, G.; Moine, D.; Descombes, P.; Charton, F.; Bourdin, G.; McCallin, S.; Ngom-Bru, C.; Neville, T.; et al. Oral Phage Therapy of Acute Bacterial Diarrhea with Two Coliphage Preparations: A Randomized Trial in Children From Bangladesh. *EBioMedicine* **2016**, *4*, 124–137. [CrossRef] [PubMed]
20. Soothill, J.S. Treatment of experimental infections of mice with bacteriophages. *J. Med. Microbiol.* **1992**, *37*, 258–261. [CrossRef] [PubMed]
21. Watanabe, R.; Matsumoto, T.; Sano, G.; Ishii, Y.; Tateda, K.; Sumiyama, Y.; Uchiyama, J.; Sakurai, S.; Matsuzaki, S.; Imai, S. Efficacy of bacteriophage therapy against gut-derived sepsis caused by Pseudomonas aeruginosa in mice. *Antimicrob. Agents Chemother.* **2007**, *51*, 446–452. [CrossRef] [PubMed]
22. Hawkins, C.; Harper, D.; Burch, D.; Änggård, E.; Soothill, J. Topical treatment of *Pseudomonas aeruginosa* otitis of dogs with a bacteriophage mixture: A before/after clinical trial. *Vet. Microbiol.* **2010**, *146*, 309–313. [CrossRef] [PubMed]
23. Marza, J.A.; Soothill, J.S.; Boydell, P.; Collyns, T.A. Multiplication of therapeutically administered bacteriophages in *Pseudomonas aeruginosa* infected patients. *Burns* **2006**, *32*, 644–646. [CrossRef] [PubMed]
24. Phagoburn. Available online: http://www.phagoburn.eu/ (accessed on 9 March 2018).
25. Rhoads, D.D.; Wolcott, R.D.; Kuskowski, M.A.; Wolcott, B.M.; Ward, L.S.; Sulakvelidze, A. Bacteriophage therapy of venous leg ulcers in humans: Results of a phase I safety trial. *J. Wound Care* **2009**, *18*, 237–243. [CrossRef] [PubMed]

26. Rose, T.; Verbeken, G.; De Vos, D.; Merabishvili, M.; Vaneechoutte, M.; Lavigne, R.; Jennes, S.; Zizi, M.; Pirnay, J.P. Experimental phage therapy of burn wound infection: Difficult first steps. *Int. J. Burns Trauma* **2014**, *4*, 66–73. [PubMed]
27. Cole, S.T.; Eisenach, K.D.; McMurray, D.N.; Jacobs, W.R. (Eds.) *Tuberculosis and the Tubercle Bacillus*; ASM Press: Washington, DC, USA, 2005; ISBN 1-55581-295-3.
28. PubMed Health. Closed Comedones. Available online: https://www.ncbi.nlm.nih.gov/pubmedhealth/PMHT0025363/ (accessed on 9 March 2018).
29. Payne, R.J.H.; Vincent, A.A. Evidence for a Phage Proliferation Threshold? *J. Virol.* **2002**, *76*, 13123–13124. [CrossRef] [PubMed]
30. Vinner, G.K.; Vladisavljević, G.T.; Clokie, M.R.J.; Malik, D.J. Microencapsulation of Clostridium difficile specific bacteriophages using microfluidic glass capillary devices for colon delivery using pH triggered release. *PLoS ONE* **2017**, *12*, e0186239. [CrossRef] [PubMed]
31. Chibani-Chennoufi, S.; Sidoti, J.; Bruttin, A.; Kutter, E.; Sarker, S.; Brüssow, H. In vitro and in vivo bacteriolytic activities of *Escherichia coli* phages: Implications for phage therapy. *Antimicrob. Agents Chemother.* **2004**, *48*, 2558–2569. [CrossRef] [PubMed]
32. Ryan, E.M.; Gorman, S.P.; Donnelly, R.F.; Gilmore, B.F. Recent advances in bacteriophage therapy: How delivery routes, formulation, concentration and timing influence the success of phage therapy. *J. Pharm. Pharmacol.* **2011**, *63*, 1253–1264. [CrossRef] [PubMed]
33. Jończyk-Matysiak, E.; Weber-Dąbrowska, B.; Owczarek, B.; Międzybrodzki, R.; Łusiak-Szelachowska, M.; Łodej, N.; Górski, A. Phage-Phagocyte Interactions and Their Implications for Phage Application as Therapeutics. *Viruses* **2017**, *9*, 150. [CrossRef] [PubMed]
34. Łusiak-Szelachowska, M.; Żaczek, M.; Weber-Dąbrowska, B.; Międzybrodzki, R.M.; Letkiewicz, S.; Fortuna, W.; Rogóż, P.; Szufnarowski, K.; Jończyk-Matysiak, E.; Olchawa, E.; et al. Antiphage activity of sera during phage therapy in relation to its outcome. *Future Microbiol.* **2017**, *12*, 109–117.
35. Ledford, H. Myriad ruling causes confusion. *Nature* **2013**, *498*, 281–282. [CrossRef] [PubMed]
36. Schooley, R.T.; Biswas, B.; Gill, J.J.; Hernandez-Morales, A.; Lancaster, J.; Lessor, L.; Barr, J.J.; Reed, S.L.; Rohwer, F.; Benler, S.; et al. Development and Use of Personalized Bacteriophage-Based Therapeutic Cocktails to Treat a Patient with a Disseminated Resistant Acinetobacter baumannii Infection. *Antimicrob. Agents Chemother.* **2017**, *61*, e00954-17. [CrossRef] [PubMed]
37. Dalmasso, M.; de Haas, E.; Neve, H. Isolation of a Novel Phage with Activity against Streptococcus mutans Biofilms. *PLoS ONE* **2015**, *10*, e0138651. [CrossRef] [PubMed]
38. Abedon, S.T.; Thomas-Abedon, C. Phage therapy pharmacology. *Curr. Pharm. Biotechnol.* **2010**, *11*, 28–47. [CrossRef] [PubMed]
39. Pirnay, J.P.; De Vos, D.; Verbeken, G.; Merabishvili, M.; Chanishvili, N.; Vaneechoutte, M.; Zizi, M.; Laire, G.; Lavigne, R.; Huys, I.; et al. The phage therapy paradigm: Prêt-à-porter or sur-mesure? *Pharm. Res.* **2011**, *28*, 934–937. [CrossRef] [PubMed]
40. Feiner, R.; Argov, T.; Rabinovich, L.; Sigal, N.; Borovok, I.; Herskovits, A.A. A new perspective on lysogeny: Prophages as active regulatory switches of bacteria. *Nat. Rev. Microbiol.* **2015**, *13*, 641–650. [CrossRef] [PubMed]
41. Hyman, P.; Abedon, S.T. Bacteriophage host range and bacterial resistance. *Adv. Appl. Microbiol.* **2010**, *70*, 217–248. [PubMed]
42. Nale, J.Y.; Spencer, J.; Hargreaves, K.R.; Buckley, A.M.; Trzepiński, P.; Douce, G.R.; Clokie, M.R. Bacteriophage Combinations Significantly Reduce Clostridium difficile Growth in Vitro and Proliferation in Vivo. *Antimicrob. Agents Chemother.* **2015**, *60*, 968–981. [CrossRef] [PubMed]
43. Hargreaves, K.R.; Clokie, M.R. Clostridium difficile phages: Still difficult? *Front. Microbiol.* **2014**, *28*, 184. [CrossRef] [PubMed]
44. Colavecchio, A.; Cadieux, B.; Lo, A.; Goodridge, L.D. Bacteriophages Contribute to the Spread of Antibiotic Resistance Genes among Foodborne Pathogens of the *Enterobacteriaceae* Family—A Review. *Front. Microbiol.* **2017**, *20*, 1108. [CrossRef] [PubMed]
45. Strauch, E.; Lurz, R.; Beutin, L. Characterization of a Shiga toxin-encoding temperate bacteriophage of Shigella sonnei. *Infect. Immun.* **2001**, *69*, 7588–7595. [CrossRef] [PubMed]
46. Christie, G.E.; Dokland, T. Pirates of the Caudovirales. *Virology* **2012**, *434*, 210–221. [CrossRef] [PubMed]

47. Ackermann, H.-W.; Tremblay, D.; Moineau, S. Long-term bacteriophage preservation. *W.F.C.C. Newsl.* **2004**, *38*, 35–40.
48. European Pharmacopoeia Online. Available online: http://online.edqm.eu/EN/entry.htm (accessed on 9 March 2018).
49. USP-NF. Available online: http://www.uspnf.com/?_ga=2.80419031.1739394632.1520820978-1625466886.1520820978 (accessed on 9 March 2018).
50. Verbeken, G.; Pirnay, J.P.; De Vos, D.; Jennes, S.; Zizi, M.; Lavigne, R.; Casteels, M.; Huys, I. Optimizing the European regulatory framework for sustainable bacteriophage therapy in human medicine. *Arch. Immunol. Ther. Exp. (Warsz.)* **2012**, *60*, 161–172. [CrossRef] [PubMed]
51. Verbeken, G.; Pirnay, J.P.; Lavigne, R.; Jennes, S.; De Vos, D.; Casteels, M.; Huys, I. Call for a dedicated European legal framework for bacteriophage therapy. *Arch. Immunol. Ther. Exp. (Warsz.)* **2014**, *62*, 117–129. [CrossRef] [PubMed]
52. Huys, I.; Pirnay, J.P.; Lavigne, R.; Jennes, S.; De Vos, D.; Casteels, M.; Verbeken, G. Paving a regulatory pathway for phage therapy. Europe should muster the resources to financially, technically and legally support the introduction of phage therapy. *EMBO Rep.* **2013**, *14*, 951–954. [CrossRef] [PubMed]
53. Defoirdt, T. Quorum-Sensing Systems as Targets for Antivirulence Therapy. *Trends Microbiol.* **2017**, *26*, 313–328. [CrossRef] [PubMed]
54. Harper, D.R.; Enright, M.C. Bacteriophages for the treatment of Pseudomonas aeruginosa infections. *J. Appl. Microbiol.* **2010**, *111*, 1–7. [CrossRef] [PubMed]
55. Soothill, J.S.; Hawkins, C.; Anggard, E.A.; Harper, D.R. Therapeutic use of bacteriophages (letter). *Lancet Infect. Dis.* **2004**, *4*, 544–545. [CrossRef]

9

The Magistral Phage

Jean-Paul Pirnay [1,*], Gilbert Verbeken [1], Pieter-Jan Ceyssens [2], Isabelle Huys [3], Daniel De Vos [1], Charlotte Ameloot [4] and Alan Fauconnier [4,5]

1 Laboratory for Molecular and Cellular Technology, Queen Astrid Military Hospital, Bruynstraat 1, 1120 Brussel, Belgium; gilbert.verbeken@mil.be (G.V.); danielmarie.devos@mil.be (D.D.V.)
2 Bacterial Diseases, Unit Antibiotic Resistance, Scientific Institute of Public Health, Rue Engelandstraat 642, 1180 Brussel, Belgium; pieterjan.ceyssens@wiv-isp.be
3 Department of Pharmaceutical and Pharmacological Sciences, KU Leuven, O&N2, Herestraat 49, Box 521, 3000 Leuven, Belgium; isabelle.huys@pharm.kuleuven.be
4 Federal Agency for Medicines and Health Products, Place Victor Horta 40/40, 1060 Brussels, Belgium; charlotte.ameloot@fagg-afmps.be (C.A.); alan.fauconnier@invivo.be (A.F.)
5 Culture In Vivo ASBL, rue du Progrès, 4, boîte 7, 1400 Nivelles, Belgium
* Correspondence: jean-paul.pirnay@mil.be

Abstract: Since time immemorial, phages—the viral parasites of bacteria—have been protecting Earth's biosphere against bacterial overgrowth. Today, phages could help address the antibiotic resistance crisis that affects all of society. The greatest hurdle to the introduction of phage therapy in Western medicine is the lack of an appropriate legal and regulatory framework. Belgium is now implementing a pragmatic phage therapy framework that centers on the magistral preparation (compounding pharmacy in the US) of tailor-made phage medicines.

Keywords: antibiotic; antimicrobial resistance; magistral preparation; compounding pharmacy; phage therapy; regulatory framework; personalized medicine

---

1. The Age of the Superbug

On 21 September 2016, the UN General Assembly convened a meeting on antimicrobial resistance (AMR) at the UN headquarters in New York. It was only the fourth time the General Assembly addressed a health emergency. This high-level meeting resulted in a UN resolution focused on combatting the AMR health threat. World leaders acknowledged that global AMR poses a fundamental long-term threat to human health, the production of food, and sustainable development. Based on scenarios of rising drug resistance for six pathogens, experts estimated that by 2050 the burden of AMR could rise to 10 million people dying every year and an economic cost of $100 trillion [1].

Commercial antibiotics that are currently used in public health, animal, food, agriculture and aquaculture sectors, are immutable chemicals that are based on natural antibiotics produced by soil bacteria or fungi to—depending on their concentration—either combat competitors, communicate with other organisms, or act as pleiotropic effectors of metabolic pathways. It was, therefore, to be expected that bacteria would be extremely proficient at evolving resistance to such antibiotics, especially when these are excessively and often unnecessarily used. Selective pressures imposed by humans have resulted in the emergence of "superbugs", or bacteria that are resistant to virtually all commercial antibiotics. Experts fear that society could return to a pre-antibiotic era, when simple infections could wipe out entire populations and surgical interventions were life threatening. Today, it seems that all "easy" antibiotics have been exploited and industry has been reluctant to put new efforts into the discovery and development of new classes of antibiotics. These are expensive to develop and are bound to offer a poor return on investment as they are only taken for a short period and their use is likely to be restricted in the future.

Therefore, the UN committed to work at national, regional and global levels to support the development of new antimicrobial agents and therapies [2].

2. Phage Therapy

One of the promising "new" treatments that is increasingly highlighted—*inter alia* during the recent UN General Assembly—is phage therapy, the therapeutic use of bacteriophages (phages in short)—the viruses of bacteria—to treat bacterial infections [3]. Since time immemorial, phages control their hosts, the bacteria, on our planet. When discovered in the early twentieth century, they were immediately applied in medicine. It soon appeared that phages are exquisitely host-specific. Most phages can only lyse a subset of a bacterial species. Physicians must thus first know which bacteria cause the infections before they can treat the patients.

As could be expected, it was shown that bacteria could also evolve to evade phage infection, even when potent phages are applied simultaneously [4]. However, the main advantage of phages over antibiotics is their ability to mutate at least as fast as their hosts, enabling them to evolve new infectivity and thus regain the "upper hand" over bacteria. Bacteria and phage are thus involved in a continuous arms race of co-evolving infectivity and defense mechanisms.

The advent of broad-spectrum antibiotics, which target a wide range of bacterial infections and could thus be used empirically, heralded the decline of phage therapy in the Western world. The success stories of the many phage applications in the past, mainly on the east side of the Iron Curtain, where phage therapy remained an established treatment, together with the increasing number of virtually untreatable bacterial infections, has created a growing demand for phage therapy. Some successful intravenous applications of phages to treat terminally ill patients in the Western world have recently been published in the scientific literature [5,6].

The Promise of the Phage Therapy Medicinal Product

At their reintroduction in the Western world, phage preparations were classified as medicinal products (European Union) or drugs (US), based on the literal implementation of definitions. Namely, any substance presented as having properties for treating or preventing disease in human beings is considered to be a medicinal product or a drug. As a result, a large body of costly and time-consuming requirements and procedures for manufacturing and for obtaining marketing authorization for medicinal products (drugs in the US) for human use were imposed on phage therapy medicinal products (PTMPs).

On the one hand, it turns out that the established pharmaceutical industry is not interested in PTMPs, mainly because of limitations in intellectual property protection of natural entities such as genes or phages and because of phage specificity and bacterial resistance issues, which compromise widespread and long-term use of immutable pre-defined PTMPs. On the other hand, it is becoming clear that medicinal product provisions, which were originally developed to cater for widely used and mass-produced chemical molecules such as aspirin and antibiotics, are not compatible with sustainable (non-empirical) or customized phage therapy approaches in which phages need to be selected and produced ad hoc [7]. Pre-defined PTMPs, could make it through the medicinal product funnel, but such preparations are less flexible to deal with changes in the incidences of infecting bacterial species in certain settings or geographical areas, or with the emergence of mutated bacterial strains. The long-term use of immutable PTMPs is also bound to elicit considerable bacterial phage resistance, although not much is known about the rate at which this would occur in clinical settings. Overall, the efficacy of PTMPs is likely to decrease over time and they would need to be regularly adapted and re-approved for use.

Some of these issues crystallized during PhagoBurn (www.phagoburn.eu), the first major trial under modern medicinal product regulatory standards in the European Union [8]. Cocktails of 12 and 13 phages were needed to ensure a certain activity against a collection of *Pseudomonas aeruginosa* and *E. coli* isolates, respectively. Manufacturing of one batch of the investigational products ended up taking

20 months and the largest part of the study budget. In addition, phage specificity issues hampered the recruitment of patients. Because each of the two study products, which couldn't be applied simultaneously, targeted only one of the multiple bacterial species that are known to (simultaneously) infect or colonize burn wounds, physicians were reluctant to include patients [8]. Regardless of the final clinical outcome of PhagoBurn, the preliminary phase of the study showed at least that dedicated and realistic production and documentation requirements are urgently needed to enable the timely supply of secure phage preparations. This would enable clinicians to conduct the desperately needed safety and efficacy studies and to deal with urgent individual or local infection issues or public health threats (e.g., the 2011 *E. coli* O104:H4 outbreak in Germany).

Meanwhile, sporadic phage applications are carried out in the West, often under the umbrella of Article 37 (Unproven Interventions in Clinical Practice) of the Declaration of Helsinki (www.wma.net). In addition, several European and US patients suffering from chronic, extremely resistant or difficult to treat bacterial infections are known to have travelled to a phage therapy center in Tbilisi, Georgia (www.eliavaphagetherapy.com, www.phagetherapycenter.com), for treatment.

3. Enter the Magistral Phage

On 5 July 2016, during a meeting of the Belgian Chamber of Representatives and in response to two parliamentary questions related to the implementation of phage therapy [9], the Belgian Minister of Social Affairs and Public Health acknowledged that phage therapy has no specific regulation in Europe and that there is a consensus that phage preparations are medicinal products. However, according to the Minister it is difficult to determine whether we should deal with industrially-prepared medicinal products or rather with magistral preparations, the former being subject to constraints related to their production and marketing authorization, unlike the latter.

3.1. Magistral Preparations

In European and Belgian law, the notion of a magistral preparation (compounded prescription drug product in the US) is defined as "any medicinal product prepared in a pharmacy in accordance with a medical prescription for an individual patient" (Article 3 of Directive 2001/83 and Article 6 quater, § 3 of the Law of 25 March 1964). Magistral preparations are mixed from their constituent ingredients by a pharmacist (or at least under his/her supervision), for a given patient according to a prescription by a physician and following the technical and scientific standards of the pharmaceutical art. The magistral formula is a practical way for a medical doctor to personalize patient treatments to specific needs and to make medications available that do not exist commercially. Some medicines, such as natural hormone combination products and allergens, are not produced by commercial manufacturers because they lack patent protection and hence return on investment for pharmaceutical companies, but are actually delivered as magistral preparations. Owing to the emergence of innovative medicines for rare diseases or for personalized therapies, magistral preparations are increasingly in demand.

3.2. The Belgian Magistral Phage Medicine Strategy

The Community code leaves the door open for some flexibility to implement certain national solutions relating to medicines for human use [10]. As such, the Belgian Minister of Public Health asked the Federal Agency for Medicines and Health Products (FAMHP, the Belgian competent authority for medicines) to help set up a national strategy for magistral phage medicines. In general, active ingredients of magistral preparations must meet the requirements of the European Pharmacopoeia, of the Belgian Pharmacopoeia or of an official pharmacopoeia [10]. If no such document exists, then the active ingredients must be authorized by the Minister of Public Health, following a favorable opinion of the national Pharmacopoeia Commission [10]. In addition, non-authorized ingredients may also be used in magistral preparations, providing that they are accompanied by a certificate of analysis issued by a Belgian Approved Laboratory [10]. The so-called "Belgian Approved Laboratories" are quality control laboratories which are granted an accreditation by the Belgian regulatory authorities. This status allows them to perform the batch release testing of medicinal products. This national accreditation is equivalent to—and gradually replaced by—the GMP certification for the batch release testing of medicinal products. Belgian Approved Laboratories can be either private (e.g., subcontractor of the pharmaceutical industry) or partially or entirely public (e.g., academic laboratories and scientific institutes). Some of them belong to the European Official Medicines Control Laboratories (OMCL) network, which is made up of independent public laboratories that have been appointed by their respective national authority.

The option of the "non-authorized ingredient" was chosen in this case because of the enormous variety of phages that could qualify as active ingredients and should then, each individually, obtain an authorization issued by the Minister of Public Health [9]. The Scientific Institute of Public Health was identified as a suitable Belgian Approved Laboratory for issuing valid certificates of analysis for batches of phage active ingredients. Although the standard procedure for unauthorized active ingredients only involves the medical doctor, his patient, the manufacturer of the active substances, the approved laboratory and the pharmacist, it was decided—in joint consultation and because of the innovative and very specific character of phage therapy—to involve the FAMHP in the elaboration of a Belgian magistral phage medicine procedure.

In practice, and to consolidate the opening left by the Minister of Public Health, a formal question and answer session was initiated between the military hospital and the FAMHP within the context of the existing national Scientific-Technical Advice (STA) procedure. On 26 October 2016, it was formally agreed that natural phages whose derivative finished products are not fully compliant with the requirements relating to medicinal products for human use (Directive 2001/83), and for which there is no monograph in an official pharmacopoeia, can be processed by a pharmacist as active pharmaceutical ingredients (APIs) in magistral preparations, providing compliance to a number of logical provisions:

- Phages should be delivered in the form of a magistral preparation to a specific (nominal) patient.
- Magistral preparations should always be delivered under the direct responsibility of a medical doctor and a pharmacist.
- The relevant characteristics and qualities of the phage APIs should be defined in an internal monograph (prepared by the supplier).
- Before the pharmacist can use the unlicensed material, he/she must ascertain—based on certificates of analysis issued by a Belgian Approved Laboratory—that the raw materials conform to the provisions of the internal monograph.
- Even if not legally required, it is recommended that the supplier submits the monograph for assessment by the FAMHP.

The general concept of the Belgian magistral phage medicine strategy is depicted in Figure 1. A single characterized phage seed lot is selected from a phage bank. To prevent the unwanted drift of properties resulting from repeated subcultures, the production of medicines obtained by microbial culture is best based on a system of banked master and working seed lots. From this phage seed lot, a phage API is produced according to a monograph. A Belgian Approved Laboratory performs External Quality Assessments to evaluate the API's properties and quality. Each batch of these phage APIs will have a batch record, which describes the production process for that batch in detail. Phage APIs can be produced by both private companies and public institutions. The phage API, accompanied by its batch record protocol and the results of the External Quality Assessments, is then transferred to the hospital pharmacy for possible incorporation in magistral formulas. Ideally, active phage APIs are selected against the target bacteria. In comparison to an antibiogram (to test antibiotic sensitivity), as it were, a "phagogram" is performed. Today, no formal guidelines exist with regard to the clinical use (e.g., medical indications, formulations and posology) of magistral phage medicines. However, it is the intention to draft these guidelines as quickly as possible, at the Belgian level and possibly at the European level.

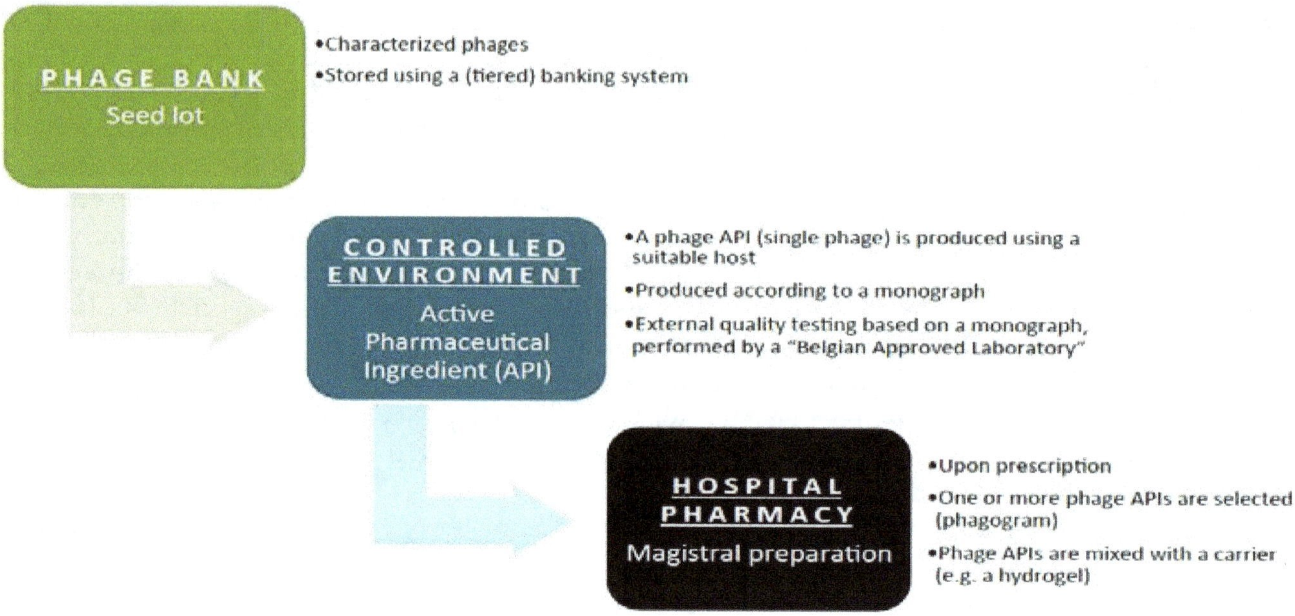

Figure 1. General flowchart of the magistral phage medicine process.

3.3. *Phage API Monograph*

Next, experts of the Queen Astrid military hospital in Brussels, the FAMHP and the Belgian Scientific Institute of Public Health elaborated a pragmatic supplier monograph for phage APIs with a limited use (to hospital pharmacies) status. This document was conceived as a general (applicable to most phages) and evolving document. On 10 January 2018, version 1.0 of the monograph (Supplementary Document 1) received a formal positive advice by the FAMHP.

3.4. *Pricing and Reimbursement*

In terms of pricing, the total cost of a magistral preparation is a reflection of the costs for the products in the preparation, eventually the costs of the prescribed excipients or recipients and an honorarium for the pharmacist for the magistral preparation. Reimbursement of a magistral preparation in Belgium is subject to several criteria: (1) the pharmacist receives a prescription from a physician; (2) this pharmacist makes the magistral preparation and delivers it; (3) products in the magistral preparation are listed on a predefined list of products eligible for reimbursement; and (4) the conditions for reimbursement need to be respected. Bacteriophages are at the moment not listed as products eligible for reimbursement. Therefore, depending on the ultimate price set for a phage magistral preparation, this might (or not) influence the access of phage therapy to patients.

4. Conclusions

It seems to be a matter of time before phage therapy regains its status as an established antibacterial tool. However, this will not only depend on the credibility of "phage researchers", but also on the political context in which they are working. Phage therapy is not sustainable without reimbursement of the researchers providing the therapeutic phages, and so far, phage research is underfunded. Just as drug companies are allowed to profit for some time after developing a drug, there must be some form of compensation for the investigators isolating, characterizing, and optimizing the phages that will be included in future therapeutic phage banks, all before a pharmacist gains access to them for combination. Phage researchers should not be expected to automatically be "altruists", and compensation must be given for their efforts at developing phage therapy as a medicine.

Believing that Belgium could do some pioneering work in the phage therapy field, the Belgian Minister of Public Health and the FAMHP opened the door to phage medicines that take into account the unique characteristics of phages and the need for personalized "sur-mesure" and sustainable phage therapy approaches [7]. There is every reason to believe that the resulting Belgian "magistral phage medicine" framework will be flexible enough to exploit and further explore the specific nature of phages as co-evolving antibacterials whilst giving precedence to patients' safety. Importantly, this Belgian solution avoids the application of certain medicinal product requirements that restrain flexible phage therapy approaches, such as compliance to Good Manufacturing Practice (GMP). There are indications that other (EU) countries might also adopt this phage therapy framework in the near future, in anticipation of a European solution. Recently, the biological master file concept was put forward as a European solution to overcome the regulatory challenges of personalized medicines in general and phage medicines more specifically [11].

Author Contributions: Jean-Paul Pirnay, Gilbert Verbeken, Pieter-Jan Ceyssens, Isabelle Huys, Daniel De Vos, Charlotte Ameloot and Alan Fauconnier contributed to the conception and writing of this paper.

References

1. Tackling Drug-Resistant Infections Globally: Final Report and Recommendations. The Review on Antimicrobial Resistance. 2016 Release. Available online: https://amr-review.org/sites/default/files/160525_Final%20paper_with%20cover.pdf (accessed on 4 February 2018).
2. United Nations. Draft Political Declaration of the High-Level Meeting of the General Assembly on Antimicrobial Resistance (16-16108 (E)). 2016 Release. Available online: http://www.un.org/pga/71/wp-content/uploads/sites/40/2016/09/DGACM_GAEAD_ESCAB-AMR-Draft-Political-Declaration-1616108E.pdf (accessed on 17 December 2017).
3. Thiel, K. Old dogma, new tricks—21st Century phage therapy. *Nat. Biotechnol.* **2004**, *22*, 31–36. [CrossRef] [PubMed]
4. Hall, A.R.; De Vos, D.; Friman, V.P.; Pirnay, J.P.; Buckling, A. Effects of sequential and simultaneous applications of bacteriophages on populations of *Pseudomonas aeruginosa* in vitro and in wax moth larvae. *Appl. Environ. Microbiol.* **2012**, *78*, 5646–5652. [CrossRef] [PubMed]
5. Jennes, S.; Merabishvili, M.; Soentjens, P.; Pang, K.W.; Rose, T.; Keersebilck, E.; Soete, O.; François, P.M.; Teodorescu, S.; Verween, G.; et al. Use of bacteriophages in the treatment of colistin-only-sensitive *Pseudomonas aeruginosa* septicaemia in a patient with acute kidney injury—A case report. *Crit. Care* **2017**, *21*, 129. [CrossRef] [PubMed]
6. Schooley, R.T.; Biswas, B.; Gill, J.J.; Hernandez-Morales, A.; Lancaster, J.; Lessor, L.; Barr, J.J.; Reed, S.L.; Rohwer, F.; Benler, S.; et al. Development and use of personalized bacteriophage-based therapeutic cocktails to treat a patient with a disseminated resistant *Acinetobacter baumannii* Infection. *Antimicrob. Agents Chemother.* **2017**, *61*, e00954-17. [CrossRef] [PubMed]
7. Pirnay, J.P.; De Vos, D.; Verbeken, G.; Merabishvili, M.; Chanishvili, N.; Vaneechoutte, M.; Zizi, M.; Laire, G.; Lavigne, R.; Huys, I.; et al. The phage therapy paradigm: Prêt-à-porter or sur-mesure? *Pharm. Res.* **2011**, *28*, 934–937. [CrossRef] [PubMed]
8. Servick, K. Beleaguered phage therapy trial presses on. *Science* **2016**, *352*, 1506. [CrossRef] [PubMed]
9. Commission De La Santé Publique, De L'environnement Et Du Renouveau De La Société. Questions Jointes De Mme Muriel Gerkens Et M. Philippe Blanchart À La Ministre Des Affaires Sociales Et De La Santé Publique Sur "La Phagothérapie" À La Ministre Des Affaires Sociales Et De La Santé Publique" (N° 11955 and N° 12911). 2016 Release. Available online: https://www.dekamer.be/doc/CCRA/pdf/54/ac464.pdf (accessed on 17 December 2017).
10. Fauconnier, A. Guidelines for Bacteriophage Product Certification. *Methods Mol. Biol.* **2018**, *1693*, 253–268. [PubMed]
11. Fauconnier, A. Regulating phage therapy: The biological master file concept could help to overcome regulatory challenge of personalized medicines. *EMBO Rep.* **2017**, *18*, 198–200. [CrossRef] [PubMed]

10

Expert Opinion on Three Phage Therapy Related Topics: Bacterial Phage Resistance, Phage Training and Prophages in Bacterial Production Strains

Christine Rohde [1,†,‡], Grégory Resch [2,†,‡], Jean-Paul Pirnay [3,†,‡], Bob G. Blasdel [4,†], Laurent Debarbieux [5], Daniel Gelman [6], Andrzej Górski [7,8], Ronen Hazan [6], Isabelle Huys [9], Elene Kakabadze [10], Małgorzata Łobocka [11,12], Alice Maestri [13], Gabriel Magno de Freitas Almeida [14], Khatuna Makalatia [10], Danish J. Malik [15], Ivana Mašlaňová [16], Maia Merabishvili [3,17], Roman Pantucek [16], Thomas Rose [3], Dana Štveráková [16,18], Hilde Van Raemdonck [3], Gilbert Verbeken [3] and Nina Chanishvili [10,*]

1 Department of Microorganisms, Leibniz Institute DSMZ—German Collection of Microorganisms and Cell Cultures, 38100 Braunschweig, Germany; Christine.Rohde@dsmz.de
2 Department of Fundamental Microbiology, University of Lausanne, 1015 Lausanne, Switzerland; Gregory.Resch@unil.ch
3 Laboratory for Molecular and Cellular Technology, Queen Astrid Military Hospital, 1120 Brussels, Belgium; jean-paul.pirnay@mil.be (J.-P.P.); maya.merabishvili@pha.ge (M.M.); thomas.rose@mil.be (T.R.); hilde.vanraemdonck@mil.be (H.V.R.); Gilbert.Verbeken@mil.be (G.V.)
4 Laboratory of Gene Technology, Department of Biosystems, 3000 Leuven, Belgium; blasdelb@gmail.com
5 Department of Microbiology, Institut Pasteur, 75015 Paris, France; laurent.debarbieux@pasteur.fr
6 Faculty of Dental Medicine, The Hebrew University of Jerusalem, Jerusalem 9112001, Israel; daniel.gelman@mail.huji.ac.il (D.G.); ronenh@ekmd.huji.ac.il (R.H.)
7 Bacteriophage Laboratory, Hirszfeld Institute of Immunology and Experimental Therapy, Polish Academy of Sciences, 53-114 Wroclaw, Poland; agorski@ikp.pl
8 Department of Clinical Immunology, Transplantation Institute, Medical University of Warsaw, 02-006 Warsaw, Poland
9 Department of Pharmaceutical and Pharmacological Sciences, KU Leuven, 3000 Leuven, Belgium; isabelle.huys@kuleuven.be
10 Eliava Institute of Bacteriophage, Microbiology and Virology, Gotua Street 3, 0160 Tbilisi, Georgia; elene.kakabadze@pha.ge (E.K.); khatuna.makalatia@pha.ge (K.M.)
11 Institute of Biochemistry and Biophysics, Polish Academy of Sciences, 00-901 Warsaw, Poland; lobocka@ibb.waw.pl
12 Autonomous Department of Microorganisms' Biology, Faculty of Agriculture and Biology, Warsaw University of Life Sciences—SGGW, 02-787 Warsaw, Poland
13 University of Turin, 10124 Turin, Italy; alice.maestri@edu.unito.it
14 Centre of Excellence in Biological Interactions, Department of Biological and Environmental Science, Nanoscience Center, University of Jyväskylä, Survontie 9C, FI-40014 Jyväskylä, Finland; gabriel.m.almeida@jyu.fi
15 Chemical Engineering Department, Loughborough University, Leicestershire LE11 3TU, UK; d.j.malik@lboro.ac.uk
16 Department of Experimental Biology, Faculty of Science, Masaryk University, 60000 Brno, Czech Republic; iva.maslanova@gmail.com (I.M.); pantucek@sci.muni.cz (R.P.); stverakova@mbph.cz (D.Š.)
17 Laboratory for Bacteriology Research, Faculty Medicine & Health Sciences, Ghent University, 9000 Ghent, Belgium
18 MB Pharma, 120 00 Prague 2 Vinohrady, Czech Republic
* Correspondence: nina.chanishvili@pha.ge
† These authors contributed equally to this work.
‡ Chair persons of the round tables.

Abstract: Phage therapy is increasingly put forward as a "new" potential tool in the fight against antibiotic resistant infections. During the "Centennial Celebration of Bacteriophage Research" conference in Tbilisi, Georgia on 26–29 June 2017, an international group of phage researchers committed to elaborate an expert opinion on three contentious phage therapy related issues that are hampering clinical progress in the field of phage therapy. This paper explores and discusses bacterial phage resistance, phage training and the presence of prophages in bacterial production strains while reviewing relevant research findings and experiences. Our purpose is to inform phage therapy stakeholders such as policy makers, officials of the competent authorities for medicines, phage researchers and phage producers, and members of the pharmaceutical industry. This brief also points out potential avenues for future phage therapy research and development as it specifically addresses those overarching questions that currently call for attention whenever phages go into purification processes for application.

Keywords: Bacteriophage; phage therapy; resistance; adaptation; prophage; production; regulation

---

1. Foreword

This article is a reflection of three roundtable discussions in question–answer format held at the "Centennial Celebration of Bacteriophage Research" conference, which took place in Tbilisi, Georgia, on 26–29 June 2017. The goal was to elaborate a concerted expert opinion, based on clinical experience and scientific knowledge, on three commonly identified knowledge gaps with regard to phage therapy and the manufacturing of adequate phage therapy products: bacterial phage resistance, phage training and the presence of prophages in bacterial production strains. Whenever phages are foreseen for application, they need to undergo a careful pre-selection after intensive application-oriented biological investigation; only such phages should go into a purification process chain. However, the combination of single phages into cocktails creates additional more complex investigation. The goal of this brief is to inform phage therapy stakeholders from the academic, industrial, medical and regulatory areas on these three contentious issues in the context of an increasing demand for human and veterinary phage applications.

2. Bacterial Resistance to Phages

The antagonistic co-evolution between bacterial hosts and their infecting phages is considered to be an important driver of ecological and evolutionary processes in microbial communities [1]. In the light of a renewed interest in using phages to treat bacterial infections, in vitro studies indicate that bacteria–phage co-evolution could be an important factor in the success (or failure) of certain phage therapy applications. The evolution of bacterial resistance to individual phages is often (if not always) observed in vitro, but with considerable variance. However, phages have evolved multiple strategies to overcome the antiviral mechanisms they encounter when infecting bacterial cells [2], such as anti-CRISPR (Clustered Regularly Interspaced Short Palindromic Repeats) proteins [3]. On the other hand, BREX and DISARM are phage resistance systems widespread in bacterial genomes that have been recently discovered [4,5].

In experimental settings, phage-resistant bacteria are observed to emerge rapidly, but often at significant fitness costs, commonly including a reduced growth rate in the absence of phages [6]. Evolved (pre-adapted or "trained") phages were shown to be more effective in reducing the densities of chronic bacterial isolates [7]. The in vivo evolution of bacterial resistance to phages in human clinical practice seems inevitable, but this has been poorly documented in the scientific literature to date. When rats with aortic experimental endocarditis (EE) were treated with an anti-*Pseudomonas* phage cocktail, phage-resistant mutants with impaired infectivity were shown to emerge in vitro but not in vivo, presumably because resistance mutations in bacteria involved bacterial surface determinants necessary for infectivity (e.g., genes involved in pilus motility and lipopolysaccharide (LPS) formation) [8]. In a recent long-term study that followed co-evolution between phages and bacteria in a natural environment, *Flavobacterium columnare* isolates were found to be generally resistant to phages from the past and susceptible to phages isolated in years after bacterial isolation. Bacterial resistance had selected for increased phage infectivity and host range. Bacterial resistance was correlated to the appearance of new anti-phage spacers in CRISPR loci, and on several occasions the corresponding protospacer regions in the genome of phages isolated in the following samplings were found to be modified in response. This study shows that, in natural conditions (e.g., natural phage/bacteria ratios and diversities), phages and bacteria co-evolve in a continuous arms race [9].

One expert further notes that the in vivo growth rates as well as the metabolic status of hosts in a polymicrobial biofilm may typically be quite different compared to observations in in vitro studies where the host is in the log growth phase in a nutrient rich environment.

2.1. Strategies to Minimize Bacterial Phage Resistance

Most of the round table participants had no idea of the frequency of emergence of bacterial phage resistance in clinical practice. According to one group's experience, however, the number of patients in whom a pathogen acquired resistance to the phage used during therapy may vary from 17% (*Staphylococcus aureus* phages) to 85% (*Escherichia coli* phages) [10]. The majority of the participants feel that it is difficult to develop a phage cocktail to which bacteria would not be able to evolve resistance during therapy. In contrast, three participants, including two biopharmaceutical researchers, presume that it might, however, be possible to develop resistance-proof therapeutic phage cocktails, using phages with a broad host range and targeting highly conserved structures that are essential for bacterial survival and/or infectivity. Two of them note that the phage resistance problem is not caused by the de novo emergence of phage resistant clones, but by the selection of naturally present phage resistant isolates harboring antiviral mechanisms such as restriction modification systems and CRISPR/Cas (CRISPR associated proteins) systems. It is not hard to imagine that the spread of these mechanisms through horizontal gene transfer may indeed be the main driver of bacterial phage resistance occurrence in natural environments, with large population diversities and dynamics, but little is known if this is also the case in the patient's infection site. These phage-resistance-proof cocktails would need to be updated regularly to target newly selected phage resistant clones. One expert stresses that, in the experience at the Eliava Phage Therapy Center, even when a phage (cocktail) shows no in vitro lytic activity against an infecting bacterial strain (e.g., using the spot test), this phage (cocktail) might still be clinically effective in vivo. A reason for this might be that these phage resistant bacteria display an impaired virulence to support an ongoing infection and may be more easily managed by the immune system [8].

All participants do believe that it is possible to minimize the occurrence of bacterial phage resistance. Phages should be selected that belong to different families/groups and that individually show important infectious ability, such as a broad host range, high efficiency of plating (EOP), high adsorption rates, short latent periods, large burst sizes and a low inclination to select resistance (e.g., as determined by the Appelmans method [11]), and which act synergistically when mixed into one cocktail. Ideally, phage cocktails should be composed of phages that adsorb to different highly conserved bacterial cell wall structures or virulence factors and exert a selective pressure on different antiviral resistance mechanisms in the same target bacterium. Based on an extensive experience as phage researcher in the Eliava Institute, one expert stresses that there is a limit to the number of phages that can be successfully combined into a single phage cocktail, as some phages are bound to be incompatible or to compete for the same bacterial host. In addition, some experts feel that these cocktails might need to be tailored to a specific patient and when necessary adapted in vitro during therapy to reduce the risk of generating persistent bacterial phage resistance. Knowing which bacterial structures phages interact with, as well as a better understanding of the resistance mechanisms they elicit, are crucial for the success of this approach. One participant states that bacterial resistance against any phage cocktail will inevitably occur at some point during treatment, but that by then the amount of pathogenic bacteria might have been sufficiently reduced (the equilibrium is restored) for the patient's immune system (or other antibacterials) to resolve the infection. It was suggested earlier that synergy between phages and the patient's immune system might be required for the resolution of the bacterial disease in certain indications [12].

Should sequential strategies in which individual active phages are applied one after the other, so that treatment does not simultaneously select for broad resistance in the targeted bacteria, be considered [6]? Most participants believe that this approach could be (more) effective, but would be very difficult to implement in clinical practice. Especially in severe acute infections, this approach would require large collections of different lytic phage clones and rapid (automated) phage selection and adaptation techniques. Rapid sequencing technologies and algorithm based phage selection of phages from libraries may allow rational selection of phage cocktails targeting different conserved receptors. In addition, sequential strategies are only feasible for hospitalized patients or ambulant patients visiting the hospital on a regular basis (e.g., every day). It would also require the use of significantly more diagnostic tools than is currently the habit of medical doctors and veterinarians when administering broad-spectrum antibacterials. One expert notes that sequential approaches could also be achieved using burst release and time delayed release systems [13]. Another participant fears that the sequential approach will give bacteria the opportunity to develop resistance against one active phage at the time. Two participants assume that decreases of phage efficiency are partly due to the patient's immune response and that sequential approaches could therefore be more effective.

In vitro studies indicate that pre-adapting lytic phages to a pathogen leads to increased pathogen clearance and lowered resistance evolution [7], but will it lower the occurrence of bacterial phage resistance in clinical practice? Most participants presume that it may, as properly pre-adapted phages could harbor mutations (e.g., single-nucleotide polymorphisms (SNPs) or short deletions), which would allow them to escape antiviral mechanisms, but they would like to see clinical evidence of this. In addition, pre-adaptation could also result in phages with broader host ranges and increased infectious abilities (see Section 3). Two participants claim that pre-adapting phages will likely only result in a faster co-evolution process and will have no impact on bacterial phage resistance.

One participant points out that phage resistance is sometimes due to an interruption of the lytic cycle and therefore advocates the use of phage endolysins. Some experts propose to combine the use of phage cocktails and antibiotics, while choosing phages that interact with relevant antibiotic resistance determinants. As such, bacterial phage resistance could lead to (regained) increased susceptibility to antibiotics [14], leading to synergistic selective pressure. More studies are needed to investigate the significance of this synergistic effect in vivo.

2.2. *Phages in Agriculture, Fisheries and Food*

Phage products are on the market for the decontamination of food pathogens and phage probiotics as well as products for farms are in development [15]. However, what do we know about the impact of the large-scale and empirical use of phages in agriculture and food on bacterial resistance to phages or on the shape and diversity of bacterial populations in the environment or in field trials?

Most participants believe that, in a way analogous to antibiotics, the uncontrolled widespread use of phages in agriculture and food decontamination might become a contributor to phage resistant bacterial diseases if phage therapy is to be (re-)integrated in human medicine. Some participants fear that bacterial phage resistance determinants will spread (e.g., through horizontal gene transfer should this transfer pathway definitely play a major role) and persist in the environment. In addition, since complex interactions between phages and bacteria already play significant roles in the composition of environmental microbial communities (e.g., bacterial adaptation to stress via phage transduction), there could be important and unpredictable impacts on the ecosystem.

One expert in aquaculture-associated phage research suggests that phage resistant bacteria might not be able to persist in the environment in the absence of the applied phage, due to the fitness cost of typical mutations that confer phage resistance. It is, however, not clear how phage resistance would differ from antibiotic resistance in this perspective. Three participants argue that the use of phages in agriculture, fisheries and food will likely increase bacterial phage resistance, but they are confident that the host–parasite co-evolutionary arms race will always result in the emergence of successful phages [16]. One expert points out that many bacterial serotypes that cause cattle/fish/plant diseases are different from those causing human disease, but that this does not exclude the emergence of cross-resistance.

With the exception of two participants, who do not believe that bacterial phage resistance will persist in the environment, most experts suggest restricting the use of phages to a greater or lesser extent to prophylactically limit the potential spread of bacterial phage resistance in anticipation of relevant data. The majority proposes avoiding the empirical (without previous diagnosis) use of phages and to control and limit the scale of phage applications especially in agriculture, fisheries and food. A few participants would like to reserve the use of phages for serious (antibiotic resistant) human infections at first priority, with phages obtained only upon medical prescription. Finally, all participants feel that phage products should not be produced, marketed and used as if they were a new class of antibiotics and suggest that phage therapy should have its own regulatory platform, allowing flexible approaches including the timely production, composition, and adaptation of phage products. Two experts stress that it is important that the production of phage preparations should comply with Good Manufacturing Practices (GMP). To summarize, more fundamental research is required in order to differentiate between bacterial phage resistance mechanisms, between in vitro and in vivo resistance phenomena and to quantify these more precisely. This is necessary to better understand therapeutic phage efficacy. Finally, and in the context of the patient's immune response, such comparative data assessments will shed light on the truth of bacterial phage resistance.

3. Phage Training

3.1. Phage Therapy and the Problem of Heterogeneity in Bacterial Populations

It is well known that bacterial populations are heterogeneous and that this heterogeneity can originate either genetically or phenotypically [17–19]. Heterogeneity is already considered problematic from a therapeutic point of view when it concerns bacterial susceptibility to antibiotics [20–22]. Similarly, it could challenge phage therapy since it is known that phage-resistant variants pre-exist within bacterial populations and can be relatively easily selected in vitro through bet hedging [8,17,23]. A very recent case of a patient suffering from an *Acinetobacter baumannii* disseminated infection treated with phage therapy highlighted the clinical relevance of such phage-resistant variants [24]. Indeed, phage-resistant clones were selected in the patient during the treatment course, which necessitated adjustment of the phage cocktail composition twice. In this case, it stands to the credit of the involved teams that they were able to sequentially produce tailored cocktails of natural phages (i.e., non-trained) able to kill the resistant clones, within the very limited amount of time available to the patient.

3.2. Phage Training?

In parallel to the adaptation of the bacterial host to the attacking phage, phages in turn naturally adapt to their hosts during co-evolution in common habitats following an arms race or fluctuating selection processes [25–27], explaining why both bacteria (the prey) and phages (the predator) are still present on the surface of our planet after billions of years of co-habitation. As a result, phages that have been evolved to better fit the context of phage therapy can be selected for in vitro and in vivo. Various forms of phage training, also known as phage adaptation or phage pre-adaptation, have been developed to select for these evolved phages through experimental procedures performed in a laboratory. It is generally acknowledged that phage training protocols originated from the so-called Appelmans experiment reported in 1921 [11]. At first, Appelmans designed his classical eponymous experiment to titer a phage solution more precisely than d'Hérelle performed at that time. In order to do so, Appelmans was inspired by an approach of serial dilutions to quantify bacteria in water samples as described in chapter III of Miquel's "*Manuel Pratique d'analyse bactériologique des eaux*" published in 1891. The principle is relatively simple and is still used today with some modifications.

In this original study, Appelmans exposed a liquid culture of a susceptible bacterium to serial dilutions of the phage (up to 10^{-12}), an experiment very similar to what is currently done in the macro-dilution method for the determination of the Minimum Inhibitory Concentration (MIC) of antibiotics. After incubation (incubation time is only indicated in Appelmans' paper as "immediate" or "lately"), the tubes in which bacteria were able to grow were considered to be devoid of phages and the tubes in which no growth was observed were considered as containing phages. Taking into consideration the dilution factor, Appelmans was able to precisely determine the phage titer in the undiluted solution. This experiment also allowed him to further validate d'Hérelle's hypothesis about the nature of phage amplification on bacteria. Moreover, Appelmans decided to perform an additional series of experiments in which he serially diluted the phage into 50% alcohol or 5% phenol. Indeed, at that time it had already been published that the phage Appelmans used in his study was stable when exposed to both agents. However, stability was only tested in a highly concentrated phage solution. Surprisingly, Appelmans, with his dilution approach, highlighted the fact that not all phages in the solution were equally resistant to both agents. Indeed, while the non-exposed phage solution was still active at a 10^{-10} dilution, the corresponding phage solution exposed to 50% alcohol remained active only when diluted up to 10^{-6} independent of the incubation time (6 h, 24 h, 3 days, 10 days or 20 days). An additional dilution of this solution led to its inactivity, arguing for the presence of a fixed number of phages insensitive to the agent in the test tube. Appelmans made the same observation with 5% phenol except that the number of phages able to resist this treatment was much lower (dilution 10^{-3} still active). In other words, this experiment demonstrated selection through dilution of phage variants able to resist to some chemicals otherwise toxic for the majority of individuals in the phage population. This is indeed exactly the principle of phage training in which phage variants able to very efficiently lyse a bacterial population are selected through dilution. There are indications that Félix d'Herelle introduced the concept of serial passages that were not performed in the original Appelmans experiments [28].

Two primary protocols of phage training for expanded host range have been reported in the literature [7,29,30]. Firstly, a phage/bacteria mixture is simply diluted into fresh growth medium after a period of co-incubation [7,30]. In the second, a fixed concentration of bacteria is co-incubated with serial dilution of a phage stock in growth medium for 16–24 h. The next morning, the mixture in the tube in which lysis occurred at the lowest phage concentration is further chloroformed and filtered before being serially re-diluted and mixed with sample of a fresh culture of the ancestor bacteria [31]. In both protocols the procedure can be repeated for several "passages".

3.3. Outcome of Phage Training

Experts pointed out that while several mechanisms of phage adaptation ensuring phage propagation on co-evolving hosts were previously described [32]; it is only more recently that the benefits of experimental phage training started to be investigated in controlled assays. In a first study [33], the training *P. aeruginosa* phage PAK_P3, which initially showed only slight lysis on strain CHA, led to the selection of phage P3-CHA with significantly increased in vitro efficiency of plating. This in vitro result was confirmed in vivo in a mouse model of lung infection with 100% versus 20% survival rate achieved by P3-CHA and PAK_P3, respectively. Strikingly, this improved in vivo activity was reported to be due to only two single nucleotide changes in different putative open reading frames (ORFs). This result highlights how quickly a new therapeutic phage with tremendously increased infectivity can emerge in a natural co-evolution process, and could therefore be artificially selected for by phage training. In another study it has been shown that four evolved *P. aeruginosa* phages obtained within two passages over four days were more efficient than ancestral phages in reducing in vitro mean bacterial densities of ten *P. aeruginosa* strains [7]. Accordingly, *P. aeruginosa* phages LKD16 and 14/1 pre-adapted over six serial passages were shown to target clones within a bacterial population of the strain PAO1 that were originally resistant to the ancestor phages. Indeed, the proportion of susceptibility over 20 different clones increased from 80% to 85% for the ancestral phages to 100% for the evolved phages [26]. Therefore, increased infectivity of evolved over ancestral phages is usually attributed to a decreased capacity of the ancestral bacterial strains to evolve resistance towards the evolved phages.

3.4. Relevance and Implementation of Phage Training in the Clinic

While one expert described how phage training has been common practice for more than 80 years at the Eliava Institute, all tend to think that there is no doubt that relying on evolved phages able to sidestep bacterial heterogeneity would have been highly desirable for the case discussed above (see Section 3.1) and would therefore be relevant in the clinic in general. Although a pre-clinical study has reported the benefit of a trained phage relative to its original counterpart in vivo, comparable studies should be set up to shed additional light on this biological phenomenon [33].

The implementation of phage training in clinical protocols is appealing for at least two reasons. First, having access to phages covering 100% of the clones within the population of a given strain could dramatically increase the success of phage therapy in a given patient. For instance, *P. aeruginosa* populations in the lungs of patients with cystic fibrosis (CF) harbor a very high phenotypic diversity [34]. Therefore, training for phages that would render them able to cover this phenotypic diversity in CF patients could be clinically significant. Secondly, having access to single phages covering close to 100% of the circulating strains of a given pathogen would allow usage of a very limited number of phages (or, in rare cases, even a single phage) for many patients, thus simplifying the production process.

All experts further distinguished two situations, i.e., acute and chronic infections. If phage training is demonstrated in the future to be an efficient way to significantly improve therapeutic outcomes, several experts noticed that implementation in chronic situations where time is not such an issue would in principle be considerably easier. However, the addition of phage training steps to a treatment protocol would be time consuming and feasible only if sufficient qualified personnel were available. In such a situation, experts pointed out that phage training could be done by either following (i) a one-size-fits-all strategy by training phages on already available representatives of local strains, which will help with setting up and regularly updating specialized phage collections, or (ii) a tailored strategy by training phages on the patient's strain as soon as it became available in a form of highly personalized medicine. Of note, this latter strategy is applied at the Eliava Institute in the process of development of so-called "autophages".

Accordingly, many experts agreed that in intensive care units (ICUs), where patients need to be treated within minutes or hours, implementation of a tailored strategy would be difficult due to time limitations. Indeed, as discussed before, phage training protocols usually require a week to be performed or at minimum 24–48 h in case of a single passage [29]. Nevertheless, an expert pointed out that often the strain that will cause the life-threatening condition, often including sepsis, in ICU patients is known days before as the dominant colonizing strain. In such a situation, patients could be decolonized with available phages (see above) and autophages could then be developed to adjust the treatment and cover potential phage-resistant variants selected by the former phages, in a way that is similar to what occurred in the case discussed in Section 3.1). This strategy is very similar to the situation where patients are first treated with broad-spectrum antibiotics and treatment is adjusted later according to an antibiogram. However, in acute situations where the strain would not be available in advance, experts agree that the emergency use of broad-host range phage cocktails could be a viable strategy. As a conclusion, while all experts rather agree on the clinical importance of developing trained phages, some think that detailed pre-clinical and clinical studies still need to be performed to properly evaluate "cost vs. benefits" and decide if it is worthwhile to invest into the time- and resources-consuming development of trained phage collections. If such a strategy were shown to be a viable option, phage training could either be implemented as a one-size-fits-all or a tailored strategy depending on the patient's condition.

3.5. *Regulatory Considerations Regarding Trained Phages*

In answer to the question "should trained phages be considered as natural phages?" if one would use them in clinical trials, a large majority of experts answered "yes". Indeed, phage training is based on a naturally occurring event and does not rely on "human-guided" modification of the phage genome through for instance synthetic biology or any other tools. A trained phage is a phage in which random mutations have been introduced by co-evolution with bacteria as it happens in nature. In other words, a trained phage is a phage variant that pre-exists in nature and is selected and amplified in the laboratory through natural, but accelerated, co-evolution. Since adapted phages are variants selected from a population of natural phages, their status regarding regulatory agencies should be similar to the original phage.

4. Prophages in Bacterial Production Strains

4.1. *Relevance of Prophages to the Production of Therapeutic Phages*

Temperate phages are champions of evolution, but unwanted during pharmaceutical phage production. Why do we address the "prophage issue" here and discuss it in depth? It is a matter of course to consider all relevant questions and parameters before therapeutic phage preparations are produced. As discussed earlier by international experts, production of phage preparations for medical application must follow defined procedures and quality assessments [35–38]. It is important to understand the biology of the two different types of phages that are in fact two different forms of life: obligately lytic, virulent phages are attractive potent alternatives to antibacterial drugs as these phages kill their bacterial host cells upon infection. Temperate phages lysogenize their bacterial host cells, exist as prophages after integration into the bacterial chromosomes or as plasmid-like extra-chromosomal elements. When "induced", they then change their life cycle and behave like virulent phages while lysing bacterial hosts. The term "temperate phage" thus refers to the character of this form of phage life whereas "prophage" describes a status in the complex life cycle of such a phage. Temperate phages exist in most bacteria as prophages, often abundantly, being normal parts of bacterial genomes.

Indeed, prophages are extremely abundant elements in the biosphere. Consequently, they also belong to our own microbiome and are part of its virome, and can be described as a phageome [39]. It has even been found that prophages in our microbiome are communicating via signaling peptides though the "arbitrium code" system [40]. Lysogeny clearly plays an enormous evolutionary role, with temperate phages substantially involved in co-evolution processes of both bacteria and phages [41]. This is relevant also in the context of this article: we are carrying countless prophages. Both, the microbiome and the individual macro-organism represent the holobiont, this rather recent and Solomonic perception of life includes all forms of life that contribute to an individual's existence and health [42].

Prophage induction occurs when expression of the transcriptional repressor keeping host lethal genes involved in lytic infection shut off is impaired to such an extent that lytic infection begins. Classically, this impairment is known to be caused by stresses such as UV irradiation, mutagens, quorum-sensing signaling molecules, fluoroquinolones, oxidative stresses (such as hydrogen peroxide) or a temperature shift that generates sufficient transient damage to the bacterial cell. In addition, it has also been long known that infection by lytic phages, like happens as an inherent part of the lytic phage production process, also strongly induces the excision of prophages. Indeed, five of seven *P. aeruginosa* phages examined by Blasdel et al. (including lytic phages being currently used for therapy) induce the transcription of at least part of at least one prophage element in their PAO1 host [43]. If prophage induction successfully highjacks the phage infection during production, then the prophage will be released into the medium, and possibly contaminate the therapeutic preparation that should exclusively contain the lytic phage. Finally, the induction of active prophages can also occur spontaneously with various frequencies [44], typically one in 10^3–10^5 cells, but sometimes one in 10^2 cells [45], and certain toxin-encoding phages were shown to be induced spontaneously with higher frequency than their non-toxin-encoding relatives [46]. As a consequence, populations of lysogens are typically contaminated with free temperate phages [47].

According to pharmaceutical standards, such a contamination of therapeutic phages with temperate phages is out of the question. Selection of the strain and a carefully adapted experimental quality control procedure is crucial as both phage types, the therapeutic phage and a temperate contaminant phage, cannot be separated chemically or physically as they share biochemical and structural similarities. Prophages are common in probably all taxonomic groups of bacteria, and knowledge about them is growing as more strains are sequenced and bioinformatics tools are getting more sophisticated. Comparative genomics is a fundamentally important scientific development. Indeed, many prophages are associated with pathogenicity, such as in *E. coli*, *Streptococcus pyogenes*, *Salmonella enterica*, *Staphylococcus aureus* and can encode for exotoxins like in *E. coli* EHEC or *Vibrio cholera* as well as a rather broad spectrum of enzymes significant for bacterial virulence [48].

However, bacterial genomes often bear non-complete (cryptic) prophages that cannot be induced or released from the cell. Due to the intensive relatedness to the human microbiome, most clinically important bacterial isolates, especially those belonging to the ESKAPE group (Enterococci (VRE), *S. aureus* (MRSA), *Klebsiella pneumoniae* (Carbapenem resistant), *A. baumannii*, *P. aeruginosa*, *Enterobacteriaceae* (ESBL)) contain both intact and cryptic prophage sequences in their genomes. It is our own rich and dense microbiome habitat that inevitably causes constant genetic exchange and co-evolution of bacteria and their phages. Especially for clinical isolates, it is a selective advantage to carry many prophages, which often encode genetic cassettes that benefit their hosts such as virulence factors [49,50]. Extreme examples are the food pathogen *E. coli* EHEC O157:H7 strain Sakai carrying 18 prophages which amount to 16% of the total genome or *S. pyogenes* with up to six prophages comprising 12% of the bacterial genome [51,52]. Stable prophages that are typically observed in isolated bacterial cultures have a long-lasting bond with their hosts comparable to a symbiosis finally supporting duration of both. However, it is important to note that prophages can either cause loss of host fitness or, just the opposite by adding new functions to the cell via lysogenic conversion comparable to a "gain-of-function". Still another type of host–phage interaction is active lysogeny: prophages may integrate in critical bacterial genes such that they function as regulatory switches [50]. Stable prophages tend to protect their bacterial hosts until "no other choice but escape" is left. In this context, it is important to distinguish precisely between different genetic transfer mechanisms like general and specialized transduction and lysogenic conversion. Bacteria may benefit from lysogenic conversion by obtaining novel virulence factors (toxins, super-antigens, immune evasion, invasivity, adherence, resistance to phages) [53,54]. It might be postulated that cryptic prophages and active lysogeny are part of bacterial regulatory systems. The interaction between such prophages and lytic phages could be considered as interaction between bacterial genomes and phages or, between lysogenic and lytic phages. Such questions are required to get in focus of fundamental research. For the purpose of this article, it is important to understand the biology of obligately lytic and of temperate phages. There are many fascinating and as yet unexplored aspects of the microbial and phage world, however, conditions outside the laboratory or production facility are not a priority for this article.

4.2. Detection of Prophages in Bacterial Genomes

There is consensus among experts that host strain genome sequencing is an essential initial investigation before starting phage production processes as it allows the identification of prophage genes like integrases, repressors, excisases, recombinases, terminases. Having this sequence available thus makes predictions for prophage properties like virulence factors or for prophage incompleteness possible. Induction ability might be experimentally studied by using Mitomycin C or UV irradiation but these induction methods are not successful enough and require indicator strains that are not always available. Due to the increasing importance of phage applications, entering prophage genomes in databases is necessary when bacterial genomes are analyzed. Algorithms for finding prophages are available like PhiSpy [55], PHAST (http://phast.wishartlab.com) and PHASTER [56] and genome annotations will shed light on prophage properties and this is getting less complicated the more sequence data are entered into databases. We strongly encourage researchers to make such data publically available.

4.3. Prophages in Bacterial Strains Used to Produce Therapeutic Phages

Finding production strains that are completely free of prophages is generally difficult, especially in the case of some pathogens. Therefore, inducibility and the genetic outfit of a prophage should be considered, definitions are necessary to deal with this issue. Genome sequencing is indispensable as prophages might be carriers of pathogenicity factors, as well as antibiotic and phage resistance determinants. Isolation of new phages aiming at therapeutic preparations cannot initially exclude temperate phages but further characterization steps should definitely eliminate them. Regarding the production strain and production process, the individual situation has to be assessed: is a strain available (and effective!) that is lacking prophages? If not, do bioinformatic genome analyses describe the prophage's genetic outfit sufficiently to confirm a cryptic nature? Is there a potential of infectious particles being released into the medium during production and if so, how probable is this event? If all these evaluations conclude that the production strain does not present likelihood of a problem, the final point should be considered that in a special situation the preparation may be the only viable alternative left, this is especially the case for magistral purposes. It is also important to note that a phage production strain must efficiently produce phages, meaning the EOP has to be satisfactory. Expert consensus was that production strains should ideally not carry prophages or should no other suitable strain exist then the risk needs to be controlled to minimize prophage expression [35].

We suggest that the significance of this concern must be put into perspective and seen in comparison to the global multidrug resistance crisis and the human crisis in individual cases. Improvement of phage production is important but it is fortunate that (1) lytic phages for clinical isolates of the ESKAPE bacteria (see above) are not difficult to isolate and (2) a rather good number of production strains within the ESKAPE bacteria should be available. Careful monitoring of the production process and where possible, a pre-adaptation of the therapeutic phage candidates to suitable production strains is a way forward. Repeated phage genome sequencing during the production process seems mandatory. Gene modification of production strains is discussed, but may only be one way out in extremely challenging cases in the future whereas currently, experts agree that eliminating prophages from the bacterial genome should not become a prerequisite. Q-PCR or sequencing can confirm purity of the DNA of the lytic phage and exclude prophage DNA. According to one expert, one possible way to assess the capacity of prophage elements to successfully induce under production conditions involves the use of Q-RT-PCR to track the concentration of DNA for each prophage relative to other genomic DNA during infection with primers specific to each prophage element as was done by Ceyssens et al. [57]. If replication of prophage DNA relative to other genomic DNA does not occur, this would definitively exclude successful prophage induction.

As a conclusion, it is obvious that more phage research is required going hand-in-hand with applied therapy approaches since an easy solution to the "prophage problem" is not obvious. Indeed, this is even more problematic if a phage should be amplified on a freshly isolated patient strain (see magistral application [38]). If compared to a threshold endotoxin limit in phage preparations, it might be feasible to define such a limit for prophage presence. Mathematical modeling of phage–bacterium pharmacodynamics may allow simulation of whether such concentrations are significant in terms of propagation of the temperate phages; low concentration of temperate phages may bear a very low statistical probability of significant amplification as the phage binding process is concentration dependent. Such thoughts seem theoretical but might be key for the design of strategies in the near future and for negotiating with licensing authorities.

4.4. Prophages in Production Strains: What Does It Mean for the Licensing Pathway?

It must be stated that intact prophages are not necessarily induced and released at high frequency. If a production strain contains a frequently inducible intact prophage it should not bear antibiotic resistance genes, toxin genes or other virulence factors to reduce the risk of gene transfer. The presence of temperate phages in a therapeutic preparation should normally not affect its efficacy (see above). Lytic phages can in principal also contribute to horizontal gene transfer via generalized transduction, but a risk–benefit evaluation must be rational, and a pragmatic common-sense approach is needed; just look at the human microbiome and its virome where prophages are the most frequent inhabitants! For commercially available phage preparations in the future it should be compulsory that production strains are free of functional prophages whereas exceptions might be made for highly experimental treatments. Generally, functional-prophage-free production strains should be the primary choice, however, other parameters need consideration including determining the suitability of a production strain e.g., efficacy and prophage-independent pathogenicity factors etc. For regulatory pathways, some kind of "prophage acceptance threshold" should be defined, it would contribute to a constructive timely European approach to design the regulatory framework for safe phage therapy. Furthermore, the establishment of collections/banks of prophage-free potential production strains, especially those of the ESKAPE bacteria, is urgently needed. Such strains can sometimes be acquired by natural means, such as prophage induction and prophage-free cell selection, without the use of genetic modifications [58].

5. Concluding Remarks

5.1. Bacterial Phage Resistance

It is commonly accepted that combining phages with different infection strategies into cocktails will help reduce the selection of phage resistant bacterial clones, but this point has only been studied on a few occasions both in vitro and in vivo. Sequential strategies might be interesting when there is no sense of urgency (e.g., long-term phage therapy of chronic infections), but more research is needed here. In acute life-threatening infections, and in anticipation of rapid (automated) bacterial identification and phage selection and adaptation techniques, well-thought-out broad-spectrum phage cocktails are warranted. More in vivo studies are needed to document the impact of phage pre-adaptation on bacterial phage resistance reduction. More research is needed to determine if the theoretical bacterial phage resistance issue (if phage therapy would be applied intensively, which, even in Georgia, is not the case today) will be comparable to the persistent bacterial multidrug resistance problem we are facing today. Meanwhile, most experts suggest restricting the use of phages, to a greater or lesser extent, to limit the potential spread of bacterial phage resistance in anticipation of relevant data.

5.2. Phage Training

Phage training is an experimental co-evolution approach considerably accelerating the pace at which "increased" phages are selected, thanks to the short doubling time of many bacterial species. Ultimately, naturally pre-adapted phages could be very interesting alternatives to original phages if their improved abilities translate from the preclinical situation to the clinic. Therefore, we believe that trained phages should be included in products to be tested in clinical trials, provided that their safety and superior efficacy compared to the ancestral phage have been documented in in vitro pre-clinical studies. In addition to their potential increased efficacy, broad host and/or variant range of trained phages could offer a significant economic advantage regarding the costs of production in GMP, which is a pre-requisite to prospective clinical trials.

5.3. Prophages in Bacterial Production Strains

Temperate phages/prophages present a problem in phage production processes, but are so abundant in all habitats including our own microbiome that we should not blindly demand their elimination from phage production processes. Instead, we broadly advise that an intensive discussion be had on how to deal with situations when no prophage-free production strains are available. We have explained which properties prophages might carry and what their unwanted features are, how abundant they are in opportunistic common ESKAPE bacteria, how genome analyses precisely characterize them and what to calculate if a production strain carries a prophage. We advocate that researchers enter bacterial and (pro)phage genome data into public databases because rich databases will provide the platform that is needed to deal with these particular pressing questions and because phage therapy will be a potent alternative therapy in the global multidrug resistance threat. Resolute and concurrent activities are urgently needed and harmonized licensing pathways are desirable. They might include best practice guidance for those few gaps that cannot be completely solved when a biological therapy approach is used; this may include the prophage issue.

Acknowledgments: This work was supported through the PHAGEFORWARD project of the fourth European Joint Programming Initiative on Antimicrobial Resistance (JPIAMR) call: "AMR Networks/Working Groups".

References

1. Koskella, B.; Brockhurst, M.A. Bacteria-phage coevolution as a driver of ecological and evolutionary processes in microbial communities. *FEMS Microbiol. Rev.* **2014**, *38*, 916–931. [CrossRef] [PubMed]
2. Labrie, S.J.; Samson, J.E.; Moineau, S. Bacteriophage resistance mechanisms. *Nat. Rev. Microbiol.* **2010**, *8*, 317–327. [CrossRef] [PubMed]
3. Maxwell, K.L. Phages fight back: Inactivation of the CRISPR-Cas bacterial immune system by anti-CRISPR proteins. *PLoS Pathog.* **2016**, *12*, e1005282. [CrossRef] [PubMed]
4. Goldfarb, T.; Sberro, H.; Weinstock, E.; Cohen, O.; Doron, S.; Yoav Charpak-Amikam, Y.; Afik, S.; Ofir, G.; Sorek, R. BREX is a novel phage resistance system widespread in microbial genomes. *EMBO J.* **2015**, *34*, 169–183. [CrossRef] [PubMed]
5. Ofir, G.; Melamed, S.; Sberro, H.; Mukamel, Z.; Silverman, S.; Yaakov, G.; Doron, S.; Sorek, R. DISARM is a widespread bacterial defence system with broad anti-phage activities. *Nat. Microbiol.* **2018**, *3*, 90–98. [CrossRef] [PubMed]
6. Hall, A.R.; de Vos, D.; Friman, V.P.; Pirnay, J.P.; Buckling, A. Effects of sequential and simultaneous applications of bacteriophages on populations of *Pseudomonas aeruginosa* in vitro and in wax moth larvae. *Appl. Environ. Microb.* **2012**, *78*, 5646–5652. [CrossRef] [PubMed]
7. Friman, V.P.; Soanes-Brown, D.; Sierocinski, P.; Molin, S.; Johansen, H.K.; Merabishvili, M.; Pirnay, J.P.; de Vos, D.; Buckling, A. Pre-adapting parasitic phages to a pathogen leads to increased pathogen clearance and lowered resistance evolution with *Pseudomonas aeruginosa* cystic fibrosis bacterial isolates. *J. Evolut. Biol.* **2016**, *29*, 188–198. [CrossRef] [PubMed]
8. Oechslin, F.; Piccardi, P.; Mancini, S.; Gabard, J.; Moreillon, P.; Entenza, J.M.; Resch, G.; Que, Y.-A. Synergistic interaction between phage therapy and antibiotics clears *Pseudomonas aeruginosa* infection in endocarditis and Reduces Virulence. *J. Infect. Dis.* **2017**, *215*, 703–712. [CrossRef] [PubMed]
9. Laanto, E.; Hoikkala, V.; Ravantti, J.; Sundberg, L.R. Long-term genomic coevolution of host-parasite interaction in the natural environment. *Nat. Commun.* **2017**, *8*. [CrossRef] [PubMed]
10. Międzybrodzki, R.; Borysowski, J.; Weber-Dąbrowska, B.; Fortuna, W.; Letkiewicz, S.; Szufnarowski, K.; Pawełczyk, Z.; Rogóż, P.; Kłak, M.; Wojtasik, E.; et al. Clinical aspects of phage therapy. *Adv. Virus Res.* **2012**, *83*, 73–121. [PubMed]
11. Appelmans, R. Le dosage du bactériophage. *C. R. Soc. Biol. Fil.* **1921**, *89*, 1098.
12. Roach, D.R.; Leung, C.Y.; Henry, M.; Morello, E.; Singh, D.; Di Santo, J.P.; Weitz, J.S.; Debarbieux, L. Synergy between the host immune system and bacteriophage is essential for successful phage therapy against an acute respiratory pathogen. *Cell Host Microbe* **2017**, *22*, 38–47. [CrossRef] [PubMed]
13. Malik, D.J.; Sokolov, I.J.; Vinner, G.K.; Mancuso, F.; Cinquerrui, S.; Vladisavljevic, G.T.; Clokie, M.R.J.; Stapley, A.G.F.; Kirpichnikova, A. Formulation, stabilisation and encapsulation of bacteriophage for phage therapy. *Adv. Colloid Interface Sci.* **2017**, *249*, 100–133. [CrossRef] [PubMed]
14. Chan, B.K.; Sistrom, M.; Wertz, J.E.; Kortright, K.E.; Narayan, D.; Turner, P.E. Phage selection restores antibiotic sensitivity in MDR *Pseudomonas aeruginosa*. *Sci. Rep.* **2016**, *6*, 26717. [CrossRef] [PubMed]

15. Cooper, I.R. A review of current methods using bacteriophages in live animals, food and animal products intended for human consumption. *J. Microbiol. Meth.* **2016**, *130*, 38–47. [CrossRef] [PubMed]
16. Ormala, A.M.; Jalasvuori, M. Phage therapy: Should bacterial resistance to phages be a concern, even in the long run? *Bacteriophage* **2013**, *3*, e24219. [CrossRef] [PubMed]
17. Davis, K.M.; Isberg, R.R. Defining heterogeneity within bacterial populations via single cell approaches. *BioEssays* **2016**, *38*, 782–790. [CrossRef] [PubMed]
18. Magdanova, L.A.; Goliasnaia, N.V. Heterogeneity as an adaptive trait of the bacterial community. *Mikrobiologiia* **2013**, *82*, 3–13. [PubMed]
19. Veening, J.W.; Smits, W.K.; Kuipers, O.P. Bistability, epigenetics, and bet-hedging in bacteria. *Annu. Rev. Microbiol.* **2008**, *62*, 193–210. [CrossRef] [PubMed]
20. Woodford, N.; Ellington, M.J. The emergence of antibiotic resistance by mutation. *Clin. Microbiol. Infect.* **2007**, *13*, 5–18. [CrossRef] [PubMed]
21. Babouee Flury, B.; Ellington, M.J.; Hopkins, K.L.; Turton, J.F.; Doumith, M.; Loy, R.; Staves, P.; Hinic, V.; Frei, R.; Woodford, N. Association of novel nonsynonymous single nucleotide polymorphisms in *ampD* with cephalosporin resistance and phylogenetic variations in *ampC*, *ampR*, *ompF*, and *ompC* in *Enterobacter cloacae* isolates that are highly resistant to carbapenems. *Antimicrob. Agents Chempother.* **2016**, *60*, 2383–2390. [CrossRef] [PubMed]
22. Proctor, R.A.; Kahl, B.; von Eiff, C.; Vaudaux, P.E.; Lew, D.P.; Peters, G. Staphylococcal small colony variants have novel mechanisms for antibiotic resistance. *Clin. Infect. Dis.* **1998**, *27* (Suppl. 1), S68–S74. [CrossRef] [PubMed]
23. Beaumont, H.J.; Gallie, J.; Kost, C.; Ferguson, G.C.; Rainey, P.B. Experimental evolution of bet hedging. *Nature* **2009**, *462*, 90–93. [CrossRef] [PubMed]
24. Schooley, R.T.; Biswas, B.; Gill, J.J.; Hernandez-Morales, A.; Lancaster, J.; Lessor, L.; Barr, J.J.; Reed, S.L.; Rohwer, F.; Benler, S.; et al. Development and use of personalized bacteriophage-based therapeutic cocktails to treat a patient with a disseminated resistant *Acinetobacter baumannii* infection. *Antimicrob. Agents Chemother.* **2017**, *61*. [CrossRef] [PubMed]
25. Stern, A.; Sorek, R. The phage-host arms race: Shaping the evolution of microbes. *BioEssays* **2011**, *33*, 43–51. [CrossRef] [PubMed]
26. Betts, A.; Kaltz, O.; Hochberg, M.E. Contrasted coevolutionary dynamics between a bacterial pathogen and its bacteriophages. *Proc. Natl. Acad. Sci. USA* **2014**, *111*, 11109–11114. [CrossRef] [PubMed]
27. De Sordi, L.; Khanna, V.; Debarbieux, L. The gut microbiota facilitates drifts in the genetic diversity and infectivity of bacterial viruses. *Cell Host Microbe* **2017**, *22*, 801–808. [CrossRef] [PubMed]
28. D'Herelle, F. On an invisible microbe antagonistic toward dysenteric bacilli: Brief note by Mr. F. D'Herelle, presented by Mr. Roux. 1917. *Res. Microbiol.* **2007**, *158*, 553–554. [PubMed]
29. Merabishvili, M.; Pirnay, J.P.; de Vos, D. Guidelines to compose an ideal bacteriophage cocktail. *Methods Mol. Biol.* **2018**, *1693*, 99–110. [CrossRef] [PubMed]
30. Betts, A.; Vasse, M.; Kaltz, O.; Hochberg, M.E. Back to the future: Evolving bacteriophages to increase their effectiveness against the pathogen *Pseudomonas aeruginosa* PAO1. *Evolut. Appl.* **2013**, *6*, 1054–1063. [CrossRef]
31. Merabishvili, M.; Pirnay, J.P.; de Vos, D. Guidelines to compose an ideal bacteriophage cocktail. In *Bacteriophage Therapy: From Lab to Clinical Practice*, 1st ed.; Azaredo, J., Sillankorva, S., Eds.; Humana Press: New York, NY, USA, 2017; Volume 1, pp. 107–108, ISBN 9781493973941 1493973940.
32. Samson, J.E.; Magadan, A.H.; Sabri, M.; Moineau, S. Revenge of the phages: Defeating bacterial defences. *Nat. Rev. Microbiol.* **2013**, *11*, 675–687. [CrossRef] [PubMed]
33. Morello, E.; Saussereau, E.; Maura, D.; Huerre, M.; Touqui, L.; Debarbieux, L. Pulmonary bacteriophage therapy on *Pseudomonas aeruginosa* cystic fibrosis strains: First steps towards treatment and prevention. *PLoS ONE* **2011**, *6*, e16963. [CrossRef] [PubMed]
34. Clark, S.T.; Diaz Caballero, J.; Cheang, M.; Coburn, B.; Wang, P.W.; Donaldson, S.L.; Zhang, Y.; Liu, M.; Keshavjee, S.; Yau, Y.C.; et al. Phenotypic diversity within a *Pseudomonas aeruginosa* population infecting an adult with cystic fibrosis. *Sci. Rep.* **2015**, *5*, 10932. [CrossRef] [PubMed]
35. Pirnay, J.P.; Blasdel, B.G.; Bretaudeau, L.; Buckling, A.; Chanishvili, N.; Clark, J.R.; Corte-Real, S.; Debarbieux, L.; Dublanchet, A.; de Vos, D.; et al. Quality and safety requirements for sustainable phage therapy products. *Pharm. Res.* **2015**, *32*, 2173–2179. [CrossRef] [PubMed]

36. Expert Round Table on Acceptance and Re-implementation of Bacteriophage Therapy. Silk route to the acceptance and re-implementation of bacteriophage therapy. *Biotechnol. J.* **2016**, *11*, 595–600. [CrossRef]
37. Cooper, C.J.; Khan Mirzaei, M.; Nilsson, A.S. Adapting drug approval pathways for bacteriophage-based therapeutics. *Front. Microbiol.* **2016**, *7*, 1209. [CrossRef] [PubMed]
38. Pirnay, J.P.; Verbeken, G.; Ceyssens, P.-J.; Huys, I.; de Vos, D.; Ameloot, C.; Fauconnier, A. The magistral phage. *Viruses* **2018**, *10*, 64. [CrossRef] [PubMed]
39. Manrique, P.; Bolduc, B.; Walk, S.T.; van der Oost, J.; de Vos, W.M.; Young, M.J. Healthy human gut phageome. *Proc. Natl. Acad. Sci. USA* **2016**, *113*, 10400–10405. [CrossRef] [PubMed]
40. Erez, Z.; Steinberger-Levy, I.; Shamir, M.; Doron, S.; Stokar-Avihail, A.; Peleg, Y.; Melamed, S.; Leavitt, A.; Savidor, A.; Albeck, S.; et al. Communication between viruses guides lysis-lysogeny decisions. *Nature* **2017**, *541*, 488–493. [CrossRef] [PubMed]
41. Howard-Varona, C.; Hargreaves, K.R.; Abedon, S.T.; Sullivan, M.B. Lysogeny in nature: Mechanisms, impact and ecology of temperate phages. *ISME J.* **2017**, *11*, 1511–1520. [CrossRef] [PubMed]
42. Thomas, S.; Izard, J.; Walsh, E.; Batich, K.; Chongsathidkiet, P.; Clarke, G.; Sela, D.A.; Muller, A.J.; Mullin, J.M.; Albert, K.; et al. The host microbiome regulates and maintains human health: A primer and perspective for non-microbiologists. *Cancer Res.* **2017**, *77*, 1783–1812. [CrossRef] [PubMed]
43. Blasdel, B.G.; Ceyssens, P.J.; Chevallereau, A.; Debarbieux, L.; Lavigne, R. Comparative transcriptomics reveals a conserved Bacterial Adaptive Phage Response (BAPR) to viral predation. *bioRxiv* **2018**. [CrossRef]
44. Lwoff, A. Lysogeny. *Bacteriol. Rev.* **1953**, *17*, 269–337. [PubMed]
45. Nanda, A.M.; Heyer, A.; Krämer, C.; Grünberger, A.; Kohlheyer, D.; Frunzke, J. Analysis of SOS-induced spontaneous prophage induction in *Corynebacterium glutamicum* at the single-cell level. *J. Bacteriol.* **2014**, *196*, 180–188. [CrossRef] [PubMed]
46. Colon, M.P.; Chakraborty, D.; Pevzner, Y.; Koudelka, G.B. Mechanisms that determine the differential stability of Stx(+) and Stx(−) lysogens. *Toxins* **2016**, *8*, 96. [CrossRef] [PubMed]
47. Łobocka, M.; Hejnowicz, M.S.; Dąbrowski, K.; Izak, D.; Gozdek, A.; Głowacka, A.; Gawor, J.; Kosakowski, J.; Gromadka, R.; Weber-Dąbrowska, B.; et al. *Staphylococcus aureus* Strains for the Production of Monoclonal Bacteriophage Preparations Deprived of Contamination with Plasmid DNA. U.S. Patent WO 2016/030871 A1, 16 March 2016.
48. Fortier, L.C.; Sekulovic, O. Importance of prophages to evolution and virulence of bacterial pathogens. *Virulence* **2013**, *4*, 354–365. [CrossRef] [PubMed]
49. Colavecchio, A.; Cadieux, B.; Lo, A.; Goodridge, L.D. Bacteriophages contribute to the spread of antibiotic resistance genes among foodborne pathogens of the *Enterobacteriaceae* family—A review. *Front. Microbiol.* **2017**, *8*, 1108. [CrossRef] [PubMed]
50. Feiner, R.; Argov, T.; Rabinovich, L.; Sigal, N.; Borovok, L.; Herskovits, A.A. A new perspective on lysogeny: Prophages as active regulatory switches of bacteria. *Nat. Rev. Microbiol.* **2015**, *13*, 641–650. [CrossRef] [PubMed]
51. Canchaya, C.; Desiere, F.; Mcshan, W.M.; Ferretti, J.J.; Parkhill, J.; Brüssow, H. Genome analysis of an inducible prophage and prophage remnants integrated in the *Streptococcus pyogenes* strain SF370. *Virology* **2002**, *302*, 245–258. [CrossRef] [PubMed]
52. Touchon, M.; Bernheim, A.; Rocha, E.P. Genetic and life-history traits associated with the distribution of prophages in bacteria. *ISME J.* **2016**, *10*, 2744–2754. [CrossRef] [PubMed]
53. Maslanova, I.; Stribna, S.; Doskar, J.; Pantucek, R. Efficient plasmid transduction to *Staphylococcus aureus* strains insensitive to the lytic action of transducing phage. *FEMS Microbiol. Lett.* **2016**, *363*. [CrossRef] [PubMed]
54. Haaber, J.; Leisner, J.L.; Cohn, M.T.; Catalan-Moreno, A.; Nielsen, J.B.; Westh, H.; Penadés, J.R.; Ingmer, H. Bacterial viruses enable their host to acquire antibiotic resistance genes from neighbouring cells. *Nat. Commun.* **2016**, *7*, 13333. [CrossRef] [PubMed]
55. Akhter, S.; Aziz, R.K.; Edwards, R.A. PhiSpy: A novel algorithm for finding prophages in bacterial genomes that combines similarity- and composition-based strategies. *Nucleic Acids Res.* **2012**, *40*, e126. [CrossRef] [PubMed]
56. Arndt, D.; Grant, J.R.; Marcu, A.; Sajed, T.; Pon, A.; Liang, Y.; Wishart, D.S. PHASTER: A better, faster version of the PHAST phage search tool. *Nucleic Acids Res.* **2016**, *44*, W16–W21. [CrossRef] [PubMed]

57. Ceyssens, P.J.; Minakhin, L.; Van den Bossche, A.; Yakunina, M.; Klimuk, E.; Blasdel, B.G.; de Smet, J.; Noben, J.P.; Bläsi, U.; Severinov, K.; et al. Development of giant bacteriophage ϕKZ is independent of the host transcription apparatus. *J. Virol.* **2018**, *88*, 10501–10510. [CrossRef] [PubMed]

58. Łobocka, M.; Hejnowicz, M.S.; Gągała, U.; Weber-Dąbrowska, B.; Węgrzyn, G.; Dadlez, M. The first step to bacteriophage therapy—How to choose the correct phage. In *Phage Therapy: Current Research and Applications*; Borysowski, J., Międzybrodzki, R., Górski, A., Eds.; Caister Academic Press: Poole, UK, 2004; pp. 23–69.

11

Resistance Development to Bacteriophages Occurring during Bacteriophage Therapy

Frank Oechslin

Department of Fundamental Microbiology (DMF), University of Lausanne, CH-1015 Lausanne, Switzerland; frank.oechslin@gmail.com

Abstract: Bacteriophage (phage) therapy, i.e., the use of viruses that infect bacteria as antimicrobial agents, is a promising alternative to conventional antibiotics. Indeed, resistance to antibiotics has become a major public health problem after decades of extensive usage. However, one of the main questions regarding phage therapy is the possible rapid emergence of phage-resistant bacterial variants, which could impede favourable treatment outcomes. Experimental data has shown that phage-resistant variants occurred in up to 80% of studies targeting the intestinal milieu and 50% of studies using sepsis models. Phage-resistant variants have also been observed in human studies, as described in three out of four clinical trials that recorded the emergence of phage resistance. On the other hand, recent animal studies suggest that bacterial mutations that confer phage-resistance may result in fitness costs in the resistant bacterium, which, in turn, could benefit the host. Thus, phage resistance should not be underestimated and efforts should be made to develop methodologies for monitoring and preventing it. Moreover, understanding and taking advantage of the resistance-induced fitness costs in bacterial pathogens is a potentially promising avenue.

Keywords: bacteriophage; phage; phage therapy; phage-resistance

---

1. Introduction

Antimicrobial resistance is a major public health problem that could possibly cause an estimated 10 million mortalities per year by 2050 [1]. For this reason, novel therapeutic strategies, beside traditional antibiotics, must be rapidly developed. One of these strategies is the use of bacteriophages (phages). Phages are nature's most abundant bacterial predators. They can be used alone or in combination with antibiotics against difficult-to-treat infections. Phage therapy has been used since the 1920s in the Soviet Union, and is still currently used in ex-Soviet countries like Poland, Russia, and Georgia [2]. Phage therapy is currently being revisited as a potential alternative to antibiotics in Western countries. However, challenging issues still exist, such as selecting the most adequate phage(s) against a given infection, the risk of phage resistance development, the immune response to phages by the host, as well as novel regulatory requirements [3,4].

Bacteria can resist phage attack through different mechanisms, including spontaneous mutations, restriction modification systems, and adaptive immunity via the CRISPR-Cas system [5]. Spontaneous mutations are the main mechanisms driving both phage resistance and phage–bacterial coevolution [6]. Spontaneous mutations may confer phage resistance by modifying the structure of bacterial surface components that act as phage receptors and that also determine phage specificity. These include lipopolysaccharides (LPS), outer membrane proteins, cell wall teichoic acids, capsules, and other bacterial appendices, such as flagella, many of which may all be part of virulence factors (e.g., LPS) [7].

However, phage resistance may also induce trade-off costs. Phage-resistant bacteria may become less virulent in case of mutations in surface virulence factors, such as LPS [8]. Likewise, the maintenance of anti-viral defence systems, such as for DNA restriction-modification enzymes and CRISPR-Cas adaptive immunity, also has its own cost [9,10].

This review discusses the implications of the development of phage resistance in the perspective of implementing phage therapy. Phage resistance is first considered in the context of population and phage–bacterial evolutionary dynamics. It is then considered in the frame of experimental therapy (summarized in Table 1), in order to determine its role in treatment failure or salvage therapy strategies.

Table 1. Principal in vivo studies investigating the relation between phage therapy and phage resistance.

	Bacterium	Model	Phage Type	Treatment Outcome	Resistant Found in after Treatment?	Impact of Resistance on Virulence	Receptor	Ref.
Intestinal colonization	*Campylobacter jejuni*	Chicken intestinal colonization	CP8 and CP34	Bacterial decrease between 0.5 and 5 log10 CFU/g of caecal contents compared to untreated controls over a 5-day period post-administration.	Yes, at a freq. of 4%	Less infective at low dose. Rapid phenotypic reversion when reintroduced in chicken.	ND	[11, 12]
	Campylobacter jejuni	Chicken intestinal colonization	phiCcoIBB35, phiCcoIBB37, and phiCcoIBB12	Phage cocktail decreases the titre of *C. jejuni* in faeces by approximately 2 log10 CFU/g when administered orally.	Yes, at a freq. of 13%	Not less infective. No phenotypic reversion when reintroduced in chicken.	ND	[13]
	Escherichia coli	Calf, piglet, lamb Ta diarrhoea	B44/1, B44/2, B44/3, P433/1, and P433/2	Protected calves against a potentially lethal infection, cured diarrhoea in piglets, improved the course of disease in lambs.	Most calves that did not respond to phage treatment had a high number of phage-resistant variants. No phage-resistant mutants were isolated from lambs.	Decreased virulence	Capsular polysaccharides	[14]
	Escherichia coli	Calf diarrhoea	B41/1	Rapid reduction of bacterial titres to numbers that are harmless.	Yes	Reduced virulence	Capsular polysaccharides	[15]
	Escherichia coli	Sheep, mouse, steer intestinal colonization	KH1 and SH1	Oral phage treatment did not decrease intestinal *E. coli* in sheep. Decreased the number of *E. coli* CFU in cattle. Phage therapy cleared the bacteria in a mouse model of intestinal *E. coli* O157 carriage.	No	-	ND	[16]
	Escherichia coli	Mouse intestinal colonization	T4 phage, oral	ND	Phage resistant bacterial strains dominated gut after 92 days.	ND	ND	[17]
	Escherichia coli	Mouse intestinal colonization	cocktail made of phages CLB_P1, CLB_P2, and CLB_P3	No bacterial level change in the faeces after treatment.	No	-	ND	[18]
	Enterococcus faecalis	Gnotobiotic mouse intestinal colonization	φ VPE25	Threefold drop in *E. faecalis* total intestinal load after 24 h of VPE25 treatment.	Phage resistant variant replaced WT during treatment.	Resistant variants can colonize intestine.	Integral membrane protein PIPEF	[19]
	Salmonella enterica	Chicken intestinal colonization	cocktail of phages, EP2, MUT3, M4, and YP	Significant difference between phage-treated and untreated groups.	Yes	ND	ND	[20]
	Salmonella enterica	Chicken intestinal colonization	φ10, φ25, and φ151	Phages reduced caecal colonization.	Phage-resistance occurred at a frequency commensurate with the titre of phage being administered.	Colonization levels of resistant variants in the ceca did not differ from the controls. Reversion observed after infection.	ND	[21]
	Vibrio cholerae	Infant mouse and rabbit cholera model	ICP1, ICP2, and ICP3	Oral administration of phages up to 24 h before *V. cholerae* challenge reduced colonization of the intestinal tract and prevented cholera-like diarrhoea.	Yes	Variants can colonize intestine.	O-Antigen	[22]

Table 1. *Cont.*

	Bacterium	Model	Phage Type	Treatment Outcome	Resistant Found in after Treatment?	Impact of Resistance on Virulence	Receptor	Ref.
Meningitis	*Escherichia coli*	Mouse meningitis	phage R	One dose of phage was at least equivalent to multiple doses of antibiotics, whether administered intramuscularly or intrathecally.	Yes	Supposably reduced virulence as described in [14].	Capsular polysaccharides	[23]
Endocarditis	*Pseudomonas aeruginosa*	Rat infective endocarditis	cocktail made of phages 12 bacteriophages	3 log reduction or valve sterilisation when combined with antibiotics.	No	Reduced virulence	LPS and pilus	[24]
Sepsis	*Escherichia coli*	Rat neonatal sepsis	phage EC200^{PP}	Phage administered 7 h postinfection rescued 100% of the animals and 50% after 24 h.	Phage resistant variant were found when phage treatment was delayed for 24 h.	Avirulence	ND	[25]
	Klebsiella pneumoniae	Mouse liver abscess and bacteraemia	Phage φNK5	Intraperitoneal and intragastric administration of phage 30 min after infection protected mice from death in a dose-dependent manner. Decreased bacterial burden and liver damage.	No	Reduced virulence	ND	[26]
	Staphylococcus aureus	Experimental cow mastitis	Bacteriophage K	Decreased bacterial load after treatment.	Yes	ND	ND	[27]
	Pseudomonas plecoglossicida	Fish haemorrhagic ascites	PPpW-3 and PPpW-4. Oral	Protective effects of phage treatment with lower and delayed mortality 1 or 24 h after bacterial challenge.	No	Reduced virulence	ND	[28]
	Klebsiella pneumoniae	Mice acute bacteraemia	GH-K1, GH-K2, and GH-K3	Phage cocktail significantly enhanced the protection of bacteremic mice against lethal infection.	ND	Reduced virulence	ND	[29]
	Salmonella enterica Parathyphi B	Mouse sepsis	phage φ1	Phage given concurrently with a lethal dose of bacteria rescued 100% of the animals.	ND	Avirulence	O-Antigen	[30]
pneumonia	*Pseudomonas aeruginosa*	Mouse acute pneumonia	PAK_P1	Treatment failed to prevent fatality due to subsequent bacterial outgrowth after 24 h in immunocompromised mice. 100% of bacteria recovered from phage-treated at 24 h were resistant.	Yes, in immunocompromised mice	ND	ND	[31]

Table 1. *Cont.*

	Bacterium	Model	Phage Type	Treatment Outcome	Resistant Found in after Treatment?	Impact of Resistance on Virulence	Receptor	Ref.
Phage resistant variants for vaccine production and studying virulence factors	*Vibrio cholerae*	Infant mouse cholera model	ICP1	ND	ND	Attenuated in vivo.	O-Antigen	[32]
	Vibrio cholerae	Infant mouse cholera model	K139	ND	ND	Significantly reduced in its ability to colonize the mouse small intestine.	Core oligosaccharide	[33]
	Vibrio cholerae	Infant mouse cholera model	phage JA1	ND	ND	Impaired colonization	Capsule/O-antigen	[34]
	Staphylococcus aureus	Mouse vaccination	M^{Sa} phage	ND	ND	Avirulence	Teichoic acids	[35]
	Yersinia pestis	Mouse vaccination	L-413C, P2 vir1, φ JA1a, φ A1122, T7, $T7Yp^{e}$, Pokrovskaya, Y, PST, R^{h}	ND	ND	Atenuated or avirulent.	LPS	[36]
	Flavobacterium columnare	Zebrafish	FCL-1 and FCL-2	ND	ND	Avirulence	ND	[37]
	Bacillus thuringiensis	Cecropia moth	φ42, φ51,and φ64	ND	ND	Decreased virulence	ND	[38]
	Serratia marcescens	Cecropia moth, Drosophila	Phages φJ and φK	ND	ND	Decreased virulence	ND	[39]
	Serratia marcescens	Cecropia moth	Phages φJ	ND	ND	Decreased virulence	ND	[40]

2. The Evolution Dynamics of Resistance

Phage–bacteria coevolution can be defined as a process of reciprocal adaptation and counter-adaptation between the phage and its bacterial host. It is an important driving force for the ecology and evolution of microbial communities [6]. Phage–bacteria interactions are mediated first by phages using their tail fibres to adsorb onto the bacterial surface, through a lock-key mechanism. Since the complete phage replication life cycle, namely the lytic cycle, relies on the killing and lysis of the host bacteria, a strong reciprocal selection pressure evolves toward increased infectivity on the side of the phage, and phage-resistance on the side of the bacterium [41]. Bacteria can evolve phage-resistance by de novo chromosomal mutations, as well as through an arsenal of antiviral mechanisms targeting virtually all steps of the phage life cycle (reviewed in [5]). For example, bacteria can prevent phage adsorption by modifying the structure of their surface phage receptors, or by hindering the access of the phage to the receptor through the production of an excess of the extracellular matrix, or even by producing competitive inhibitors [42–44].

The development of phage-resistant bacteria was already described almost a century ago in a seminal paper by Luria and Delbrück, who observed that the initial phage-induced lysis of a bacterial population was followed by bacterial regrowth, due to the selection of a phage-resistant sub-populations [45]. Phage-resistant bacterial variants that were already present in the initial bacterial culture (at a rate of ca. 10^{-8}) were selected and led to the replacement of the entire culture with the resistant variant. This extreme situation leads to an evolutionary dead-end, for instance if the phage receptor is lost, and phage do not have the opportunity to develop a counter-resistance. A large number of studies concluded similarly on the absence of phage–bacterial coevolution following the emergence of phage-resistant bacteria (reviewed in [46]). This was the case in chemostat experiments using *Escherichia coli* infected with series of T or lambda phages. Phages could not interact anymore with the resistant *E. coli* variants [47]. However, phage-susceptible parent bacteria could still be recovered from sanctuary niches such as biofilms present on the chemostat's walls. These survivors allowed maintaining low levels of phage persistence.

Other studies observed more persistent cycles of coevolution between phages and the host bacteria. This was the case for *E. coli* O157:H7 and phage PP01 in a continuous chemostat culture [48]. In this experiment, phages could coexist with phage-resistant variants and evolve different host ranges for the phage-escape bacterial mutants. Phage-resistance was associated with a dual bacterial population carrying either LPS alterations or OmpC surface protein silencing. Moreover, a third type of mucoid colony mutant emerged and could coexist with phages until the end of the experiment. Eventually, phage mutants with different host ranges also appeared.

One possible explanation was that none of the three phage-resistant bacterial mutants were completely immune to phage infection and, thus, entered a phage coevolution cycle permitting parallel phage and bacterial expansion and selection for phage variants with broader host range.

In other experiments, using lambda phages, an arms race was observed when using minimal media and maltose as the only carbon source [49]. Since the lambda phage uses the maltose outer membrane porin, LamB, as a bacterial receptor, decreasing LamB synthesis decreased phage susceptibility. However, this also decreased bacterial fitness in the presence of a lactose-only carbon source. In parallel, phages selected variants with increased LamB affinity or new variants able to infect via alternative receptors. Phages shifted from using the LamB to OmpF receptor through amino acid substitutions in their tail fibre J protein [50]. This mutual counter-selection process between the phage and the bacterium that enabled each of them to survive, without eliminating the other.

Further confirmation of the arms race came from observations with *Pseudomonas fluroescens* and the Podovirus $\phi 2$ [51,52]. In this case, reciprocal evolution of infectivity and resistance was followed during >100 bacterial generations, with phages becoming more broadly infectious and bacteria more broadly resistant over time [41,52]. However, the arms race became progressively weaker, with increasing fitness cost due to generalist adaptive mutations on both sides [53].

A common paradigm in evolutionary biology is that evolution tends to maximize the adaptation ability (in this case phage-resistance) by allocating resources preferentially when they are limited. If resources are dedicated to phage-resistance, a fitness cost may be associated with a mutation conferring phage resistance that arises during coevolution, as demonstrated for the altered integrity of LPS and OmpC resulting in heterogeneous populations in the example of *E. coli* O157:H7 and phage PP01 [48], and altered maltose uptake with porin LamB mutation in the example of lambda phage and maltose restriction [49]. Numerous other examples exist regarding various phage–bacteria coevolution systems (see [54–57]). Environmental conditions can also greatly impact the coevolution of virulence and resistance by imposing limits to the arm race, as exemplified by the LamB example where maltose becomes a limiting factor [49]. This may result in different coevolution routes in natural settings from what is observed in the test tube. Such exogenous factors can include UV light-induced mutagenesis, which may induce phage-resistance mutations, but also cause additional mutations affecting in parallel [57]. Other examples include the influence of still or shaking culture conditions on population structures, which may influence particle collisions between phages and bacterial preys, or niche resource availability [58–60].

A recent work with *P. fluorescens* SBW25 showed that phage–bacterial interaction increased the bacterial mutation rates as well as its chance to adapt and survive both predation and altered environmental conditions. This indicates that phage-driven evolution may be ultimately beneficial for the bacteria [61].

Interestingly, while this phage-stimulated mutation rate of *P. fluorescens* SBW25 was observed in laboratory conditions [61], it was not observed for *P. fluorescens* communities living in the soil [62], most probably because selection for phage-resistance is higher in the soil than in vitro [63]. It is then assumed that, unlike in vitro coevolution that is characterized by the so-called arms race of increased resistance versus infectivity over time, coevolution in natural environments is largely driven by fluctuating selection, where cycles of phage-susceptible and phage-resistant bacterial populations intertwine with parent phages and evolved phages (mutant phages) that regain infectivity against the resistant bacteria [41].

3. Emergences of Phage Resistance in Animal Models

3.1. E. coli Diarrhoea in Cattle

Controlled studies on phage therapy and the emergence of phage resistance started in Western countries with a series of farm animal trials against experimental diarrhoea with enteropathogenic *E. coli* strains. In a first trial, oral phage therapy prevented *E. coli*-induced diarrhoea in colostrum-fed calves even when given 8 h after bacterial inoculation [14]. No phage-resistant variants were isolated from the calves. In another trial, phage therapy was administered at the onset of diarrhoeal symptoms, but resolved the intestinal symptoms in only half of the animals (14 out of 21 calves died). Phage-resistant variants were recovered from the small intestine of all calves failing clinical improvement. In parallel, the faecal bacterial content of 11 calves that responded to phage therapy was examined over a period of 14 days. *E. coli* titres progressively decreased over time and phage numbers increased during the first 48 h, therefore indicating phage replication. Phage-resistant bacteria emerged after 19 h, peaked at 2 days and decreased to undetectable levels after 10 days. Of note, these resistant mutants did not proliferate in the small intestine and did not cause diarrhoea when reinoculated to healthy colostrum-fed calves. The reduced virulence was associated with loss of the K antigen, which is known to be a virulence factor for enteropathogenic strains [64].

Prevention of diarrhoea by oral phages was also observed in piglets and lambs infected with *E. coli* [14]. Resistant variants were also isolated in the piglet faeces, but at relatively low rates. In contrast, no phage-resistant variants were observed in lambs. Similar results regarding the potential of phage therapy to prevent or treat *E. coli* diarrhoea were described in a second study done by Smith and Huggin [15]. This time, K-positive phage-resistant *E. coli* variants were isolated in addition to the already-observed K-negative variants. However, unlike the K-negative resistant variants, K-positive resistant variants were as virulent as the parent strain. These resistant variants were isolated only in vivo from the calves and not in vitro from a broth culture.

In another study in Holstein steers, phage therapy could reduce the average number of *E. coli* O157:H7 CFU in the faeces compared to controls, although it did not eliminate the bacteria from the majority of animals [16]. No phage-resistant *E. coli* O157:H7 mutants were observed.

Thus, phage-resistant variants are readily selected during phage therapy in vivo, but their pathological significance is unclear.

3.2. *E. coli and Enterococcus faecalis Intestinal Colonization in Mice*

Three studies using mouse models of *E. coli* intestinal colonization have also investigated the effect of phage therapy on the emergence of phage-resistance. In the first study, *E. coli* O157:H7 intestinal carriage could be eliminated within 48 h using three repeated phage oral doses. No resistant colonies were recovered and untreated control mice remained culture-positive for 10 days [16].

In the second study, an oral cocktail composed of three different phages was administered to mice colonized with enteroaggregative *E. coli* O104:H4 [18]. The bacterial titres did not decrease as compared to controls as expected and remained stable for 21 days, although phages were observed to replicate continuously during the time of the experiment. In addition, bacteria recovered on day 21 were still susceptible to each of the bacteriophages present in the cocktail when tested separately.

The third murine gut colonization study was a long-term 240 day protocol using oral T4 phages. Phage-resistant *E. coli* emerged only on day 92 and resistant variants constituted 100% of bacterial colonies isolated from phage-treated mice [17]. In comparison, only 20% of untreated mice carried phage-resistant variants. Moreover, when phage therapy was stopped at day 92, the presence of phage-resistant *E. coli* persisted over the 240 experimental days. The mechanism of phage-resistance was not described.

In an additional work, Duerkop et al. inoculated germ-free mice with *E. faecalis* V583 before starting phage therapy, which was first administered by oral gavage 6 h after colonization followed by administration in drinking water [19]. Phage therapy slightly decreased faecal bacterial loads by three-fold after 24 h. However, the level of colonization was not different from control animals after 48 h, even if phages were added to the drinking water. While 100% of the *E. faecalis* isolates remained phage-susceptible after 6 h of treatment, only 15% were still susceptible at 24 h and 100% were resistant at two days. Sequencing of 20 resistant bacterial variants revealed that they all had various mutations in the integral membrane protein PIPef, which was observed to promote phage infection.

Finally, using a model of gnotobiotic mouse intestinal colonization, Reyes et al. analysed the impact of viral predation on a consortium of 14 human bacterial symbionts [65]. When the community was subjected to virus-like particles purified from the faecal microbiota of human healthy donors, changes in the relative bacterial abundance was observed, but not with heat-killed viral-particle preparations. Especially, *Bacillus caccae* bacterial communities were observed to first decrease after phage attack, although they recovered later on. Evidence that phage resistance occurred due to genetic changes, like acquisition of CRISPR elements, could not be observed. The authors hypothesized that resistance was more the result of the expansion of an unexposed fraction of the population that could be protected in intestine microhabitat.

3.3. *Control of Poultry Pathogens*

A large part of the phage therapy application to control pathogenic bacteria in animals has been done in poultry, in order to prevent *Salmonella* spp. and *Campylobacter* spp. gut colonization and infection. *Salmonella enterica* is one of the major causes of foodborne infection in humans due to its symptomless carriage by chickens [66]. Up to now, the use of phage therapy to control *S. enterica* in poultry could reduce, but not eliminate, the bacteria. Sklar and Joerger reported that phage therapy did not significantly decrease *S. enterica* intestinal carriage in three animal trials [20].

Although phage resistance was observed after treatment, the authors speculate that other factors, like the salmonella intracellular lifestyle, could have contributed to the therapeutic failure. Atterbury et al. observed that low phage concentrations were not efficient in significantly decreasing bacterial loads [21]. They proposed that the low salmonella concentration in the chicken gut, associated with the complexity of the intestinal milieu—including physicochemical conditions, such as viscosity—was not suitable for phage amplification. Increasing the phage titre of phage preparations increase efficacy, but did not result in bacterial eradication. Interestingly, phage-resistance rates were higher following higher phage titres, indicating phage–bacteria interactions took place. Moreover, phage-resistant bacteria were not hampered in their ability to colonize the gut, and they often reverted to the susceptible parent phenotype. These observations were further confirmed by Carvalho et al., including the fact that phage-resistant mutants were able to colonize the gut, possibly by quick reversion to the parent phenotype [13].

Carrillo et al. reported somewhat analogous results with *Campylobacter jejuni* [11]. Phage treatment resulted in a decrease in the bacterial load ranging from 0.5 to 5 log CFU/g depending on the amount of phage and time of administration. As for *S. enterica*, certain phage-resistant isolates were observed to have decreased colonization abilities, but quickly recovered by reverting to the phage sensitive phenotype. Interestingly, phage-resistance in *C. jejuni* entailed a large (90 kb) genomic inversion at Mu-like prophage DNA sequences. The resulting cells demonstrated resistance to virulent phages, inefficient gut colonization and production of infectious bacteriophage CampMu particles [12]. Recovering gut colonization capability was associated with re-inversion of the DNA fragment. The observation revealed unprecedented phase-variation resistance mechanisms that could also occur in other bacteria. Later observations by Sørensen et al. suggested that phage-resistance phase variation was associated with excess capsular polysaccharide production in the case of chicken co-infection with *C. jejuni* and phage F336 [67]. However, resistant variants had kept their gut colonization capability.

Taken together, these different studies raise the question of the selection of phage-resistance in the gut environment and its implication for phage therapy. Indeed, the complexity of the gut environment, kinetics of resistance development with phage concentration dependency [21], resistance phenotype reversion [11,13] and selection for phase variable receptor structure leading to continuing co-evolution [12] must be taken into account when developing future phage strategies. One optimistic view is that, in contrast to antibiotic resistance, phage-resistance will be naturally kept under control via coevolution. In a longitudinal study on bacteria and phage interactions in a broiler house, Connerton et al. observed that although phage-resistant bacteria did emerge, they never outgrew and dominated the susceptible ones [68].

3.4. *Vibrio Cholerae*

Phages play a critical role in the evolution of pathogenic bacteria and especially that of *V. cholerae*, the causative agent of cholera epidemic diarrhoea. This is, for example, the case for the transmission of the cholera toxin into a nontoxigenic strain via integration of the lysogenic filamentous phage CTX_3 [69].

Phage-resistance appears to plays a central role in the evolution and regulation of this species in its natural environment. In a landmark three-year study in Bangladesh, Faruque et al. showed that the presence of phages infecting a given serogroup of *V. cholerae* was inversely correlated with the presence of viable *V. cholerae* of the same serogroup in the aquatic environment [70]. In addition, if a strain of a specific serogroup was observed in water samples with a phage infecting strains of the same serogroup, the strain was resistant to the coincidentally isolated phage in 73% of the case. During that period, the number of cholera patients correlated seasonally with the presence of *V. cholerae* in water samples devoid of cholera phages, and inter-epidemic periods correlated with water samples containing only cholera phages. These observations strongly confirmed the concept of fluctuating waves of different environmental *V. cholerae* serogroups existing in the aquatic environment, with successive rounds of phage amplification and selection of new resistant serogroups. The timing of phage peaks in the environment was also correlated with phage peaks in the stools of the patients, with increasing amount of phage particles in patients as the epidemic progressed [71]. In addition, phages excreted in cholera stools were the same as those found in the environment during the late stage of the epidemic and were expected to mediate *V. cholerae* elimination and antagonize its transmissibility. Indeed, *V. cholerae* populations recovered from phage-positive patient stools were significantly less infective than phage-negative stools in an animal model [72].

Interestingly, when phage-positive stools were cultured in rich nutrient medium, but not environmental water, a rapid emergence of phage-resistant variants that had lost the O1 antigen was observed. Since the O1 antigen is important for protection from the environmental stress and to escape host immune defences, it was suggested that the dominance of phage-resistant variants should not be able to sustain an ongoing epidemic. Indeed, phage-resistant *V. cholerae* variants having altered O1 antigens were significantly less able to colonize the small intestine of mice [33]. O1 antigen alteration was also observed to be phase variable due to single nucleotide deletions in two genes critical for O1 antigenic variation [32]. Indeed, modulation of O1 antigen in *V. cholerae* is important to escape O1 antigen specific phages in nature. Although O1 phage variants were attenuated in a mouse model of intestinal colonization, positive selection of revertants was shown in the intestinal tract. As a consequence, the intestinal environment favours O1 revertant that are infectious, but simultaneously susceptible to phages [32,72].

The phage content of patients' stools was analysed during a 10-year survey in Dhaka, Bangladesh [73]. One phage, ICP1, was present in all stools from cholera patient and used the O1 antigen of lipopolysaccharide as receptor. This suggests that ICP1 is extremely well adapted to its host with a high selective pressure to maintain its genomic structure. Two other phages (ICP2 and ICP3) were only transiently observed. ICP2 and ICP3 are not O1-specific, which explains why they were less frequent, since *V. cholerae* O1 is the predominant serotype.

The surface receptor of phage ICP2 is the OmpU outer membrane protein. *V. cholerae* resistant variants with decreased OmpU expression were described, and had attenuated virulence in an infant mouse colonization model in vivo [74].

Since a cocktail composed of phage targeting different bacterial receptor would reduce the chance of phage bacterial multi-resistance, Yen et al. reasoned that a cocktail composed of the three different ICP phages could be used to prevent cholera infection [22]. The tree-ICP cocktail could kill *V. cholerae* in vitro and prevent intestine colonization or cholera-like diarrhoea of infant mice and rabbit models. All isolates from mice having received the phage cocktail 6 or 12 h after bacterial challenge were sensitive to all three phages. Resistance was, however, observed for mice having received the cocktail 24 h before bacterial infection, raising the question of phage partial washout prior to bacterial inoculation, and thus incomplete efficacy. These resistant variants had a mutation in the O antigen gene for phage ICP 1 and ICP 3 resistant variants, and OmpU for phage ICP 2 resistant variants. None of the isolates were resistant to all three phages.

3.5. Experimental Meningitis and Endocarditis

The intrinsic bactericidal properties of anti-infective compounds such as phages can be reliably studied in models where host defences are poorly involved. Such models of therapeutic sanctuaries include experimental meningitis and experimental endocarditis (EE). Experimental meningitis implicates a special anatomical setting where drug distribution depends on the blood–brain barrier. In contrast, EE mirrors the general situation encountered in many deep-seated infections where pathogens on the cardiac valves surround themselves with amorphous aggregates of platelet-fibrin clots, which cellular host defences cannot penetrate (for review see [14]). Thus, the capability of antimicrobials to cross the blood-brain barrier for meningitis or to penetrate into cardiac valve lesions (also called vegetations) are critical issues in these models.

Early studies by Smith and Huggins used a mouse model of meningitis. Mice were infected with *E. coli* 018:K1:H7ColV+ and treated 16 h later with one intramuscular dose of anti K phage or 12 doses of tetracycline, ampicillin, chloramphenicol, or a mixture of trimethoprim and sulfamethoxazole. The mortality was significantly lower in phage-treated mice than in the different antibiotics groups. Isolates recovered from mouse brains were tested for phage and antibiotic resistance. No antibiotic resistance was detected. In contrast, 6 out of 360 independent colonies (observed in 5/36 of the mice) recovered from phage-treated mice were phage resistant. All six phage-resistant isolates were K1 antigen negative, predicting decreased infectivity.

Oechslin et al. examined the efficacy of an antipseudomonal cocktail of 12 phages, used alone or in combination with antibiotics, in a dual in vitro and in vivo model of *P. aeruginosa* experimental endocarditis [24]. First, ex vivo fibrin-platelet clots were inoculated with 10^8 log CFU of *P. aeruginosa*. Phage treatment rapidly decreased bacterial counts by 6 log CFU in 6 h. However, bacterial regrowth was observed after 24 h due to the selection of resistant variants. The rate of phage-resistance mutation in the original inoculum was of ca. 10^{-7}, and resistant mutants expectedly took over after initial phage-induced killing, as described by Luria and Delbrück [45]. Bacterial regrowth after 6 h was prevented by the addition of sub-inhibitory concentrations of antibiotics, namely ciprofloxacin or meropenem.

In rats with experimental aortic endocarditis, phage therapy decreased vegetation bacterial counts by 2.3 to 3 log CFU, depending on the mode of administration. Phage therapy alone was comparable to ciprofloxacin. However, combining both treatments resulted in a highly synergistic effect with 7/11 (64%) of rats having culture-negative vegetations after only 6 h, an unprecedented efficacy in this very experimental setting.

Most importantly, phage-resistant *pseudomonas* variants were not observed in in vivo endocarditis therapy, either before or after treatment, therefore suggesting that phage-resistance could result in altered virulence or altered fitness of bacteria in animals. The hypothesis was investigated by characterizing two phage-resistant variants recovered from the ex vivo fibrin clot experiments, which displayed either transient resistance to all phages present in the cocktail or total resistance against 10 of the 12 phages. Total genomic sequencing and comparison disclosed that one of the variants had a 15 bp deletion in the *pilt* ATPase gene involved in pilus retraction, thus resulting in altered twitching motility. The other phage-resistant variant had lost the O-antigen and LPS core due to a large 350 kb deletion encompassing the *galU* gene, which is involved in LPS synthesis. Both resistant variants were less able to infect sterile vegetations than the parent strain. Since both pilus and LPS are virulence factors, it was concluded that mutations conferring phage-resistance come at a high physiological cost in fitness and virulence.

3.6. Sepsis and Acute Infections

Pouillot et al. evaluated phage therapy in a murine model of fatal neonatal sepsis [25]. Rat pups received intraperitoneal injections with a virulent strain of *E. coli* O25b:H4-ST131 and were treated 7 h or 24 h post infection with subcutaneous injections of monophage $EC200^{PP}$. Phage therapy administered 7 h post infection rescued all the rats, whereas delaying therapy until 24 h rescued only 50% of the animals. Phage-resistant colonies with rough morphologies were recovered from the treatment failures. However, these variants were more susceptible to serum-induced killing and their virulence was dramatically attenuated in a sepsis model. Smith and Huggins made similar observations when injecting mice in one gastrocnemius muscle with *E. coli* 018:K1:H7 and injecting phages in the contralateral muscle [23]. Phages were efficient in decreasing bacterial muscle densities, and only very few phage-resistant variants were recovered at the inoculation site. These isolates were K1 antigen negative, which was previously shown to decrease virulence in mice [75].

Hung et al. used an experimental mouse model of *Klebsiella pneumoniae* liver abscess. Both intraperitoneal and intragastric administration of a single phage NK5 protected mice from death in a dose-dependent manner [26]. *K. pneumoniae*-induced liver injury and inflammatory cytokine production were significantly decreased by phage therapy. As in the experimental endocarditis study [24], phage-resistant variants emerged after 6 h or 12 h during phage time-kill curves in vitro, but no phage-resistant variants were observed in vivo. The resistant variants selected in vitro had lost the hypermucoviscosity characteristic of *K. pneumoniae* NK-5. Five individual resistant variants were tested for virulence in an intragastric model of infection and were significantly less virulent than the parent strain. The phage-resistant variants were more susceptible to phagocyte-induced killing. Gu et al. also observed the emergence of phage-resistant *K. pneumoniae* variants in vitro that were less virulent in vivo [29]. These variants exhibited colony morphology variations with a rough phenotype, as compared to the large and smooth wild-type colonies. This morphological feature of variant strains remained stable even after repeated subculture and storage at –80 °C. Variants also displayed much weaker virulence when intraperitoneally injected into mice.

Using a different type of model, Park et al. observed the effect of oral administration of phage-impregnated food (mixture of two different phages PPpW-3 and PPpW-4) to ayu fish infected by *Pseudomonas plecoglossicida* [28]. *P. plecoglossicida* were always detected in the kidneys of non-treated control fishes, while they were rapidly eradicated in fishes receiving phage therapy. Bacteria recovered from dying non-treated controls were susceptible to both phages. In contrast, phage-resistant variants were observed in liquid cultures after exposure to phages PPpW-3 and PPpW-4. Four individual variant isolates (three resistant to both phages and one resistant to phage PPpW-4 only) were tested in vivo by intramuscular injection. While the parent strain was highly virulent, all four resistant variants were avirulent, even at high inocula. In addition, one peculiar strain of *P. plecoglossicida*, which was highly virulent following intramuscular injection in ayu fish, was also tested and became poorly virulent after selection for phage-resistance. Moreover, bacterial growth in freshwater was observed to be lower in the presence of phages, and the number of phage PFUs increased rapidly, indicating phage predation and replication. These results are reminiscent of the *V. cholerae* phage ecology, and suggest that it might be possible to use phages to control *P. plecoglossicida*-induced disease in fish.

Finally, Lerodelle and Poutrel evaluated the potential of phage therapy to cure sub-clinical mastitis due to *Staphylococcus aureus* in lactating cows [27]. Udders were inoculated with *S. aureus* 106-6 and 107-59 via the mammary ducts and bacteriophage K lysates were administered by the same route once sub-clinical mastitis was confirmed. Phage therapy decreased *S. aureus* bacterial loads in 60% to 100% of the animals within 48 h of treatment, but could not sterilize all the udders. Treatment failures were attributed to the deep-seated and intracellular localization of *S. aureus* in mastitis, which hide bacteria from extracellular phages. Phage resistance was not responsible for treatment failure, as virtually no resistant variants were recovered.

4. Phage Resistant Variants for Vaccine Production and Studying Virulence Factors

The potential of phages to select for resistant variants with decreased in vivo virulence was used to generate vaccines against *S. enterica* or *S. aureus*. Capparelli et al. isolated a phage-resistant variant of *S. enterica* serovar Paratyphi B selected with phage φ1. The resistant variants formed smaller colonies and had lost their O-antigen; this phenotype was stable over many subculture passages. In addition, phage-resistance was also associated with impaired transcription of six virulence factors, resulting in an avirulent phenotype when inoculated intravenously into mice. Remarkably, immunization of mice with the resistant variant protected the animals against infection with the lethal parent strain, with 100% efficacy. As a control, vaccination with the heat-killed parent strain did not elicit protection.

The authors also observed that immunization of mice with phage-resistant *S. aureus* mutants conferred broad-spectrum immunity against this pathogen [35]. Acquisition of phage-resistance against phage M^{SA} resulted in several altered properties from the *S. aureus* parent strain, including teichoic acid alteration—which was responsible for resistance—reduced growth rate, decreased expression of several virulence factors, and increased production of capsular polysaccharides. All these features were stable during prolonged subculturing. Intramuscular administration of the phage-resistant variant protected mice from lethal doses of the wild-type parent strain in 90% of the animals.

Regarding virulence factor studies, Filippov et al. used site-directed mutagenesis of different LPS genes involved in the inner and outer core synthesis, followed by trans-complementation, to determine six *Yersinia pestis* phage receptors [36]. Phage-resistant mutants had attenuated virulence with increased LD50 and time-to-death in mice, including five mutants that became totally avirulent. Likewise, Lannto et al. reported loss of virulence driven by phage-resistant *Flavobacterium columnare* in a zebrafish model of infection [37]. Phage-resistant variants produced rough colony morphotypes and exhibited impaired gliding motility, a phenotype that was maintained over ten serial passages in liquid culture. Virulence of the parental morphotype was compared to the phage-resistant R type in a zebrafish infection model. The R type mutant became completely avirulent.

Heierson et al. reported that phage-resistant mutants of *Bacillus thuringiensis* had a decreased virulence phenotype in pupae of the Cecropia moths, which correlated with flagella loss and an increased susceptibility to methicillin [38]. In two studies performed by Flyg et al., phage-resistant variants of the insect pathogen *Serratia marcescens* were also observed to have decreased resistance to insect immunity and decreased virulence in a drosophila infection model, although the exact reason for this virulence decrease was not described [39,40]. Finally, Regeimbal et al. also observed that *Acinetobacter baumannii* phage-resistant variants that had lost their capsule became avirulent in a *Galleria mellonella* model [76].

While alterations of virulence features related to phage resistance might be useful for vaccination, they also help understand bacterial pathogenesis. In this regard, the above-mentioned studies support the fact that phage resistance may be accompanied by fitness costs for the bacteria that may benefit the host. As a result, the emergence of phage resistance during phage therapy is not always synonymous with treatment failure.

5. The Biological Cost of Antibiotic Resistance and the Combined Action of Phage and Antibiotics

As for phage–bacteria coevolution, antimicrobial resistance is an ancient process that results from the complex interaction between many microorganisms in their natural environment. Indeed, most antibiotics are naturally-produced toxic molecules against which bacteria had to evolve protective mechanisms in order to survive [77]. Antibiotic-resistant bacteria are an increasing problem in human and veterinary medicine, as well as in the farming industry, due to the overuse of antibiotics over the last half century. Antibiotic resistance may be intrinsic (i.e., bacteria may be naturally resistant to certain antibiotics) or may result from spontaneous mutations or from the acquisition of horizontally-transferred resistance genes [78]. Foreign gene acquisition may involve DNA transformation, cell-cell conjugation, and phage-mediated transduction.

Resistance mechanisms include structural alteration or decreased expression of the antibiotic target, decreased drug accumulation (via decreased permeability or increased drug efflux), or changes in global metabolic pathways (for review on the topic see [79]).

Since antibiotics target important physiological functions, such as protein synthesis, cell wall synthesis, or DNA replication, antibiotic resistance often implies a certain fitness cost (for a review on the topic see [80]). However, the fitness cost associated with resistance may sometimes become counterbalanced by compensatory mutations. This was the case in *E. coli*, were streptomycin resistance conferred by mutations in the ribosomal protein RpsL first decreased the speed of protein synthesis, but were compensated after several passages (evolved cultures) by neighbouring mutations that restored the speed of protein synthesis [81]. Likewise, acquisition of the tetracycline and chloramphenicol resistance plasmid pACYC184 by *E. coli* decreased its growth rate. The growth speed was recovered, and even surpassed in evolved cultures, thanks to adaptive mutations present on the bacterial chromosome (not on the plasmid), which took advantage of the tetracycline-resistance efflux pump [82]. Thus, it was the bacterium that took advantage of the presence of the plasmid, not the plasmid that took advantage of the bacterium. Numerous other examples of adaptive mutations exist both in vitro and in vivo [83,84]. In addition, the acquisition of mobile genetic elements can also lead to co-selection to more than one antibiotic resistance if different resistance genes are genetically linked [85], and such multi-resistance is not incompatible with the restoration of fitness, as exemplified in the pACYC184 experiments [82]. Therefore, as with phages, bacteria undergo dynamic evolutionary processes when challenged with antibiotics.

On the other hand, combining both phages and antibiotics could act in synergism to prevent resistance or increase therapeutic efficacy (for review on the topic see [86]). Verma et al. showed that combining ciprofloxacin and phages prevented the emergence of phage-resistant variants during treatment of *K. pneumoniae* biofilms, although no direct bactericidal synergism between phages and antibiotics was observed [87]. The emergence of phage-resistance was also prevented by treating *S. aureus* (in continuous culture) with a combination of phages and gentamicin [88]. Torres-Barcelo et al. confirmed the potential benefit of combining phages and antibiotics (in this case, streptomycin) against *P. aeruginosa* [89]. The phenomenon of phage-antibiotic synergism was also observed in animal experiments of *P. aeruginosa* endocarditis [24], as well as with the multi-resistant bacterium *Burkholderia cepacia* [90].

In addition, Chan et al. showed that selection of phage-resistance could also restore antibiotic susceptibility [91]. When using a lytic phage specifically targeting bacterial receptors that are part of the multidrug efflux systems, MexAB and MexXY—for instance, the outer membrane porin OprM—phage-resistance restored antibiotic susceptibility because the efflux pump, which confers resistance to several antibiotic classes, was no longer functional.

However, phage-antibiotic synergism may be dependent on experimental systems, and especially antibiotic dosages. Cairns et al. showed that using sub-inhibitory concentrations of streptomycin, as might be found in natural environments or sewage, could increase the rate of phage-resistance mutations in *Pseudomonas fluorescens*, and, conversely, phage exposure increased the rate of mutation to streptomycin resistance [92], which is compatible with phage-induced bacterial mutations described by Pal et al. [61]. Nevertheless, looking at the association between antibiotic and phage-resistance in a large collection of laboratory or clinical *E. coli* isolates, Allen et al. did not find a positive or systematic correlation between drug-resistance and phage-resistance, suggesting that antibiotics used in medicine or agriculture are unlikely to induce changes in phage resistance or phage-antibiotic cross-resistance in the environment [93].

Taken together, while different kinds of positive or negative phage–bacteria interactions can be observed in the laboratory or under natural conditions, potentially useful synergistic interactions do exist and could be valuable to use in specific clinical situations.

6. Phage-Resistance in the Setting of Phage Therapy

While the use of phages as therapeutic agents is conceptually simple, complex questions still exist regarding host range, route of administration, pharmacokinetic/pharmacodynamic parameters, and managing the risk of resistance. One of the main differences between phages and antibiotics is the ability of phages to self-replicate at the infection site. Therefore, the pharmacokinetics of phage therapy is closer to the population dynamics of predator-prey models described in co-evolutionary studies (see Section 1) than classical peak-distribution-elimination phases classically measured for antibiotics. Levin and Bull proposed theoretical predictions for modelling interactions between phages and bacteria during phage therapy of acute infections [94]. Assuming that there is a bacterial density threshold beyond which the patient dies, and a limit in host defences, below which bacterial growth cannot be controlled, the absence of therapy may lead to a situation where host defences cannot keep bacteria in check in order to prevent death. By combining host defence and phage therapy, the bacterial growth rate becomes negative before it reaches the lethal density threshold. In addition, the remaining host defences are likely to more easily hinder the delayed growth of phage-resistant bacteria before they reach the lethal threshold. In a recent study done by Roach et al., the effect of host immunity and phage-mediated bacterial clearance was investigated in a mouse model of acute *P. aeruginosa* pneumonia [31]. Phage therapy using healthy mice and mice with various immune defects revealed that neutrophil-phage synergism was essential for the resolution of disease. Indeed, phage therapy failed to prevent fatal outcomes in mice with neutrophil signalling defects due to the outgrowth of phage-resistant variants. In silico analysis also predicted that neutrophils were important to prevent the emergence of phage-resistant variants and to efficiently clear infection. Thus, without immune activation, phage-resistant mutants overwhelm the basal immune defences and lead to a resurgence of a phage-resistant population that ultimately causes mortality.

Two general models of phage therapy implementation were proposed in order to manage the risk of phage-resistance. First using phage cocktails and second adapting single phages to each patient condition, referred to as personalized phage therapy.

The main reason for combining multiple phages in cocktails is to broaden the phage host range and improve effectiveness by increasing the number of potential target pathogens. This results in a greater potential for empirical treatment [95,96]. Regarding the emergence of resistance, the different phages present in the cocktail are expected to synergize by targeting different receptors on the bacterial surface, resulting in a lower statistical chance of bacterial co-resistance, as with combined phage-antibiotic therapy. This was supported by Gu et al. who observed significantly lower frequencies of phage-resistant *K. pneumoniae* mutants using a cocktail of three phages, compared to monotherapy [29]. Similar observations were made with *E. coli*, where phage cocktails decreased the frequency of phage-resistance or delayed the emergence of phage-resistant variants [97,98]. This broad spectrum antimicrobial strategy is reminiscent of the model developed by pharmaceutical companies for antibiotics, with the risk of treatment failure in case of a lack of susceptible bacteria, as well as the risk of selecting resistance in fortuitous innocuous bacterial bystanders [96]. This approach is used in countries such as Georgia, where phage cocktails are administered as an empiric treatment, although the phage content may change over time in order to adapt to the most prevalent pathogens [99]. Alternatively, existing phages can also be adapted to existing phage-resistant strains [100].

The personalized phage strategy uses single phages or targeted phage cocktails directly formulated from a phage bank according to the pathogen isolated from the patient [96,100]. Although this strategy entails a higher cost associated with personalized treatment, it offers much more flexibility regarding the spectrum of the phage and can counter the emergence of bacterial resistance more efficiently. In one of the few well-documented phage therapy clinical trials that took the emergence of phage-resistance into account, Międzybrodzki et al. achieved ca. 40% of a positive clinical outcome with 20% pathogen eradication using phage monotherapy [101,102]. Following phage therapy, phage typing patterns of the pathogens were modified in 70% of the patients treated for *S. aureus* infection (53 patients in total), 91% for *P. aeruginosa* (11 patients in total), and 100% for *E. faecalis* (14 patients in total), and *E. coli* (14 patients in total). Resistance of the target pathogen to the therapeutic phage was also observed in up to 17% of *S. aureus* cases, 36% of *P. aeruginosa*, 43% of *E. faecalis*, and 86% of *E. coli*. The high frequency in the *E. coli* infection group was a cause of frequent change of the phage during the treatment. Complete resistance to any of the phages present in the phage collection of the Ludwik Hirszfeld Institute, Poland, was observed in 7% of the *S. aureus* cases, 27% of the *P. aeruginosa* cases, 21% *E. faecalis* cases, and 27% of the *E. coli* cases.

Emergence of resistance during phage therapy was also documented by Zhvania et al. in a recent case study of chronic *S. aureus* skin infection at the Eliava Phage Therapy Center, Georgia [103]. Treatment with two anti-staphylococcal products greatly improved the patients' symptoms starting from seven days posttreatment. However, phage-resistance to the phage cocktail (Pyobacteriophage) was observed after three months of treatment and an alternate phage cocktail had to be substituted.

The use of personalized phage therapy was also exemplified in a case report by Schooley et al., where personalized-based therapeutic phages were administered parenterally to successfully treat one patient with a disseminated multidrug resistant *A. baumannii* infection. Different phage cocktails were assembled based on time-kill assays using a library of 96 phages. In vitro tests by serial passages revealed a stepwise selection of resistance to two of the cocktails. A third phage cocktail was prepared using the resistant isolates, which was then administered to the patient until the successful outcome of the infection. Of note, the phage-resistant phenotype that arose over time was associated with increased antibiotic susceptibility when phage and antibiotics were simultaneously administered. In addition, differences in colony morphology were observed during the therapy, with the eventual loss of the capsule. The authors speculate that the capsule loss may have contributed to the phage-antibiotic synergy, which included decreased virulence that had also been observed by the same author in previous studies [76]. In addition, another case of successful personalized phage therapy was reported in a lung transplant patient suffering from multi-drug resistant *P. aeruginosa* pneumonia [104]. Different phage cocktails were administered to the patient intravenously or by inhalation. Susceptibility of the bacteria to the phage was monitored during the treatment. New phage cocktails were administered as bacteriophage resistance emerged. As above, a shift in the antibiotic susceptibility pattern was also observed during phage treatment. Thus, while phage resistance does emerge, it is not prohibitive to phage therapy as long as it is carefully monitored in order to adapt the phage composition, and additional synergistic interactions with host defences or antibiotics may occur.

Finally, Khawaldeh et al. reported a successful case of adjunctive bacteriophage therapy for a refractory *P. aeruginosa* urinary tract infection [105]. The phage cocktail used for the study was composed of six lytic bacteriophages coming from existing bacteriophage libraries at the Eliava Institute in Tbilisi and were selected based on several isolates of the infecting *P. aeruginosa*. Bacteriophage counts was observed to remain high until after the disappearance of the target organism and then diminished sharply. Urine samples remained sterile for six months after the completion of antibacterial treatment and no bacteriophage-resistant bacteria arose during the time of the treatment.

7. Conclusions and Perspectives

Early studies suggested that phage–bacterial coevolution was limited to a few rounds of infection cycles. Resistance emerges following the selection of bacterial subpopulations carrying preexisting mutations and results in alterations in envelope determinants used by phages to adsorb on the bacterial surface. Hence, phage-resistant variants were totally immune to further infection and coevolution was rapidly stopped. These initial observations raised doubts regarding the use of phages as therapeutic agents because such rapid emergence of phage-resistance could hamper treatment effectiveness. However, phage-resistance is often balanced with resulting fitness costs for the bacteria. Indeed, abiotic/biotic factors, including environmental conditions, multiple bacterial exploiters, and resource availability, can greatly impact the successful emergence or stability of phage-resistance in natural environments.

The altered fitness of phage-resistant bacteria is believed to be important in phage therapy, where resistance mechanisms have been shown to alter virulence factors. In this literature review, the cost of phage-resistance was associated with virulence reduction in 17/22 (78%) of the articles (summarized in Table 1). Phage-resistant variants emerged in up to 82% of cases during phage-induced gut decolonization (out of 11 studies). Resistant variants were also reported after treatment of acute infection such as meningitis or sepsis, in up to 50% of the studies (out of six studies). Regarding the studied organisms, only 3/28 studies assessed the emergence of phage-resistance in Gram-positive bacteria, including two in *S. aureus* and one in *E. faecalis*. This focus on Gram-negative bacteria raises the question as to whether Gram-negative bacteria are more problematic regarding resistance selection.

Several lessons can be extrapolated from the reviewed studies. First, phage-resistant variants are often recovered after experimental therapy. Second, the intestinal milieu seems to be more prone to the evolution of phage-resistance, possibly due to its complexity, including mechanical viscosity and limited host defences in the lumen. Third, although phage-resistance often has a cost for the bacteria, it is not always associated with decreased infectivity, at least in the intestinal milieu.

From the five studies that clearly linked the emergence of resistance during phage therapy with alteration of a known virulence factor, like the O-antigen or LPS [14,15,22–24], four still reported resistant variants after therapy. The question then arises as to whether these variants were mere innocuous bystanders on the way of being eliminated by host defences, or whether they could still produce infection.

In any case, the ideal experimental setting should be to apply the Koch postulate and inoculate the variants to the animals in order to re-evaluate their infectivity. Indeed, recovering phage-resistant variants from in vivo samples may not be automatically synonymous with therapeutic failure, a counter-intuitive concept that appears to apply to phage therapy.

Regarding phage therapy clinical trials in human, the emergence of resistance seems to be a serious case of therapy failure if not monitored correctly. In three out of four clinical studies that monitored resistance, phage resistance led to adaptation of the composition of administered phages. Moreover, additional factors other than spontaneous mutations could also impact clinical resistance, including the immune status of the patient, the presence of biofilm, bacterial persistors, a chronic type of disease, and the possibility that the pathogenic strain possesses acquired types of resistance, like CRISPR [5,31,94,106].

It remains unclear whether the widespread use of phages to treat infections might lead to a problematic increase in phage-resistant bacterial pathogens in an analogous way that resistance developed to antibiotics. Although fitness cost may be associated with phage-resistance, this may depend on the environment, e.g., less virulence reduction associated in the intestinal milieu. Fitness was mainly assessed in the context of virulence, not in the bacterial survival in the environment. The initial fitness cost associated with antibiotic resistance could be compensated by adaptive mutations that stabilized resistant bacteria in the environment. In addition, as for antibiotics, horizontal transfer of phage resistance by plasmid acquisition was observed, which could be a problem in the long-term [107].

The real question is whether or not phages will be as widely used as antibiotics in the future. Antibiotics are used in medicine not only to prevent and combat infection, but also for other industrial applications in agriculture, which used up to 63,000 tons of antibiotics for livestock production alone in 2010 [108]. For now, it is more likely that phage therapy will be utilized as a more personalized medicine. In this case, the emergence of resistance will be manageable thanks to careful monitoring during therapy.

It is interesting to note that in the hypothetical emergence of a phage-resistant superbug, coevolution studies suggest that new phages will always be available in nature. Indeed, from environmental perspectives, bacteria were observed to be more resistant to their contemporary phages than to past or future phages and that hard-to-infect bacteria were infected by generalist phages and not specialists [63,109].

Finally, in addition of the use of phage particles themselves, or phage-antibiotic combinations, it is also possible to use purified phage lysins as a potential therapy. Recombinant phage lysins demonstrate high antibacterial activity, although they are mainly restricted to Gram-positive pathogens (reviewed in [110]). Regarding resistance, the lysin PlyG was evaluated for the possible resistance emergence after repeated treatment of *Bacillus anthracis* [111]. Spontaneous resistant mutants could not be detected, even when a compound like ethyl methanesulfonate was used to increase the bacterial mutation rate. This suggests that phage lysins target essential cell wall components that are unlikely to be modified by the host bacteria. Similar observations were made for *Streptococcus pneumoniae* and the phage lysin Pal, where repeated exposure to low concentrations of enzyme did not lead to resistant mutants [112]. More recently, Totté et al. successfully treated three cases of chronic dermatoses due to *S. aureus* with topical applications of the Staphefekt SA.100 endolysin product [113]. For all cases, resistance induction was not observed during long-term treatment, which is usually observed with antibiotic therapy.

The reviewed studies highlight both the potential power and the limits of phage therapy. Phages and bacteria are longstanding partners that have learned how to respect each other and coevolve together. The use of phages for therapy might be highly efficacious to eradicate pathogens in well-defined and circumscribed infected niches, particularly if used in combination with antibiotics. Their great advantage over antibiotics alone is their extremely rapid killing kinetics, which surpasses any known antimicrobial molecules, and the fact that they can self-replicate at the infection site. Other advantages are that they may increase antibiotic susceptibility in specific cases, and that the emergence of phage-resistant escape mutants may be prevented by antibiotics, or may carry alterations in virulence factors. These developments are promising, but should follow a thorough step-by-step developmental process, in order to avoid creating a resistance dead-end like that of antibiotics.

On the other hand, large scale or open field utilization of phage therapy, such as gut decolonization for the agricultural industry, is less certain. The coevolution dynamics of phage and bacteria is extremely sophisticated in such complex environments. Moreover, although the fascinating example of cholera control is inspiring, it is clear that phages never eradicated *V. cholerae*, whereas *V. cholerae* never got rid of the phage. As enlightening as this example may be, it primarily underlines coevolution, but not eradication, and not even efficacious population control, as epidemics still proceed.

Acknowledgments: The author would like to thanks Philippe Moreillon and Shawna E. McCallin for their helpful comments on the manuscript.

References

1. Sugden, R.; Kelly, R.; Davies, S. Combatting antimicrobial resistance globally. *Nat. Microbiol.* **2016**, *1*, 16187. [CrossRef] [PubMed]
2. Salmond, G.P.; Fineran, P.C. A century of the phage: Past, present and future. *Nat. Rev. Microbiol.* **2015**, *13*, 777–786. [CrossRef] [PubMed]
3. Roach, D.R.; Debarbieux, L. Phage therapy: Awakening a sleeping giant. *Emerg. Top. Life Sci.* **2017**, *1*, 93. [CrossRef]
4. Harper, D.R. Criteria for selecting suitable infectious diseases for phage therapy. *Viruses* **2018**, *10*, 177. [CrossRef] [PubMed]
5. Labrie, S.J.; Samson, J.E.; Moineau, S. Bacteriophage resistance mechanisms. *Nat. Rev. Microbiol.* **2010**, *8*, 317–327. [CrossRef] [PubMed]
6. Koskella, B.; Brockhurst, M.A. Bacteria–phage coevolution as a driver of ecological and evolutionary processes in microbial communities. *FEMS Microbiol. Rev.* **2014**, *38*, 916–931. [CrossRef] [PubMed]
7. Bertozzi Silva, J.; Storms, Z.; Sauvageau, D. Host receptors for bacteriophage adsorption. *FEMS Microbiol. Lett.* **2016**, *363*. [CrossRef] [PubMed]
8. León, M.; Bastías, R. Virulence reduction in bacteriophage resistant bacteria. *Front. Microbiol.* **2015**, *6*, 343. [CrossRef] [PubMed]
9. Vasu, K.; Nagaraja, V. Diverse functions of restriction-modification systems in addition to cellular defense. *Microbiol. Mol. Biol. Rev.* **2013**, *77*, 53–72. [CrossRef] [PubMed]
10. Vale, P.F.; Lafforgue, G.; Gatchitch, F.; Gardan, R.; Moineau, S.; Gandon, S. Costs of CRISPR-Cas-mediated resistance in *Streptococcus thermophilus*. *Proc. R. Soc. B* **2015**, *282*, 20151270. [CrossRef] [PubMed]
11. Loc Carrillo, C.; Atterbury, R.J.; el-Shibiny, A.; Connerton, P.L.; Dillon, E.; Scott, A.; Connerton, I.F. Bacteriophage therapy to reduce *Campylobacter jejuni* colonization of broiler chickens. *Appl. Environ. Microbiol.* **2005**, *71*, 6554–6563. [CrossRef] [PubMed]
12. Scott, A.E.; Timms, A.R.; Connerton, P.L.; Loc Carrillo, C.; Adzfa Radzum, K.; Connerton, I.F. Genome dynamics of *Campylobacter jejuni* in response to bacteriophage predation. *PLoS Pathog.* **2007**, *3*, e119. [CrossRef] [PubMed]
13. Carvalho, C.M.; Gannon, B.W.; Halfhide, D.E.; Santos, S.B.; Hayes, C.M.; Roe, J.M.; Azeredo, J. The in vivo efficacy of two administration routes of a phage cocktail to reduce numbers of *Campylobacter coli* and *Campylobacter jejuni* in chickens. *BMC Microbiol.* **2010**, *10*, 232. [CrossRef] [PubMed]
14. Smith, H.W.; Huggins, M.B. Effectiveness of phages in treating experimental *Escherichia coli* diarrhoea in calves, piglets and lambs. *J. Gen. Microbiol.* **1983**, *129*, 2659–2675. [CrossRef] [PubMed]
15. Smith, H.W.; Huggins, M.B.; Shaw, K.M. The control of experimental *Escherichia coli* diarrhoea in calves by means of bacteriophages. *Microbiology* **1987**, *133*, 1111–1126. [CrossRef] [PubMed]
16. Sheng, H.; Knecht, H.J.; Kudva, I.T.; Hovde, C.J. Application of bacteriophages to control intestinal *Escherichia coli* o157:H7 levels in ruminants. *Appl. Environ. Microbiol.* **2006**, *72*, 5359–5366. [CrossRef] [PubMed]
17. Majewska, J.; Beta, W.; Lecion, D.; Hodyra-Stefaniak, K.; Klopot, A.; Kazmierczak, Z.; Miernikiewicz, P.; Piotrowicz, A.; Ciekot, J.; Owczarek, B.; et al. Oral application of T4 phage induces weak antibody production in the gut and in the blood. *Viruses* **2015**, *7*, 4783–4799. [CrossRef] [PubMed]
18. Maura, D.; Morello, E.; du Merle, L.; Bomme, P.; Le Bouguenec, C.; Debarbieux, L. Intestinal colonization by enteroaggregative *Escherichia coli* supports long-term bacteriophage replication in mice. *Environ. Microbiol.* **2012** *14*, 1844–1854. [CrossRef] [PubMed]

19. Duerkop, B.A.; Huo, W.; Bhardwaj, P.; Palmer, K.L.; Hooper, L.V. Molecular basis for lytic bacteriophage resistance in enterococci. *mBio* **2016**, *7*. [CrossRef] [PubMed]
20. Sklar, I.B.; Joerger, R.D. Attempts to utilize bacteriophage to combat salmonella enterica serovar entemtidis infection in chickens. *J. Food Saf.* **2001**, *21*, 15–29. [CrossRef]
21. Atterbury, R.J.; van Bergen, M.A.; Ortiz, F.; Lovell, M.A.; Harris, J.A.; de Boer, A.; Wagenaar, J.A.; Allen, V.M.; Barrow, P.A. Bacteriophage therapy to reduce salmonella colonization of broiler chickens. *Appl. Environ. Microbiol.* **2007**, *73*, 4543–4549. [CrossRef] [PubMed]
22. Yen, M.; Cairns, L.S.; Camilli, A. A cocktail of three virulent bacteriophages prevents vibrio cholerae infection in animal models. *Nat. Commun.* **2017**, *8*, 14187. [CrossRef] [PubMed]
23. Smith, H.W.; Huggins, M.B. Successful treatment of experimental escherichia coli infections in mice using phage: Its general superiority over antibiotics. *J. Gen. Microbiol.* **1982**, *128*, 307–318. [CrossRef] [PubMed]
24. Oechslin, F.; Piccardi, P.; Mancini, S.; Gabard, J.; Moreillon, P.; Entenza, J.M.; Resch, G.; Que, Y.A. Synergistic interaction between phage therapy and antibiotics clears *Pseudomonas aeruginosa* infection in endocarditis and reduces virulence. *J. Infect. Dis.* **2017**, *215*, 703–712. [CrossRef] [PubMed]
25. Pouillot, F.; Chomton, M.; Blois, H.; Courroux, C.; Noelig, J.; Bidet, P.; Bingen, E.; Bonacorsi, S. Efficacy of bacteriophage therapy in experimental sepsis and meningitis caused by a clone o25b:H4-st131 *Escherichia coli* strain producing CTX-M-15. *Antimicrob. Agents Chemother.* **2012**, *56*, 3568–3575. [CrossRef] [PubMed]
26. Hung, C.H.; Kuo, C.F.; Wang, C.H.; Wu, C.M.; Tsao, N. Experimental phage therapy in treating klebsiella pneumoniae-mediated liver abscesses and bacteremia in mice. *Antimicrob. Agents Chemother.* **2011**, *55*, 1358–1365. [CrossRef] [PubMed]
27. Lerondelle, C.; Poutrel, B. Bacteriophage treatment trials on staphylococcal udder infection in lactating cows. *Ann. Rech. Vet.* **1980**, *11*, 421–426. [PubMed]
28. Park, S.C.; Shimamura, I.; Fukunaga, M.; Mori, K.I.; Nakai, T. Isolation of bacteriophages specific to a fish pathogen, pseudomonas plecoglossicida, as a candidate for disease control. *Appl. Environ. Microbiol.* **2000**, *66*, 1416–1422. [CrossRef] [PubMed]
29. Gu, J.; Liu, X.; Li, Y.; Han, W.; Lei, L.; Yang, Y.; Zhao, H.; Gao, Y.; Song, J.; Lu, R.; et al. A method for generation phage cocktail with great therapeutic potential. *PLoS ONE* **2012**, *7*, e31698. [CrossRef] [PubMed]
30. Capparelli, R.; Nocerino, N.; Iannaccone, M.; Ercolini, D.; Parlato, M.; Chiara, M.; Iannelli, D. Bacteriophage therapy of salmonella enterica: A fresh appraisal of bacteriophage therapy. *J. Infect. Dis.* **2010**, *201*, 52–61. [CrossRef] [PubMed]
31. Roach, D.R.; Leung, C.Y.; Henry, M.; Morello, E.; Singh, D.; Di Santo, J.P.; Weitz, J.S.; Debarbieux, L. Synergy between the host immune system and bacteriophage is essential for successful phage therapy against an acute respiratory pathogen. *Cell Host Microbe* **2017**, *22*, 38–47. [CrossRef] [PubMed]
32. Seed, K.D.; Faruque, S.M.; Mekalanos, J.J.; Calderwood, S.B.; Qadri, F.; Camilli, A. Phase variable o antigen biosynthetic genes control expression of the major protective antigen and bacteriophage receptor in vibrio cholerae o1. *PLoS Pathog.* **2012**, *8*, e1002917. [CrossRef] [PubMed]
33. Nesper, J.; Kapfhammer, D.; Klose, K.E.; Merkert, H.; Reidl, J. Characterization of vibrio cholerae O1 antigen as the bacteriophage K139 receptor and identification of IS1004 insertions aborting O1 antigen biosynthesis. *J. Bacteriol.* **2000**, *182*, 5097–5104. [CrossRef] [PubMed]
34. Attridge, S.R.; Fazeli, A.; Manning, P.A.; Stroeher, U.H. Isolation and characterization of bacteriophage-resistant mutants of *Vibrio cholerae* O139. *Microb. Pathog.* **2001**, *30*, 237–246. [CrossRef] [PubMed]
35. Capparelli, R.; Nocerino, N.; Lanzetta, R.; Silipo, A.; Amoresano, A.; Giangrande, C.; Becker, K.; Blaiotta, G.; Evidente, A.; Cimmino, A.; et al. Bacteriophage-resistant *Staphylococcus aureus* mutant confers broad immunity against staphylococcal infection in mice. *PLoS ONE* **2010**, *5*, e11720. [CrossRef] [PubMed]
36. Filippov, A.A.; Sergueev, K.V.; He, Y.; Huang, X.Z.; Gnade, B.T.; Mueller, A.J.; Fernandez-Prada, C.M.; Nikolich, M.P. Bacteriophage-resistant mutants in yersinia pestis: Identification of phage receptors and attenuation for mice. *PLoS ONE* **2011**, *6*, e25486. [CrossRef] [PubMed]
37. Laanto, E.; Bamford, J.K.H.; Laakso, J.; Sundberg, L.R. Phage-driven loss of virulence in a fish pathogenic bacterium. *PLoS ONE* **2012** *7*, e53157. [CrossRef] [PubMed]
38. Heierson, A.; Sidén, I.; Kivaisi, A.; Boman, H.G. Bacteriophage-resistant mutants of *Bacillus thuringiensis* with decreased virulence in pupae of *Hyalophora cecropia*. *J. Bacteriol.* **1986**, *167*, 18–24. [CrossRef] [PubMed]

39. Flyg, C.; Kenne, K.; Boman, H.G. Insect pathogenic properties of serratia marcescens: Phage-resistant mutants with a decreased resistance to cecropia immunity and a decreased virulence to drosophila. *J. Gen. Microbiol.* **1980**, *120*, 173–181. [CrossRef] [PubMed]
40. Flyg, C.; Xanthopoulos, K.G. Insect pathogenic properties of serratia marcescens. Passive and active resistance to insect immunity studied with protease-deficient and phage-resistant mutants. *J. Gen. Microbiol.* **1983**, *129*, 453–464. [CrossRef]
41. Buckling, A.; Rainey, P.B. Antagonistic coevolution between a bacterium and a bacteriophage. *Proc. R. Soc. B* **2002**, *269*, 931–936. [CrossRef] [PubMed]
42. Riede, I.; Eschbach, M.L. Evidence that trat interacts with ompa of *Escherichia coli*. *FEBS Lett.* **1986**, *205*, 241–245. [CrossRef]
43. Hanlon, G.W.; Denyer, S.P.; Olliff, C.J.; Ibrahim, L.J. Reduction in exopolysaccharide viscosity as an aid to bacteriophage penetration through *Pseudomonas aeruginosa* biofilms. *Appl. Environ. Microbiol.* **2001**, *67*, 2746–2753. [CrossRef] [PubMed]
44. Destoumieux-Garzón, D.; Duquesne, S.; Peduzzi, J.; Goulard, C.; Desmadril, M.; Letellier, L.; Rebuffat, S.; Boulanger, P. The iron–siderophore transporter fhua is the receptor for the antimicrobial peptide microcin J25: Role of the microcin val(11)–pro(16) β-hairpin region in the recognition mechanism. *Biochem. J.* **2005**, *389*, 869–876. [CrossRef] [PubMed]
45. Luria, S.E.; Delbruck, M. Mutations of bacteria from virus sensitivity to virus resistance. *Genetics* **1943**, *28*, 491–511. [PubMed]
46. Dennehy, J.J. What can phages tell us about host-pathogen coevolution? *Int. J. Evol. Biol.* **2012**, *2012*, 12. [CrossRef] [PubMed]
47. Lenski, R.E.; Levin, B.R. Constraints on the coevolution of bacteria and virulent phage: A model, some experiments, and predictions for natural communities. *Am. Nat.* **1985**, *125*, 585–602. [CrossRef]
48. Mizoguchi, K.; Morita, M.; Fischer, C.R.; Yoichi, M.; Tanji, Y.; Unno, H. Coevolution of bacteriophage pp01 and *Escherichia coli* o157:H7 in continuous culture. *Appl. Environ. Microbiol.* **2003**, *69*, 170–176. [CrossRef] [PubMed]
49. Spanakis, E.; Horne, M.T. Co-adaptation of *Escherichia coli* and coliphage lambda vir in continuous culture. *J. Gen. Microbiol.* **1987**, *133*, 353–360. [PubMed]
50. Meyer, J.R.; Dobias, D.T.; Weitz, J.S.; Barrick, J.E.; Quick, R.T.; Lenski, R.E. Repeatability and contingency in the evolution of a key innovation in phage lambda. *Science* **2012**, *335*, 428–432. [CrossRef] [PubMed]
51. Hall, A.R.; Scanlan, P.D.; Buckling, A. Bacteria-phage coevolution and the emergence of generalist pathogens. *Am. Nat.* **2011**, *177*, 44–53. [CrossRef] [PubMed]
52. Buckling, A.; Rainey, P.B. The role of parasites in sympatric and allopatric host diversification. *Nature* **2002**, *420*, 496–499. [CrossRef] [PubMed]
53. Hall, A.R.; Scanlan, P.D.; Morgan, A.D.; Buckling, A. Host-parasite coevolutionary arms races give way to fluctuating selection. *Ecol. Lett.* **2011**, *14*, 635–642. [CrossRef] [PubMed]
54. Lennon, J.T.; Khatana, S.A.; Marston, M.F.; Martiny, J.B. Is there a cost of virus resistance in marine cyanobacteria? *ISME J.* **2007**, *1*, 300–312. [CrossRef] [PubMed]
55. Quance, M.A.; Travisano, M. Effects of temperature on the fitness cost of resistance to bacteriophage t4 in *Escherichia coli*. *Evolution* **2009**, *63*, 1406–1416. [CrossRef] [PubMed]
56. Marston, M.F.; Pierciey, F.J., Jr.; Shepard, A.; Gearin, G.; Qi, J.; Yandava, C.; Schuster, S.C.; Henn, M.R.; Martiny, J.B. Rapid diversification of coevolving marine synechococcus and a virus. *Proc. Natl. Acad. Sci. USA* **2012**, *109*, 4544–4549. [CrossRef] [PubMed]
57. Buckling, A.; Wei, Y.; Massey, R.C.; Brockhurst, M.A.; Hochberg, M.E. Antagonistic coevolution with parasites increases the cost of host deleterious mutations. *Proc. R. Soc. B* **2006**, *273*, 45–49. [CrossRef] [PubMed]
58. Gómez, P.; Ashby, B.; Buckling, A. Population mixing promotes arms race host–parasite coevolution. *Proc. R. Soc. B* **2015**, *282*, 20142297. [CrossRef] [PubMed]
59. Friman, V.P.; Buckling, A. Effects of predation on real-time host-parasite coevolutionary dynamics. *Ecol. Lett.* **2013**, *16*, 39–46. [CrossRef] [PubMed]
60. Friman, V.P.; Buckling, A. Phages can constrain protist predation-driven attenuation of *Pseudomonas aeruginosa* virulence in multienemy communities. *ISME J.* **2014**, *8*, 1820–1830. [CrossRef] [PubMed]
61. Pal, C.; Macia, M.D.; Oliver, A.; Schachar, I.; Buckling, A. Coevolution with viruses drives the evolution of bacterial mutation rates. *Nature* **2007**, *450*, 1079–1081. [CrossRef] [PubMed]

62. Gomez, P.; Buckling, A. Coevolution with phages does not influence the evolution of bacterial mutation rates in soil. *ISME J.* **2013**, *7*, 2242–2244. [CrossRef] [PubMed]
63. Gomez, P.; Buckling, A. Bacteria-phage antagonistic coevolution in soil. *Science* **2011**, *332*, 106–109. [CrossRef] [PubMed]
64. Taylor, C.M.; Roberts, I.S. Capsular polysaccharides and their role in virulence. *Contrib. Microbiol.* **2005**, *12*, 55–66. [PubMed]
65. Reyes, A.; Wu, M.; McNulty, N.P.; Rohwer, F.L.; Gordon, J.I. Gnotobiotic mouse model of phage–bacterial host dynamics in the human gut. *Proc. Natl. Acad. Sci. USA* **2013**, *110*, 20236. [CrossRef] [PubMed]
66. Andino, A.; Hanning, I. Salmonella enterica: Survival, colonization, and virulence differences among serovars. *Sci. World J.* **2015**, *2015*, 520179. [CrossRef] [PubMed]
67. Sørensen, M.C.H.; van Alphen, L.B.; Fodor, C.; Crowley, S.M.; Christensen, B.B.; Szymanski, C.M.; Brøndsted, L. Phase variable expression of capsular polysaccharide modifications allows *Campylobacter jejuni* to avoid bacteriophage infection in chickens. *Front. Cell. Infect. Microbiol.* **2012**, *2*, 11. [CrossRef] [PubMed]
68. Connerton, P.L.; Loc Carrillo, C.M.; Swift, C.; Dillon, E.; Scott, A.; Rees, C.E.; Dodd, C.E.; Frost, J.; Connerton, I.F. Longitudinal study of *Campylobacter jejuni* bacteriophages and their hosts from broiler chickens. *Appl. Environ. Microbiol.* **2004**, *70*, 3877–3883. [CrossRef] [PubMed]
69. Waldor, M.K.; Mekalanos, J.J. Lysogenic conversion by a filamentous phage encoding cholera toxin. *Science* **1996**, *272*, 1910–1914. [CrossRef] [PubMed]
70. Faruque, S.M.; Naser, I.B.; Islam, M.J.; Faruque, A.S.G.; Ghosh, A.N.; Nair, G.B.; Sack, D.A.; Mekalanos, J.J. Seasonal epidemics of cholera inversely correlate with the prevalence of environmental cholera phages. *Proc. Natl. Acad. Sci. USA* **2005**, *102*, 1702–1707. [CrossRef] [PubMed]
71. Faruque, S.M.; Islam, M.J.; Ahmad, Q.S.; Faruque, A.S.G.; Sack, D.A.; Nair, G.B.; Mekalanos, J.J. Self-limiting nature of seasonal cholera epidemics: Role of host-mediated amplification of phage. *Proc. Natl. Acad. Sci. USA* **2005**, *102*, 6119–6124. [CrossRef] [PubMed]
72. Zahid, M.S.H.; Udden, S.M.N.; Faruque, A.S.G.; Calderwood, S.B.; Mekalanos, J.J.; Faruque, S.M. Effect of phage on the infectivity of vibrio cholerae and emergence of genetic variants. *Infect. Immun.* **2008**, *76*, 5266–5273. [CrossRef] [PubMed]
73. Seed, K.D.; Bodi, K.L.; Kropinski, A.M.; Ackermann, H.-W.; Calderwood, S.B.; Qadri, F.; Camilli, A. Evidence of a dominant lineage of vibrio cholerae-specific lytic bacteriophages shed by cholera patients over a 10-year period in Dhaka, Bangladesh. *mBio* **2011**, *2*, e00334-10. [CrossRef] [PubMed]
74. Seed, K.D.; Yen, M.; Shapiro, B.J.; Hilaire, I.J.; Charles, R.C.; Teng, J.E.; Ivers, L.C.; Boncy, J.; Harris, J.B.; Camilli, A. Evolutionary consequences of intra-patient phage predation on microbial populations. *eLife* **2014**, *3*, e03497. [CrossRef] [PubMed]
75. Smith, H.W.; Huggins, M.B. The association of the O18, K1 and H7 antigens and the CO1V plasmid of a strain of *Escherichia coli* with its virulence and immunogenicity. *J. Gen. Microbiol.* **1980**, *121*, 387–400. [PubMed]
76. Regeimbal, J.M.; Jacobs, A.C.; Corey, B.W.; Henry, M.S.; Thompson, M.G.; Pavlicek, R.L.; Quinones, J.; Hannah, R.M.; Ghebremedhin, M.; Crane, N.J.; et al. Personalized therapeutic cocktail of wild environmental phages rescues mice from *Acinetobacter baumannii* wound infections. *Antimicrob. Agents Chemother.* **2016**, *60*, 5806–5816. [CrossRef] [PubMed]
77. Clardy, J.; Walsh, C. Lessons from natural molecules. *Nature* **2004**, *432*, 829–837. [CrossRef] [PubMed]
78. Van Hoek, A.H.A.M.; Mevius, D.; Guerra, B.; Mullany, P.; Roberts, A.P.; Aarts, H.J.M. Acquired antibiotic resistance genes: An overview. *Front. Microbiol.* **2011**, *2*, 203. [CrossRef] [PubMed]
79. Munita, J.M.; Arias, C.A. Mechanisms of antibiotic resistance. *Microbiol. Spectr.* **2016**, *4*. [CrossRef]
80. Beceiro, A.; Tomás, M.; Bou, G. Antimicrobial resistance and virulence: A successful or deleterious association in the bacterial world? *Clin. Microbiol. Rev.* **2013**, *26*, 185–230. [CrossRef] [PubMed]
81. Schrag, S.J.; Perrot, V.; Levin, B.R. Adaptation to the fitness costs of antibiotic resistance in *Escherichia coli*. *Proc. R. Soc. B* **1997**, *264*, 1287–1291. [CrossRef] [PubMed]
82. Bouma, J.E.; Lenski, R.E. Evolution of a bacteria/plasmid association. *Nature* **1988**, *335*, 351–352. [CrossRef] [PubMed]
83. Marcusson, L.L.; Frimodt-Møller, N.; Hughes, D. Interplay in the selection of fluoroquinolone resistance and bacterial fitness. *PLoS Pathog.* **2009**, *5*, e1000541. [CrossRef] [PubMed]
84. Partridge, S.R. Analysis of antibiotic resistance regions in gram-negative bacteria. *FEMS Microbiol. Rev.* **2011**, *35*, 820–855. [CrossRef] [PubMed]

85. Enne, V.I.; Bennett, P.M.; Livermore, D.M.; Hall, L.M. Enhancement of host fitness by the sul2-coding plasmid p9123 in the absence of selective pressure. *J. Antimicrob. Chemother.* **2004**, *53*, 958–963. [CrossRef] [PubMed]
86. Torres-Barcelo, C.; Hochberg, M.E. Evolutionary rationale for phages as complements of antibiotics. *Trends Microbiol.* **2016**, *24*, 249–256. [CrossRef] [PubMed]
87. Verma, V.; Harjai, K.; Chhibber, S. Restricting ciprofloxacin-induced resistant variant formation in biofilm of *Klebsiella pneumoniae* b5055 by complementary bacteriophage treatment. *J. Antimicrob. Chemother.* **2009**, *64*, 1212–1218. [CrossRef] [PubMed]
88. Kirby, A.E. Synergistic action of gentamicin and bacteriophage in a continuous culture population of *Staphylococcus aureus*. *PLoS ONE* **2012**, *7*, e51017. [CrossRef] [PubMed]
89. Torres-Barcelo, C.; Arias-Sanchez, F.I.; Vasse, M.; Ramsayer, J.; Kaltz, O.; Hochberg, M.E. A window of opportunity to control the bacterial pathogen *Pseudomonas aeruginosa* combining antibiotics and phages. *PLoS ONE* **2014**, *9*, e106628. [CrossRef] [PubMed]
90. Kamal, F.; Dennis, J.J. Burkholderia cepacia complex phage-antibiotic synergy (PAS): Antibiotics stimulate lytic phage activity. *Appl. Environ. Microbiol.* **2015**, *81*, 1132–1138. [CrossRef] [PubMed]
91. Chan, B.K.; Sistrom, M.; Wertz, J.E.; Kortright, K.E.; Narayan, D.; Turner, P.E. Phage selection restores antibiotic sensitivity in MDR *Pseudomonas aeruginosa*. *Sci. Rep.* **2016**, *6*, 26717. [CrossRef] [PubMed]
92. Cairns, J.; Becks, L.; Jalasvuori, M.; Hiltunen, T. Sublethal streptomycin concentrations and lytic bacteriophage together promote resistance evolution. *Philos. Trans. R. Soc. B* **2017**, *372*, 20160040. [CrossRef] [PubMed]
93. Allen, R.C.; Pfrunder-Cardozo, K.R.; Meinel, D.; Egli, A.; Hall, A.R. Associations among antibiotic and phage resistance phenotypes in natural and clinical *Escherichia coli* isolates. *mBio* **2017**, *8*. [CrossRef] [PubMed]
94. Levin, B.R.; Bull, J.J. Population and evolutionary dynamics of phage therapy. *Nat. Rev. Microbiol.* **2004**, *2*, 166–173. [CrossRef] [PubMed]
95. Chan, B.K.; Abedon, S.T. Phage therapy pharmacology phage cocktails. *Adv. Appl. Microbiol.* **2012**, *78*, 1–23. [PubMed]
96. Chan, B.K.; Abedon, S.T.; Loc-Carrillo, C. Phage cocktails and the future of phage therapy. *Future Microbiol.* **2013**, *8*, 769–783. [CrossRef] [PubMed]
97. O'Flynn, G.; Ross, R.P.; Fitzgerald, G.F.; Coffey, A. Evaluation of a cocktail of three bacteriophages for biocontrol of *Escherichia coli* o157:H7. *Appl. Environ. Microbiol.* **2004**, *70*, 3417–3424. [CrossRef] [PubMed]
98. Tanji, Y.; Shimada, T.; Yoichi, M.; Miyanaga, K.; Hori, K.; Unno, H. Toward rational control of *Escherichia coli* O157:H7 by a phage cocktail. *Appl. Microbiol. Biotechnol.* **2004**, *64*, 270–274. [CrossRef] [PubMed]
99. Abedon, S.T.; Kuhl, S.J.; Blasdel, B.G.; Kutter, E.M. Phage treatment of human infections. *Bacteriophage* **2011**, *1*, 66–85. [CrossRef] [PubMed]
100. Pirnay, J.P.; De Vos, D.; Verbeken, G.; Merabishvili, M.; Chanishvili, N.; Vaneechoutte, M.; Zizi, M.; Laire, G.; Lavigne, R.; Huys, I.; et al. The phage therapy paradigm: Pret-a-porter or sur-mesure? *Pharm. Res.* **2011**, *28*, 934–937. [CrossRef] [PubMed]
101. Międzybrodzki, R.; Borysowski, J.; Weber-Dąbrowska, B.; Fortuna, W.; Letkiewicz, S.; Szufnarowski, K.; Pawełczyk, Z.; Rogóż, P.; Kłak, M.; Wojtasik, E.; et al. Chapter 3—clinical aspects of phage therapy. In *Advances in Virus Research*; Łobocka, M., Szybalski, W., Eds.; Academic Press: Cambridge, MA, USA, 2012; Volume 83, pp. 73–121.
102. Górski, A.; Międzybrodzki, R.; Weber-Dąbrowska, B.; Fortuna, W.; Letkiewicz, S.; Rogóż, P.; Jończyk-Matysiak, E.; Dąbrowska, K.; Majewska, J.; Borysowski, J. Phage therapy: Combating infections with potential for evolving from merely a treatment for complications to targeting diseases. *Front. Microbiol.* **2016**, *7*, 1515. [CrossRef] [PubMed]
103. Zhvania, P.; Hoyle, N.S.; Nadareishvili, L.; Nizharadze, D.; Kutateladze, M. Phage therapy in a 16-year-old boy with netherton syndrome. *Front. Med.* **2017**, *4*, 94. [CrossRef] [PubMed]
104. Aslam, S.; Yung, G.; Dan, J.; Reed, S.; LeFebvre, M.; Logan, C.; Taplitz, R.; Law, N.; Golts, E.; Afshar, K.; et al. (373)—Bacteriophage treatment in a lung transplant recipient. *J. Heart Lung Transplant.* **2018**, *37*, S155–S156. [CrossRef]
105. Khawaldeh, A.; Morales, S.; Dillon, B.; Alavidze, Z.; Ginn, A.N.; Thomas, L.; Chapman, S.J.; Dublanchet, A.; Smithyman, A.; Iredell, J.R. Bacteriophage therapy for refractory *Pseudomonas aeruginosa* urinary tract infection. *J. Med. Microbiol.* **2011**, *60*, 1697–1700. [CrossRef] [PubMed]

106. Harper, D.R.; Parracho, H.M.R.T.; Walker, J.; Sharp, R.; Hughes, G.; Werthén, M.; Lehman, S.; Morales, S. Bacteriophages and biofilms. *Antibiotics* **2014**, *3*, 270–284. [CrossRef]
107. Forde, A.; Daly, C.; Fitzgerald, G.F. Identification of four phage resistance plasmids from *Lactococcus lactis* subsp. Cremoris HO2. *Appl. Environ. Microbiol.* **1999**, *65*, 1540–1547. [PubMed]
108. Van Boeckel, T.P.; Brower, C.; Gilbert, M.; Grenfell, B.T.; Levin, S.A.; Robinson, T.P.; Teillant, A.; Laxminarayan, R. Global trends in antimicrobial use in food animals. *Proc. Natl. Acad. Sci. USA* **2015**, *112*, 5649. [CrossRef] [PubMed]
109. Flores, C.O.; Meyer, J.R.; Valverde, S.; Farr, L.; Weitz, J.S. Statistical structure of host–phage interactions. *Proc. Natl. Acad. Sci. USA* **2011**, *108*, E288. [CrossRef] [PubMed]
110. Fischetti, V.A. Bacteriophage lysins as effective antibacterials. *Curr. Opin. Microbiol.* **2008**, *11*, 393–400. [CrossRef] [PubMed]
111. Schuch, R.; Nelson, D.; Fischetti, V.A. A bacteriolytic agent that detects and kills *Bacillus anthracis*. *Nature* **2002**, *418*, 884. [CrossRef] [PubMed]
112. Loeffler, J.M.; Nelson, D.; Fischetti, V.A. Rapid killing of *Streptococcus pneumoniae* with a bacteriophage cell wall hydrolase. *Science* **2001**, *294*, 2170–2172. [CrossRef] [PubMed]
113. Totte, J.E.E.; van Doorn, M.B.; Pasmans, S. Successful treatment of chronic staphylococcus aureus-related dermatoses with the topical endolysin staphefekt sa.100: A report of 3 cases. *Case Rep. Dermatol.* **2017**, *9*, 19–25. [CrossRef] [PubMed]

12

Clinical Indications and Compassionate Use of Phage Therapy: Personal Experience and Literature Review with a Focus on Osteoarticular Infections

Olivier Patey [1], Shawna McCallin [2], Hubert Mazure [3], Max Liddle [4], Anthony Smithyman [5] and Alain Dublanchet [1,*]

1. Service of Infectious and Tropical Diseases, CHI Lucie et Raymond Aubrac, 94190 Villeneuve Saint Georges, France; opatey@aol.com
2. Department of Musculoskeletal Medicine DAL, Centre Hospitalier Universitaire Vaudois CHUV, Service of Plastic, Reconstructive & Hand Surgery, Regenerative Therapy Unit (UTR), CHUV-EPCR/Croisettes 22, 1066 Epalinges, Switzerland; shawna.mccallin@gmail.com
3. HGM Consultants, 63 Rebecca Parade, Winston Hills, NSW 2153, Australia; humazure@hotmail.com
4. School of Life Sciences, University of Technology, Ultimo, NSW 2007, Australia; max.liddle17@gmail.com
5. Cellabs Pty Ltd, and Founder Special Phage Services Pty Ltd, both of 7/27 Dale St, Brookvale, NSW 2100, Australia; tonysmithyman@gmail.com

* Correspondence: adublanchet@orange.fr

Abstract: The history of phage therapy started with its first clinical application in 1919 and continues its development to this day. Phages continue to lack any market approval in Western medicine as a recognized drug, but are increasingly used as an experimental therapy for the compassionate treatment of patients experiencing antibiotic failure. The few formal experimental phage clinical trials that have been completed to date have produced inconclusive results on the efficacy of phage therapy, which contradicts the many successful treatment outcomes observed in historical accounts and recent individual case reports. It would therefore be wise to identify why such a discordance exists between trials and compassionate use in order to better develop future phage treatment and clinical applications. The multitude of observations reported over the years in the literature constitutes an invaluable experience, and we add to this by presenting a number of cases of patients treated compassionately with phages throughout the past decade with a focus on osteoarticular infections. Additionally, an abundance of scientific literature into phage-related areas is transforming our knowledge base, creating a greater understanding that should be applied for future clinical applications. Due to the increasing number of treatment failures anticipatedfrom the perspective of a possible post-antibiotic era, we believe that the introduction of bacteriophages into the therapeutic arsenal seems a scientifically sound and eminently practicable consideration today as a substitute or adjuvant to antibiotic therapy.

Keywords: bacterial infection; antibiotic resistance; bacteriophage; antibiotic therapy; phage therapy; cases report

---

1. Introduction

In 1917, Félix d'Hérelle observed a phenomenon in stool cultures from convalescent patients with bacillary dysentery [1], which took the form of perfectly round clear areas in the bacterial lawn. He made the assumption that these clear zones were caused by an "invisible microbe" capable of killing bacteria, to which he gave the name bacteriophage. Two years later (1919), he demonstrated that the oral administration of bacteriophages in humans is harmless and causes the healing of bacterial enteritis caused by *Shigella* sp. (bacillary dysentery). Based on a large number of published cases in the years that followed, the interest and use of this new treatment in various infections spread rapidly across the world, reaching nearly every continent [2,3]. This was the situation until the discovery of antibiotics; when faced with their easier use, phage therapy was gradually abandoned in Western countries until it finally disappeared completely in France with the closure in 1990 of the elast remaining sources of therapeutic bacteriophages from the two Pasteur Institutes (Paris and Lyon). However, phage therapy continued uninterrupted in the Soviet Union during this time and is still practiced in Russia, Poland, Georgia and some other former Soviet States today, in accordance with specific national regulations.

We have been witnessing the worldwide spread of multidrug-resistant (MDR) bacteria in recent years. As new and truly innovative antibiotics are rare, the increasing frequency of therapeutic failures are raising fears of a new pre-antibiotic era [4]. To respond to this worrying situation, the return of phage therapy seems to be an answer not only as an alternative [5], but also a complementary treatment, to faltering antibiotic therapy [6–8]. This renewed interest in phage therapy is manifested by the motivation to conduct several clinical trials since 2009 that have used phages for a variety of indications, including chronic otitis, burn wound or urinary tract infections (UTI), and *Escherichia coli* diarrhea [9–12]. Indeed, phage therapy must be proven to be therapeutically effective through experimental clinical trials in order to obtain marketing approval, which is required for use in Western medicine. While studies have repeatedly documented its safety, it is unfortunate that no marketing approval has been attributed to a phage product to date as a result of these resource-intensive studies; three trials were unable to statistically prove efficacy [9,11,13], even if clinical benefit was achieved for some patients, and the only trial that was successful has not been further pursued for commercialization [12].

Many researchers and medical doctors have voiced the need to revise the regulatory classification of phage therapy products in order to facilitate their clinical evaluation. Natural phages are currently classified as Medicinal Products (MP) under European Union (EU) legislation [14] and as a drug by the Food and Drug Administration (FDA) in the United States, which necessitate that phages be produced under Good Manufacturing Practice (GMP) guidelines and infrastructure. While such criteria do not completely inhibit the ability to conduct trials, they do render formal phage trials more difficult and more expensive to conduct. Substantial financial investment is required to conduct clinical trials, and an inconvenient amount of time is needed to procure results in order to address current clinical needs.

Phage therapy is now at a state where it is not officially recognized as a legitimate treatment, but has been increasingly granted emergency approvals for addressing antibiotic treatment failures. There are more than 10 published case reports [15] and a fast-growing number of undocumented compassionate cases that report successful treatment outcomes with phage therapy. Within only the last year, two experimental phage therapy centers have opened in addition to the long-established Phage Therapy Unit at the Ludwik Hirszfeld Institute in Poland (Box 1). From this perspective, and in conjunction with a century of publications on this subject for different bacterial infections treated by phage therapy, compassionate use and case reports constitute an invaluable source of knowledge that help to elucidate best practices for phage therapy. Many original and historical texts published in French or Russian have been unfortunately excluded from contributing to this large body of information and should enter into consideration. While case reports and historical accounts do not substitute for formal clinical trials, the findings and remarks they contain are useful to set up modern therapeutic protocols and hopefully to avoid conducting additional therapeutically-futile clinical trials. This is what we propose to report here, both by summarizing findings from the literature and by adding our own experience of cases, particularly for osteoarticular infections, treated under compassionate protocols, as a means to advise on the progression of phage therapy into modern medicine.

Box 1. Experimental phage therapy centers established in Western countries.

Ludwik Hirszfeld Institute of Immunology and Experimental Therapy, Polish Academy of Sciences, Phage Therapy Unit in Wroclaw, Poland (IIET PAS PTU): This is the oldest and most established experimental center in central Europe, which has been preparing phage formulations for hospital use in Poland since the 1970s, before it became a member state of the European Union (EU). Phage therapy was and is continued under the national regulatory framework as an experimental therapy for specific medical conditions and in specific centers under Article 37 of the Helsinki Declaration. They have an in-house bank of phages against 15 different bacterial pathogens (*Staphylococcus, Enterococcus, Pseudomonas, Escherichia, Klebsiella, Serratia, Proteus, Acinetobacter, Citrobacter, Enterobacter, Stenotrophomonas, Shigella, Salmonella, Burkholderia, Morganella*). Treatment is proceeded by phage susceptibility testing (phage typing procedure) and preparations are used for outpatient treatment. The PTU periodically publishes summaries of their experiences [16–20] that provide factual justification for using phage therapy and useful information for clinical applications.

Magistral preparations in Belgium (also known as a compounded prescription drug in the US) [14]. Phage therapy can be provided as a magistral preparation in Belgium since 2018, after several years of discussion involving public health and federal regulatory authorities, in order to facilitate physician-prescribed treatment for individual patients. Phages are considered active pharmaceutical ingredients (APIs) that must be produced according to an internal monograph (set of instructions) and that are subsequently certified by competent laboratories before they are mixed or put into formulation under the supervision of a pharmacist and delivered to a specific patient.

Center for Innovative Phage Applications and Therapeutics (IPATH) University of California San Diego, School of Medicine: This center announced its opening in June 2018 following several successful treatments with phage. Their first case used phage to treat an MDR systemic infection caused by *Acinetobacter baumannii*, which was initiated and coordinated by the wife of the patient, a global health professor, and his physician [21,22]. While this was the first American patient with a systemic MDR infection to be successfully treated intravenous (iv) by phage therapy, more than five patients have been treated since under the FDAs compassionate use program and IPATH is planning to conduct clinical trials in the near future.

2. General Prerequisites for the Medical Use of Bacteriophages

Due to the unfamiliarity with and particularities of phage therapy, it is worthwhile to touch upon several general aspects of clinical use: product availability, production, formulation and administration, dosage, and evaluation. The permission to use phage therapy for compassionate or experimental treatment, at the patient, physician, hospital, and health and regulatory authority levels, are beyond the scope of this publication, but are evidently necessary to proceed with treatment and requirements may vary country-to-country. Approvals are now often granted on an individual bases for emergency use or in the case of antibiotic treatment failures, mostly in France, Belgium, Poland, Australia, and the US.

2.1. Availability

The first condition for use of phage therapy is simply to have bacteriophages available for treatment, which is often complicated at this stage of phage development. This implies having access to phages that are both biologically active against the patient's bacterial isolate and satisfy regulatory requirements (purity, traceability, characterization). A single phage may be used (monophage preparation) or several phages may be combined against one or more bacterial species (phage cocktail).

As phage therapy is not currently a recognized medicine in the West and no registered products exist, phages are either being prepared specifically for a patient infection (personalized or custom approach) or treatment can be done with commercial phage preparations from Russian or Georgian suppliers, which have pre-defined phage compositions ("ready-to-use") [23]. Such commercial bacteriophage preparations that are available for purchase may, or may not, encounter importation difficulties into Western countries due to product traceability or a lack of certification or analytical information. Access can be accomplished by patients traveling to countries where phage therapy is an approved practice (medical tourism), and the Eliava Institute in Georgia treats a number of foreign patients onsite each year. This last option, however, is dependent upon patient mobility and financial ability to pay for treatment.

Alternatively, phages have been prepared for compassionate cases by small biotech and academic institutions for individual patients. Indeed, a large number of different bacteriophages are deposited in different collections that target clinically relevant bacteria, and it would be desirable that the collections held in these "phage banks" organize themselves into a network to facilitate exchanges. A networking initiative, known as the Phage Directory [24], is attempting to facilitate phage sharing for emergency or compassionate clinical needs. If an active phage is not present or available from such an organization, it is normally still possible to isolate one from the environment, although this is pathogen dependent, sufficient characterization is still required, and is difficult to achieve for acute life-threatening infections [25].

2.2. Production

Phage products must be produced with an acceptable level of purification for clinical use in order to remove remaining endotoxin and bacterial contaminants. If phage preparations are viewed as medicinal products, they will be subject to GMP compliance, which are standards intended to guarantee the quality of a medicine [26]. This requires that a procedure be defined for their manufacture and stipulates a combination of physicochemical and biological tests, as well as stringent production facilities. The quality (i.e., the stability and consistency) of a biological drug, such as phages, is harder to guarantee and control than that of a chemical, and GMP requirements have put a strain on the clinical development of phage therapy in Western medicine, as well as greatly increasing production costs. Indeed, GMP constraints both delayed patient enrollment for the Phagoburn clinical study and negatively impacted the phage titer of the final product [9]. An adaptation of the regulation is necessary [27–32] and, in particular, will have to take into account the use of individualized preparations [33] as a personalized medicine [28,34], and modification of phage components throughout treatment to counteract bacterial–phage resistance. Production considerations must take into account the sustainability of the phage treatment approach and patient safety.

Phage therapy is currently implemented for compassionate use and individual patients by by-passing GMP-requirements. Belgium has opted to facilitate phage therapy by presenting the phage as magistral preparations, which are individually prepared by prescription for individual patients by a qualified hospital pharmacist, and the quality of phage preparations are verified by accredited laboratories (Box 1) [14]. Even without such a systematic approval system, phage biotech companies (MicroGen, Eliava, Pherecydes Pharma, Advanced Phage Therapeutics, AmpliPhi Biosciences), as well as academic institutions and military research institutions, have helped in the production process and/or supply of phages for emergency use.

2.3. Formulation and Administration

The administration of a drug is dependent on the vectorization/formulation of the active phage component [35,36]. Local application is easiest to apply, and tolerance has been repeatedly documented for this route [9,37]. Phages may be applied topically either in cream/gel formulations or by contact with soaked bandages on the wound surface. Bacteriophages, being of a protein nature, raise the concern of an anaphylactic reaction following repeated administration. However, severe reactions have only been rarely reported, and today the risk is further reduced by advanced purification methods [38–40].

While oral administration is easy and without side effects, gastric acidity is a hostile barrier to ingested bacteriophages. To overcome this drawbackthere are two possible approaches: alkalinisation, by administration of an alkaline liquid (bicarbonate water, carbonated water), or gastro-resistant vectorization (i.e., in release capsules or pills). Alkaline neutralization may come with an increased risk of opportunistic infections for patients, and vectorization comes at an increased cost of production; more clinical data are required to determine the best strategy for oral phage application.

Inhalation seems to be effective in delivering lyophilized bacteriophages to the lungs in the form of powder propelled by inhalers [41]. The bronchopulmonary tree is indeed easily accessible by air, and thus, it is conceivable to spray bacteriophage suspensions (nebulization, misting) or dry forms (spray) [42]. However, few cases have been published to date [43–48], and using appropriate vectorization for inhalation remains to be evaluated.

Diffusion is rapid after systemic ie intravenous administration, though circulating phages are sequestered by the reticuloendothelial system in the spleen and liver. In the absence of bacterial target hosts, phages are quickly eliminated. On the contrary, if bacterial targets are present, phages multiply to a degree dependent on a multitude of bacterial (metabolic activity, sensitivity) and mammalian factors, making the estimation of pharmacokinetics [49] variable and difficult to estimate between patients.

2.4. Dosage

The required dosage, rhythm, and duration of treatment have been poorly studied. Theoretically, in situ multiplication requires only one application; while in practice, repetition is often the rule. Unlike conventional drug treatments, the pharmacological parameters are poorly defined and understood at present, which presents the main difficulty in being unable to predict the extent of in vivo multiplication.

2.5. Therapeutic Evaluation

Like any drug, a biomedicine must be studied experimentally to appreciate its positive and negative effects on a living organism. Although many publications (individual cases and clinical series) have shown positive results of phage therapy and presented few adverse effects, it is necessary to respond to modern requirements and to carry out randomized, double-blind controlled trials [50,51]. Nonetheless, simpler hospital observational studies, despite their drawbacks and inadequacies, would make it possible to provide highly valuable information for pressing questions while satisfying prerequisites (i.e., the number of patients likely to be included within a defined period of time) that have often been difficult for modern trials to achieve to date.

Many case studies today evaluate phage therapy by the most essential factor: the clinical improvement of the patient. However, information documenting phage activity within the patient, such as phage amplification or phage sensitivity, are often lacking, and therefore claims that phage therapy causes clinical amelioration are not data-supported. Much more information could and should be obtained from compassionate and emergency-use treatments to further our knowledge-base of phage therapy in humans.

3. Clinical Indications in the Literature

Inherently, phages are able to treat any clinical presentation of bacterial infections. Reports have been published using phage therapy for a large array of clinical indications, including gastro-intestinal [2,11,52–54], localized [3,37,55–59], burn wound [9,60], systemic [21,39,61–72], urogenital [10,73–82], respiratory [44,45,47,82–85], oto-rhino-laryngeal (ORL) [12,86–95], and osteoarticular infections (see section below). These clinical indications include infections that are acute or chronic, sensitive or resistant to antibiotics, and are caused by highly variable common or opportunistic pathogens.

Acute systemic infections, such for septicemia or meningitis, have been treated with phages with some success. It seems premature to consider such indications initially for phage therapy for at least two reasons: the urgency of treatment and the need for parenteral administration. Both aspects require readily-available, highly-purified phages, and rapid approval processes that, while not insurmountable, are not feasible for broad implementation at this time. Indeed, the few published cases of systemic treatments are the result of a few geographical competency centers and close collaboration between phage researchers and clinicians.

Chronic infections, however, are increasingly frequent and have gained attention as a target for phage therapy. Chronicity is supported by the formation of bacterial biofilms, intracellular bacterial persisters, or tolerant bacteria that are particularly problematic for UTIs, bacterial prostatitis, prosthetic joint infections (PJI), osteomyelitis, and respiratory conditions such as cystic fibrosis (CF). They require long-term antibiotic treatment that disrupts healthy microbiomes and selects for antimicrobial resistance. Such infections, if not constantly suppressed, risk development into bacterial sepsis. CF, although not an infectious disease itself, is the subject of special attention for phage therapy because of the chronic state of repetitive superinfections in these patients, which are usually caused by mucosal *Pseudomonas aeruginosa* strains resistant to many antimicrobials and capable of forming biofilms [96].

In addition to classical pathogens, opportunistic bacteria are often multidrug-resistant and cause infections that are difficult to control [96], for which the question of the interest of phage therapy is repeatedly raised. Infections with some bacteria, such as mycobacteria, present additional biological obstacles, such as preferential intracellular location of bacteria (macrophage or epithelial cells) and a slow growth rate, as in tuberculosis. Ready-to-use bacteriophage suspensions are generally not available for such situations, and a few teams have looked at some of them, although it is still too early to draw any conclusions. These include, more specifically, infections caused by *Helicobacter* [97,98]; *Borrelia* (Lyme disease [99]), as well as *Brucella*, *Yersinia pestis* and *Bacillus anthracis* [100] in the context of biological-weapon risks [101]. Other bacterial species (*Haemophilus influenzae*, *Streptococcus pneumoniae*) do not generate much interest today for phage therapy application. It should be noted that *Campylobacter* bacteriophages are mainly studied in poultry farms in a preventive context rather than therapeutically.

Osteoarticular infections are a particular form of deep-seated, localized infection that are a prime target for phage therapy given their frequency and poor response to antibiotic therapy. The diffusion of antibiotics into bone tissue is often mediocre and impaired by the presence of bacterial biofilms that form *in vivo* at the contact between bone and prosthetic material. The recurrence and transition to chronicity is more and more common for many reasons, including the presence of MDR bacteria. Today, the number of post-surgical bone infections on fracture or joint prosthesis continues to increase [102]. Conventional antibiotic treatments are long and costly, with frequent repeat surgery, and sometimes amputation is the only infection control option [103].

Phage therapy has been used very early and frequently for this type of infection, as evidenced by many publications from Northern America [104] and in Eastern European countries [105–107]. In France, the surgeon André Raiga [66,108] made several assessments of his long experience in this field. Clinical cases in Strasbourg, France were published in 1979, which document positive outcomes in bone infections with phages (Box 2) [109]. A review of Soviet literature has also indicated complete recovery from osteomyelitis using phages alone or in combination with antibiotics [110]. More recently, two cases of PJI (*Staphylococcus aureus*) and one case of *P. aeruginosa* osteomyelitis were treated with direct application of phages in France [111].

The potential of phage therapy to treat such post-accidental, surgical osteitis, or peri-prosthetic joint infections is likely rooted in phage activity against bacterial biofilms and potentially against intracellular bacteria. An experimental model [112] has demonstrated that a treatment combining bacteriophages and antibiotics helps to dissolve biofilms with a pronounced effect on biofilms of *Staphylococcus* sp. compared to those of *P. aeruginosa*. Indeed, there has been a very large number of experimental studies for several years on this subject not only in vitro, but also in vivo [113,114]. While bacterial infections begin by biofilm formation on prosthetic surfaces, they can become chronic by establishing an intracellular life-style within mammalian cells that shields them from antibiotic treatment and then causes recurrent active infections. A recent model documented the ability of phages to kill intracellular *S. aureus* [115].

All of the above provide substantial evidence that osteoarticular infections are a sound target for phage therapy. With this logic, a budget has been attributed for a future clinical trial in France, "Phagos," for PJIs caused by *S. aureus*, which will begin as soon as GMP-compliant phage suspensions are achieved [116]. Our experience with the compassionate treatment of oesteoarticular, as well as other, infections is presented herein.

Box 2. Conclusion of Lang et al. 1979 [109].

Seven orthopedic surgery cases were treated with bacteriophages between 1975 and 1976. Of the treated patients, six were male and one was female. The age of patients ranged from 19–70 years of age. The cases presented by authors were chronic, having exhausted the usual therapeutic arsenal, and phage was added to other treatments in order to maximize patient benefit.

Five treatments resulted in good clinical outcomes, which was supported by radiological and bacteriological examination. A condition was considered improved if symptoms were ameliorated and radiological examination was positive, but problems persisted with scarring and positive bacterial cultures (one case). Treatment failure with added phages occurred for one patient and caused a change in treatment plan, comprising first local and general antibiotic therapy (ampicillin, cephalosporin, gentamicin), then hyperbaric oxygen therapy, and finally surgical intervention, which ultimately resulted in a favorable outcome. In conclusion, the use of suitable bacteriophages in the treatment of antibiotic-resistant chronic bone infections seemed to be an interesting therapeutic alternative for authors, and the results of these cases encouraged continuation in this therapeutic direction.

4. Compassionate Phage Use in France and at Villeneuve Saint Georges

Phage therapy was used to treat patients compassionately during the 1970s and 80s in France, at a time when it was possible obtain suspensions of therapeutic phage for the pathogenic bacterium of a patient from the Pasteur Institute. The clinical outcomes during this time with the treatment of frequent, high-risk infections with phages have been summarized previously in a short paper outlining conclusions and new indications for phage therapy (Box 3) [117]. At that time, phage therapy was routinely performed in some hospitals, such as in Lyon, Paris, and Strasbourg. A surgical service at the latter had published a small clinical study of seven cases and concluded that phage therapy was promising, particularly in bone infections (Box 2) [109]. Several patients with bone infections in the hospital of Villeneuve Saint Georges, for whom conventional treatment had failed, also benefited from such phage therapy treatment during this time (unpublished results). However, by 1990, phage therapy and its practice in France became impossible after phage production was ceased at the Pasteur Institute. There followed a period of about 15 years during which phage therapy was totally inaccessible in France.

Box 3. Conclusion of Vieu et al. 1979. [117].

This article, published in French, highlighted how and why phage therapy was used in France at this time. In particular, the growing importance of opportunistic bacteria resistant to antibiotics in infectious pathology oriented the therapeutic applications of bacteriophages to three new areas: (1) the curative treatment of postoperative surgical infections; (2) suppression of the infectious process during gram-negative pediatric epidemics, caused notably by *Salmonella*, *Klebsiella*, *E. coli*, and *Serratia*, via oral phage administration; and (3) curative treatment of chronic UTIs. The authors noted that a close collaboration between phage scientists and clinicians was absolutely necessary to treat patients with phages, from identifying phages to following clinical progression over time. The success of phage therapy was dependent upon verifying in vitro susceptibility prior to treatment. If treatment failure occurred, it was attributable to low titers of the phage, pH environment of the GI or urinary tracts, inactivation of the phage by simultaneously-prescribed local antiseptics, or the involvement of several pathogens not identified at diagnosis outside the bacterial host range of the phage preparation. In conclusion, the authors affirmed that phage therapy was a merited treatment option due to the frequent clinical successes it produced.

In 2004, we were able to buy over-the-counter commercial preparations of bacteriophages from pharmacies in Moscow for a few dozen Euros. After an evaluation (for sterility, activity, specificity) of these preparations [118], those capable of responding to the clinical problems at hand were retained and used. The first case we treated was a particularly worrying case of an evolving infection of the external auditory canal, where a bacteriophage suspension against *S. aureus* was used to treat chronic otitis externa (Box 4; Patient 1 in Table 1). With this experience, and in the face of the increasing therapeutic failures that we were confronted with, especially in orthopedic surgery, some of us decided to reintroduce phage therapy more routinely from 2008 in the hospital in which we practiced, and it is still occasionally used as needed at the hospital of Villeneuve Saint Georges. We will briefly outline the process of using phages for compassionate use and present several clinicals cases of our experiences in phage therapy.

Box 4. Treatment of an external otitis.

A young patient was examined for chronic otitis after episodes of repeated otitis treated with various antibiotics. The specialist noted an otorrhea and decided to treat it medically (cefpodoxime and ofloxacin) before surgery. Repair of the tympanic membrane was performed. The immediate treatment outcome was obvious: symptoms (pain, drainage) rapidly disappeared with no complications or side effects.

After three months, the otorrhea reappeared. The examination was particularly difficult because of very sharp local pain, as the eardrum was inflamed and wet. The resumption of local antibiotic therapy (bacitracin) helped reduce pain. During one year, the patient experienced several treated otorrheas (ofloxacin). During an outpatient consultation with acute pain and under general anaesthesia, a specimen was collected showing the presence in pure culture of *S. aureus* (penicillin-R, methicillin-R, erythromycin-R and ofloxacin-R). Despite antibiotic therapy being immediately prescribed (not specified), the purulent flow and pain persisted, and the *Staphylococcus* was still present.

It was then decided to carry out a more precise examination and to collect multiple specimens (tympanic membrane, cutaneous coating of the external duct) before the local application of a bacteriophage suspension, active in vitro against the patient isolate, in combination with pristinamycin. Within 48 hours, the patient noticed a clear improvement: the cessation of purulent flow and pain. Subsequent consultations confirmed a favorable course: the absence of otorrhea or pain and disappearance of *Staphylococcus*. After three months, the ear examination was still very satisfactory and the treatment was stopped.

5. Protocol for Compassionate Use of Phage Therapy

Before patient admission, the decision to use phage therapy is made by a multi-disciplinary hospital team (surgeon, infectious disease specialist, microbiologist), who conduct a complete examination of the patient and patient file. In addition to the biological assessment, one or more preliminary specimens is taken to isolate the bacterium and test its sensitivity to available phages. Patients are informed about phages and the possibility of treatment. Phages are administered by a treating physician who exercises their ethical right to use an experimental treatment in the best interest of the patient, without an elaborate regulatory or administrative framework.

During therapeutic care, if necessary, the infectious foci are excised (debridement) and cleaned in the operating room. One or more intraoperative specimens are collected to confirm the initial bacteriological diagnosis. At the end of surgery and before closure of the operative field, the preparation of bacteriophages is used to flood the operative field (5 to 10 ml according to the surface of the field). Access to the treatment site (opening or drain) allows a bacteriological control and the introduction of the same phage preparation in the days following the intervention.

Antibiotic therapy reflecting the pathogen's antibiotic resistance profile is used in combination with phage therapy, and the patient is kept under surveillance for several days (less than one week) to ensure that there was no evidence of infection (local, biological, or bacteriological). The postoperative course has presented no complications, and no side effects have been reported.

Regarding follow-up, ambulatory monitoring is performed in our facility for several months at a variable frequency, as deemed necessary. The evaluation of each case is performed clinically, as well as biologically and radiologically. Some patients provide us periodically with their health status, which so far has been excellent.

All cases reported here (Table 1) have benefited from compassionate phage therapy for the duly recorded treatment failure. The phage therapy treatments were carried out between 2006 and 2018 after a long evolution, generally several years, of a conventional treatment according to official medical guidelines. All patients had benefited from multiple attempts at treatment (surgical interventions and antibiotic therapy) and had been in therapeutic failure for months or even years. Some had previously tried treatment at the Eliava Institute in Tbilisi. All presented cases were treated in France at the Villeneuve Saint Georges Hospital, unless otherwise noted. The authors have also been involved in the treatment with phage therapy for a case for a refractory UTI in Australia, published previously [78].

Table 1. Summary of patients treated with compassionate use of bacteriophages from 2006–2018.

N	Age; Sex	Symptom Onset; PT Start	Clinical Symptoms	Bacteria	Phage Therapy	Outcome
1	20; F	2004; 2006	Suppurating chronic otitis; intense pain	*S. aureus*	Commercial anti-*S. aureus* suspension; ear drop instillations (15 days)	2006 Complete cure
2	44; M	2005; 2008	Accidental fall; multiple fractures (*n* = 37); amputation considered	*S. aureus*	Commercial anti-*S. aureus* and Pyophage suspensions; administered peroperatively over several weeks	2009 Wound closure and complete cure
3	25; M	2007; 2008	Road accident causing multiple trauma; uncontrolled pelvic bone infection	*S. aureus* *P. aeruginosa*	Anti-*S. aureus* and anti-*P. aeruginosa* phage suspension; administered peroperatively and via catheter in days following operation (Belgium).	2010 Complete cure
4	40; F	1995; 2009	Fall leading to complex fracture of the right foot; Planned amputation	*S. aureus*	Commercial anti-*S. aureus* suspension administered peroperatively and via catheter in the days following operation	2009 Wound closure and complete cure
5	60; M	2008; 2009	Fistulised abdominal plaque infection; continuous suppressive antibiotic administration	Methicillin resistant *S. aureus* (MRSA)	Commercial anti-*S. aureus* suspension administered via fistula	2010 No recurrence without any antibiotic over 4 years
6	80; F	2008; 2010	Knee prosthesis infection unsuitable for surgery	*P. aeruginosa*	Commercial broad spectrum multi-bacteriophage suspension; Knee joint injection	2012 *P. aeruginosa* clearance, but appearance of *Enterococcus* sp.
7	61; F	1995/2005; 2010	Operated tongue cancer; Dental extraction, jaw fracture, osteo-synthesis and fistulised infection	*S. aureus* (MRSA)	Commercial anti-*S. aureus* suspension administered peroperatively	2011 Complete cure
8	90; F	2009/2010; 2010	Femoral fracture under hip prosthesis; Drained hematoma and antibiotherapy-infection	*S. aureus* (MRSA)	Commercial anti-*S. aureus* suspension administered peroperatively by flooding the infection site and via catheter in the 10 days following the operation	2011 Complete cure, rapid recovery without recurrence after 1 year with retention of the hip prosthesis and osteosynthesis material *in situ*
9	20; M	2012; 2012	Chronic Ulcerative Colitis with liver complications. Severe weight loss (54 kg down from 80 kg). Poor digestion of food.	*E. coli*, *Proteus* spp. *S. aureus* (Urine) *S. aureus* (skin) *E. coli*, *Proteus vulgaris*, *Proteus mirabilis* (stool)	Treatment in Tbilisi (Georgia) with 2 commercially available phage suspensions plus special customised phage suspension. Probiotics, enzymes and Camelyn immune stimulant also given. Treatment lasted 1 month.	2012 Healing with sterilisation of urine, reduction of *E. coli* and *P. vulgaris* growth from high (10^8) to low ($<10^2$) in stool. Weight gain to 72 kg by end of treatment. Digestion improved but still poor
10	72; F	2009; 2013	Left knee prosthesis infection	*Staphylococcus* sp.	Commercial anti-*S. aureus* suspension administered peroperatively by flooding the infection site	2013 Initial partial disinfection with closure of several fistula followed by stabilisation

Table 1. *Cont.*

N	Age; Sex	Symptom Onset; PT Start	Clinical Symptoms	Bacteria	Phage Therapy	Outcome
11	84; M	1943/2012; 2013	Osteomyelitis of the left tibia; Fistula next to the wound	*S. aureus* (MRSA)	Initial phage therapy treatment in Tbilisi via fistula with temporary improvement, followed by surgical follow up intervention in France in 2013; Commercial anti-*S. aureus* suspension administered peroperatively by flooding the infection site	2013 Complete cure
12	58; F	2000; 2013	Acoustic neuroma with nosocomial infection of the ENT and ophthalmic regions	*S. aureus*	Treatment in Tbilisi with locally produced phage suspensions administered locally and orally	2013 Complete cure allowing an ophthalmic intervention of the retina that had been delayed for several years
13	68; F	1973; 2015	Operated left tibia fracture, followed by re-opened bone infection 2013: Travel to Phage Therapy Center (Tbilisi)	*S. aureus*	Surgery, phage therapy with commercial staphylococcal phage suspension, and antibiotherapy	2016 Disappearance of *S. aureus* replaced by *P. aeruginosa* & *Streptococcus constellatus*, followed by complete cure without recurrence
14	84; M	2006 & 2015; 2016	Prostate adenectomy with chronic urinary infection and bacteraemia	Extended-spectrum beta-lacatamase *E. coli* (ESBL)	Anti-*E. coli* phage suspension administered per os and rectally	2018 Complete cure
15	86; M	2016; 2018	Recurring prostatitis with bacteraemia	*P. aeruginosa*	Commercial multi-phage suspension administered orally and rectally	2018 Complete cure with disappearance of any urinary infection for the first time in 2 years

The infectious sites were predominantly osteoarticular (9/15), but also included two cases that involved the prostate and other four various infections (two ENT, one abdominal, and one GI tract). The predominantly targeted bacterial species was *S. aureus* (12/15). More rarely, *P. aeruginosa* (three instances) and two instances of *E. coli* were the causative pathogens or were present in polymicrobial infections. Most often, this was a mono-microbial infection (13/15). Suspensions of bacteriophages were mainly from commercial sources (Microgen in Russia and the Eliava Institute in Georgia). In the absence of commercially available preparations, two cases were treated with personalized bacteriophage suspensions.

This small series of cases calls for some remarks. We found that the local application of bacteriophages is completely safe, and no accidents or incidents have been reported. We have also observed highly satisfactory results, and often with rapid improvement. In fact, 12/15 cases resulted in a complete recovery (a secondary problematic pathogen emerged in one case, only a stable condition was achieved for one patient, and one case of a GI infection improved after phage treatment, but for which the condition was not fully resolved). The administration of bacteriophages had always been accompanied by antibiotic therapy with the aim of obtaining a possible synergy. Note that these were chronic cases which had exhausted the usual therapeutic resources, and whose clinical condition was worrying with a poorly functional prognosis. The focus was not to try to experiment or optimize phage therapy, but instead to treat patients with all available resources.

The pathologies that have been treated are varied. In our small case study, bone infections were the most frequent and generally evolved favorably within a few weeks. If there were fistulas, they disappeared, and bone consolidation was observed both clinically and functionally and was confirmed by imaging. Bacterial pathogens became quickly undetectable by microbiology after phage therapy began. After a follow-up for some patients of over 10 years, no relapse has been observed, and it is possible to conclude that patients were completely healed. In two cases where amputation of the lower limb was being considered, this option was avoided. Treatments that prevented the ablation of prosthetic material were also clinically satisfying.

To emphasize the treatment of two prostatitis cases, which constitute the most recent that we have taken care of, infections were caused by *E. coli* in one case and *P. aeruginosa* in the other. They affected elderly people who had been undergoing antibiotic therapy for several months. Concomitant oral and rectal administration over two consecutive days in one case and over three days for the other quickly resolved the recurrent infectious problem.

6. Recent Knowledge to be Taken into Consideration for Phage Therapy

The number of phage-related in vitro and in vivo studies, combined with newer areas of research such as the microbiome, has never been greater and provides a wealth of knowledge to keep in consideration when approaching clinical application. The activity of phages against biofilms, their ability to block bacterial receptors, and their synergy with conventional antibiotics has important implications for clinical treatment. Beyond bacterial lysis, phages have also been shown to interact in different ways with the immune system of the patient and their overall microbial community. The role that phages play naturally in the microbiome ecosystem is only starting to be discovered. Awareness and incorporation of these aspects provides a greater understanding of phage therapy and its clinical utility.

Regarding antibacterial aspects, the most pertinent aspect of new knowledge is the exploration of phage-antibiotic synergy (PAS). Several recent studies both in vitro [7,8,119,120] and in vivo on numerous experimental animal models [121] have confirmed the potential of combined use by showing the synergy of specific bacteriophage–antibiotic combinations at sometimes sub-inhibitory doses [122,123]. This could be a function of reducing the development of bacterial clones resistant to traditional antibiotics, by separate killing mechanisms, or other additive functions.

In almost all compassionate use cases, phages have been used in conjunction with antibiotics. It was even shown that phage administration changed the antibiotic resistance profile during the treatment of an *A. baumanii* infection, which led to the inclusion of the antibiotic in the treatment regimen [21]. Additionally, it has been shown [124] that, to combat *S. aureus* infections, the therapeutic results can also be influenced by the sequence in which the therapeutic agents are administered: best results were obtained when phage therapy precedes antibiotic therapy. As interesting as this effect may be, methods for determining the best choice of phage(s) and antibiotic(s) are still lacking. Nevertheless, the reintroduction of phage therapy deserves to be approached with the idea that it could be not only an alternative, but also a complement, in circumstances where the diffusion of an antibiotic is weak, as is the case in bone tissue or in the presence of a biofilm for example [6].

The activity of phages against bacterial biofilms is yet another factor in support of phage therapy. The pathogenic role of biofilms appears fundamental in chronic infections, especially in the presence of foreign materials (i.e., prosthesis, catheter). The proteolytic enzymes of certain bacteriophages are capable of destroying polysaccharides in biofilms which allow bacteria to escape natural defenses and antibiotic treatments [125]. In addition to allowing the adhesion of bacteriophages on the bacterial surface, this action facilitates the diffusion of antibiotics. It should be noted that soluble degradation products of *S. aureus* biofilm components could have a deleterious role on osteoblasts [126] and thus limit the growth of bone callus, which would explain the rapid bone healing observed after bacteriophage treatment observed in the compassionate cases in Table 1.

The very interaction of phages with the surface of bacterial cells may itself have an additive effect for phage therapy. It has been shown that bacteriophages, by attaching themselves to the bacterial surface at particular sites, could block resistance mechanisms such as an efflux pump or impair the fitness or the virulence factor of a bacterium [127]. This would then make certain bacteria (i.e., *P. aeruginosa* or *K. pneumoniae*) more susceptible to traditional antibiotics and facilitate the healing of certain pathologies, such as endocarditis or vascular prosthesis infections.

Regarding the interaction with mammalian cells, facets that are directly linked to the bactericidal effects are further complemented by a larger understanding of phage interaction with human cells and physiology, particularly with the immune system. Studies indicate that, in addition to their well-known antibacterial action, bacteriophages have potent immunomodulatory properties. For some authors, the success of phage therapy, depending on the bacterial permissiveness of the phage, is related to the immunity of the subject. In particular, for Roach et al. [46], neutrophil–bacteriophage synergy demonstrated that it is essential for the cure of pneumonia. For Dabrowska [128], the impact on the immune system affects the final outcome of phage therapy. While antibody induction may play a role in eliminating bacteriophages, it has also been shown that they can induce cytokine production in mammalian immune cells.

In reference to phages and surrounding microbiota, bacteriophages are present in all micro-ecosystems found in nature, and their presence in human microbiota is becoming increasingly recognized. Human microbiomes are distinct for various anatomical niches of the body (digestive tract, vaginal cavity, mouth, airway, nares, skin, urine [129–135]) that house dense microbial communities containing not only bacteria, archaea and fungi, but also mainly viruses, of which bacteriophages are the majority and remain largely unexplored [135–137]. The notion of the microbiome must be borne in mind when a bacteriophage treatment is being considered [138]. Indeed, the introduction of a bacteriophage in a structured community is not without consequence, because it induces difficult-to-predict interactions that may facilitate or hinder the intended effect [139]. Interactions occur not only with the microbiome with which it comes in contact, but also eukaryotic tissue cells [140,141] and the immune system of the host organism, as mentioned above [142]. Consequently, a model consisting of this "ménage à trois" has been proposed and should be considered [143]. A good knowledge of these components could help improve treatment outcomes and should make phage therapy a more personalized therapy.

An interesting consideration of gastro-intestinal diseases is the interplay with surrounding gut microbiota. Indeed, many gastro-intestinal diseases are increasingly described as a dysbiosis in the microbial community rather than being caused by a discrete pathogen, and microbiome sequencing has been useful in revealing disease-associated microbial signatures [144,145]. Phages may be useful in restoring a proper balance, such as for Crohn's disease or ulcerative colitis, and a trial targeting Enteroaggregative *E. coli* (EAEC) has been initiated for Crohn's patients [146–148].

Currently in Western countries, *Clostridium difficile* is a major problem (regarding diarrhea and transmission within the community), against which conventional antibiotics are ineffective. Many authors in recent years have considered addressing this condition with bacteriophages [149–151], and a study has shown a strong adsorption of bacteriophages on human cells in vitro that would promote bacteriophage–bacterial interactions is important for treating such a condition [152]. Fecal microbiota transplantations (FMT) have been shown to be effective at treating *C. difficile*, and, more so, filtrates of FMT that are devoid of bacteria also retain therapeutic properties, which may be due to the presence or modulation of phages [153].

7. Conclusions

Noting a continuing increase in bacterial resistance to antibiotics and the scarcity of new antibiotic molecules, the World Health Organization declared in 2014 that a pre-antibiotic era was imminent [154] and that there was an urgent need worldwide to mobilize international cooperation. In view of the risk to public health, new strategies need to be considered without delay: phage therapy is one of the most successful options today, if not the most successful. The advancement of phage therapy will, however, require an entwinement of old and new, of science and medicine, of fundamental research and clinical application, that is unparalleled in other areas of medical research. A multidisciplinary approach is needed more than ever, bringing together microbiologists, ecologists, evolutionary biologists, infectious disease specialists, medical doctors, and public health professionals. The growing threat of antibiotic resistance is indeed a compelling motivation to include and evaluate as much historical, compassionate use, and pre-clinical information as possible to increase the likelihood of the effective implementation of phage therapy.

The limited knowledge of phages available when they were first used historically has been complemented by a wealth of scientific studies, and yet therapy remains largely as empiric today as it was then. Our own empirical compassionate experiences with phages have nevertheless resulted in good clinical outcomes and have led us to conclude that phage therapy has much to offer, particularly for osteoarticular infections. A clinical trial is now planned to treat osteoarticular infections as an extension of our empirical findings through compassionate treatment. Such observational evidence from individual treatments provides valuable information on how to refine treatment protocols and to guide effective clinical practice in the future.

The use of biological rather than chemical drugs, such as phages, is new and upsets conventional treatment paradigms. Moreover, this development is occurring in a more strictly regulated context than in the past, where therapeutic frameworks need to be navigated and financial support is lacking. If it is unlikely that phage therapy will ever replace antibiotic therapy, it would surely be best to combine available antimicrobial strategies to create an effective treatment, and more research is merited in this direction. In the interim of conclusive phage efficacy trials, compassionate use of phage therapy, in combination with appropriate antibiotics, should be continued to maximize positive treatment outcomes for patients suffering from antibiotic resistant or difficult-to-treat infections.

References

1. D'Hérelle, F. Sur un microbe invisible antagoniste des bacilles dysentériques. *Acad. Sci. Paris* **1917**, *165*, 373–375.
2. D'Hérelle, F. *Le Bactériophage: Son Rôle dans L'immunité*; Masson et Cie: Paris, France, 1921.
3. Bruynoghe, R.; Maisin, J. Essais de thérapeutique au moyen du bactériophage. *CR Soc. Biol.* **1922**, *85*, 1120–1121.

4. WHO. Antimicrobial Resistance: Global Report on Surveillance. Available online: http://www.thehealthwell.info/node/763364 (accessed on 14 November 2018).
5. Wittebole, X.; Roock, S.; Opal, S.M. A historical overview of bacteriophage therapy as an alternative to antibiotics for the treatment of bacterial pathogens. *Virulence* **2013**, *5*, 226–235. [CrossRef] [PubMed]
6. Pires, D.; Melo, L.; Boas, V.D.; Sillankorva, S.; Azeredo, J. Phage therapy as an alternative or complementary strategy to prevent and control biofilm-related infections. *Curr. Opin. Microbiol.* **2017**, *39*, 48–56. [CrossRef] [PubMed]
7. Torres-Barceló, C.; Arias-Sánchez, F.I.; Vasse, M.; Ramsayer, J.; Kaltz, O.; Hochberg, M.E. A window of opportunity to control the bacterial pathogen *Pseudomonas aeruginosa* combining antibiotics and phages. *PLoS ONE* **2014**, *9*, e106628. [CrossRef] [PubMed]
8. Torres-Barceló, C.; Hochberg, M.E. Evolutionary rationale for phages as complements of antibiotics. *Trends Microbiol.* **2016**, *24*, 249–256. [CrossRef] [PubMed]
9. Jault, P.; Leclerc, T.; Jennes, S.; Pirnay, J.P.; Que, Y.-A.A.; Resch, G.; Rousseau, A.F.; Ravat, F.; Carsin, H.; Floch, R.; et al. Efficacy and tolerability of a cocktail of bacteriophages to treat burn wounds infected by *Pseudomonas aeruginosa* (PhagoBurn): A randomised, controlled, double-blind phase 1/2 trial. *Lancet Infect. Dis.* **2018**, *19*, 35–45. [CrossRef]
10. Leitner, L.; Sybesma, W.; Chanishvili, N.; Goderdzishvili, M.; Chkhotua, A.; Ujmajuridze, A.; Schneider, M.P.; Sartori, A.; Mehnert, U.; Bachmann, L.M.; et al. Bacteriophages for treating urinary tract infections in patients undergoing transurethral resection of the prostate: A randomized, placebo-controlled, double-blind clinical trial. *BMC Urol.* **2017**, *17*, 90. [CrossRef]
11. Sarker, S.; Sultana, S.; Reuteler, G.; Moine, D.; Descombes, P.; Charton, F.; Bourdin, G.; McCallin, S.; Ngom-Bru, C.; Neville, T.; et al. Oral phage therapy of acute bacterial diarrhea with two coliphage preparations: A randomized trial in children from bangladesh. *EBioMedicine* **2016**, *4*, 124–137. [CrossRef]
12. Wright, A.; Hawkins, C.; Anggård, E.; Harper, D. A controlled clinical trial of a therapeutic bacteriophage preparation in chronic otitis due to antibiotic-resistant *Pseudomonas aeruginosa*; a preliminary report of efficacy. *Clin. Otolaryngol. Allied Sci.* **2009**, *34*, 349–357. [CrossRef]
13. Ujmajuridze, A.; Chanishvili, N.; Goderdzishvili, M.; Leitner, L.; Mehnert, U.; Chkhotua, A.; Kessler, T.M.; Sybesma, W. Adapted bacteriophages for treating urinary tract infections. *Front. Microbiol.* **2018**, *9*, 1832. [CrossRef] [PubMed]
14. Pirnay, J.-P.; Verbeken, G.; Ceyssens, P.-J.; Huys, I.; de Vos, D.; Ameloot, C.; Fauconnier, A. The Magistral Phage. *Viruses* **2018**, *10*, 64. [CrossRef] [PubMed]
15. Sybesma, W.; Rohde, C.; Bardy, P.; Pirnay, J.-P.; Cooper, I.; Caplin, J.; Chanishvili, N.; Coffey, A.; de Vos, D.; Scholz, A.; et al. Silk route to the acceptance and re-implementation of bacteriophage therapy-Part II. *Antibiotics* **2018**, *7*, 2.
16. Górski, A.; Jończyk-Matysiak, E.; Łusiak-Szelachowska, M.; Międzybrodzki, R.; Weber-Dąbrowska, B.; Borysowski, J.; Letkiewicz, S.; Bagińska, N.; Sfanos, K.S. Phage therapy in prostatitis: Recent prospects. *Front. Microbiol.* **2018**, *9*, 1434. [CrossRef] [PubMed]
17. Weber-Dąbrowska, B.; Jończyk-Matysiak, E.; Żaczek, M.; Łobocka, M.; Łusiak-Szelachowska, M.; Górski, A. Bacteriophage procurement for therapeutic purposes. *Front. Microbiol.* **2016**, *7*, 1177. [CrossRef] [PubMed]
18. Weber-Dabrowska, B.; Mulczyk, M.; Górski, A. Bacteriophages as an efficient therapy for antibiotic-resistant septicemia in man. *Transplant. Proc.* **2003**, *35*, 1385–1386. [CrossRef]
19. Weber-Dabrowska, B.; Mulczyk, M.; Górski, A. Bacteriophage therapy for infections in cancer patients. *Clin. Appl. Immunol. Rev.* **2001**, *1*, 131–134. [CrossRef]
20. Weber-Dabrowska, B.; Mulczyk, M.; Górski, A. Bacteriophage therapy of bacterial infections: An update of our institute's experience. *Archivum Immunologiae Therapiae Experimentalis* **2000**, *48*, 547–551.
21. Schooley, R.T.; Biswas, B.; Gill, J.J.; Hernandez-Morales, A.; Lancaster, J.; Lessor, L.; Barr, J.J.; Reed, S.L.; Rohwer, F.; Benler, S.; et al. Development and use of personalized bacteriophage-based therapeutic cocktails to treat a patient with a disseminated resistant *Acinetobacter baumannii* infection. *Antimicrob. Agents Chemother.* **2017**, *61*, AAC-00954. [CrossRef]
22. LaVergne, S.; Hamilton, T.; Biswas, B.; Kumaraswamy, M.; Schooley, R.; Wooten, D. Phage therapy for a multidrug-resistant *Acinetobacter baumannii* craniectomy site infection. *Open Forum Infect. Dis.* **2018**, *5*, ofy064. [CrossRef]

23. Pirnay, J.-P.P.; de Vos, D.; Verbeken, G.; Merabishvili, M.; Chanishvili, N.; Vaneechoutte, M.; Zizi, M.; Laire, G.; Lavigne, R.; Huys, I.; et al. The phage therapy paradigm: Prêt-à-porter or sur-mesure? *Pharm. Res.* **2011**, *28*, 934–937. [CrossRef] [PubMed]
24. Phage Directory. Available online: https://phage.directory/ (accessed on 14 November 2018).
25. Sillankorva, S. Isolation of bacteriophages for clinically relevant bacteria. *Methods Mol. Biol.* **2018**, *1693*, 23–30. [PubMed]
26. EudraLex Good Manufacturing Practice (GMP) Guidelines. European Commission. 2010. Available online: https://ec.europa.eu/health/documents/eudralex/vol-4_en (accessed on 14 November 2018).
27. Verbeken, G.; Pirnay, J.-P.; de Vos, D.; Jennes, S.; Zizi, M.; Lavigne, R.; Casteels, M.; Huys, I. Optimizing the European Regulatory Framework for Sustainable Bacteriophage Therapy in Human Medicine. *Archivum Immunologiae Therapiae Experimentalis* **2012**, *60*, 161–172. [CrossRef] [PubMed]
28. Verbeken, G.; Pirnay, J.-P.; Lavigne, R.; Jennes, S.; de Vos, D.; Casteels, M.; Huys, I. Call for a dedicated european legal framework for bacteriophage therapy. *Archivum Immunologiae Therapiae Experimentalis* **2014**, *62*, 117–129. [CrossRef] [PubMed]
29. Pirnay, J.-P.P.; Blasdel, B.G.; Bretaudeau, L.; Buckling, A.; Chanishvili, N.; Clark, J.R.; Corte-Real, S.; Debarbieux, L.; Dublanchet, A.; de Vos, D.; et al. Quality and safety requirements for sustainable phage therapy products. *Pharm. Res.* **2015**, *32*, 2173–2179. [CrossRef] [PubMed]
30. Pirnay, J.-P.; Merabishvili, M.; Raemdonck, H.; de Vos, D.; Verbeken, G. Bacteriophage production in compliance with regulatory requirements. In Bacteriophage Therapy. *Methods Mol. Biol.* **2018**, *1693*, 233–252. [PubMed]
31. Fauconnier, A. Regulating phage therapy. *EMBO Rep.* **2017**, *18*, 198–200. [CrossRef]
32. Furfaro, L.L.; Payne, M.S.; Chang, B.J. Bacteriophage therapy: Clinical trials and regulatory hurdles. *Front. Cell. Infect. Microbiol.* **2018**, *8*, 376. [CrossRef]
33. Kutter, E.M.; Gvasalia, G.; Alavidze, Z.; Brewster, E. Phage Therapy. In *Biotherapy—History, Principles and Practice*; CRC Press: Boca Raton, FL, USA, 2013; pp. 191–231.
34. Fauconnier, A. Bacteriophage Therapy. *Methods Mol. Biol.* **2018**, *1693*, 253–268.
35. Skurnik, M.; Pajunen, M.; Kiljunen, S. Biotechnological challenges of phage therapy. *Biotechnol. Lett.* **2007**, *29*, 995–1003. [CrossRef]
36. Vandenheuvel, D.; Lavigne, R.; Brussow, H. Bacteriophage therapy: Advances in formulation strategies and human clinical trials. *Annu. Rev. Virol.* **2015**, *2*, 599–618. [CrossRef] [PubMed]
37. Rhoads, D.D.; Wolcott, R.D.; Kuskowski, M.A.; Wolcott, B.M.; Ward, L.S.; Sulakvelidze, A. Bacteriophage therapy of venous leg ulcers in humans: Results of a phase I safety trial. *J. Wound Care* **2009**, *18*, 237–243. [CrossRef] [PubMed]
38. Kutter, E.; Borysowski, J.; Miedzybrodzki, R.; Gorski, A.; Weber-Dąbrowska, B.; Kutateladze, M.; Alavidze, Z.; Goderdzishvili, M.; Adamia, R. Clinical Phage Therapy. In *Phage Therapy: Current Research and Applications*; Borysowski, J., Miedzybrodzki, R., Gorski, A., Eds.; Nova Science Publishers: Norfolk, UK, 2014; Chapter 11; pp. 257–288.
39. Speck, P.; Smithyman, A. Safety and efficacy of phage therapy via the intravenous route. *FEMS Microbiol. Lett.* **2016**, *363*. [CrossRef] [PubMed]
40. Międzybrodzki, R.; Borysowski, J.; Weber-Dabrowska, B.; Fortuna, W.; Letkiewicz, S.; Szufnarowski, K.; Pawełczyk, Z.; Rogoz, P.; Kłak, M.; Wojtasik, E.B.; et al. Clinical aspects of phage therapy. *Adv. Virus Res.* **2012**, *83*, 73–121. [PubMed]
41. Vandenheuvel, D.; Singh, A.; Vandersteegen, K.; Klumpp, J.; Lavigne, R.; Van den Mooter, G. Feasibility of spray drying bacteriophages into respirable powders to combat pulmonary bacterial infections. *Eur. J. Pharm. Biopharm.* **2013**, *84*, 578–582. [CrossRef] [PubMed]
42. Matinkhoo, S.; Lynch, K.; Dennis, J.J.; Finlay, W.H.; Vehring, R. Spray-dried respirable powders containing bacteriophages for the treatment of pulmonary infections. *J. Pharm. Sci.* **2011**, *100*, 5197–5205. [CrossRef] [PubMed]
43. Golshahi, L.; Lynch, K.H.; Dennis, J.J.; Finlay, W.H. In vitro lung delivery of bacteriophages KS4-M and PhiKZ using dry powder inhalers for treatment of *Burkholderia cepacia* complex and *Pseudomonas aeruginosa* infections in cystic fibrosis. *J. Appl. Microbiol.* **2011**, *110*, 106–117. [CrossRef]

44. Morello, E.; Saussereau, E.; Maura, D.; Huerre, M.; Touqui, L.; Debarbieux, L. Pulmonary bacteriophage therapy on *Pseudomonas aeruginosa* cystic fibrosis strains: First steps towards treatment and prevention. *PLoS ONE* **2011**, *6*, e16963. [CrossRef]
45. Abedon, S.T. Phage therapy of pulmonary infections. *Bacteriophage* **2015**, *5*, e1020260. [CrossRef]
46. Roach, D.R.; Leung, C.; Henry, M.; Morello, E.; Singh, D.; Santo, J.P.; Weitz, J.S.; Debarbieux, L. Synergy between the host immune system and bacteriophage is essential for successful phage therapy against an acute respiratory pathogen. *Cell Host Microbe* **2017**, *22*, 38–47. [CrossRef]
47. Semler, D.D.; Lynch, K.H.; Dennis, J.J. The promise of bacteriophage therapy for *Burkholderia cepacia* complex respiratory infections. *Front. Cell Infect. Microbiol.* **2012**, *1*, 27. [CrossRef] [PubMed]
48. Hoe, S.; Semler, D.D.; Goudie, A.D.; Lynch, K.H.; Matinkhoo, S.; Finlay, W.H.; Dennis, J.J.; Vehring, R. Respirable bacteriophages for the treatment of bacterial lung infections. *J. Aerosol Med. Pulm. Drug Deliv.* **2013**, *26*, 317–335. [CrossRef]
49. Abedon, S.T. Phage therapy: Eco-physiological pharmacology. *Scientifica* **2014**, *2014*, 581639. [CrossRef]
50. Parracho, H.M.; Burrowes, B.H.; Enright, M.C.; McConville, M.L.; Harper, D.R. The role of regulated clinical trials in the development of bacteriophage therapeutics. *J. Mol. Genet. Med.* **2012**, *6*, 279–286. [CrossRef]
51. McCallin, S.; Brüssow, H. Clinical Trials of Bacteriophage Therapeutics. In *Bacteriophages*; Harper, D., Abedon, S., Burrowes, B., McConville, M., Eds.; Springer: Cham, Switzerland, 2017; pp. 1–29.
52. Leszczynski, P.; Weber-Dabrowska, B.; Kohutnicka, M.; Luczak, M.; Gorecki, A.; Gorski, A. Successful eradication of methicillin-resistant *Staphylococcus aureus* (MRSA) intestinal carrier status in a healthcare worker-case report. *Folia Microbiol.* **2006**, *51*, 236–238. [CrossRef]
53. Marcuk, L.M.; Nikiforov, V.N.; Scerbak, J.F.; Levitov, T.A.; Kotljarova, R.I.; Naumgina, M.S.; Davydov, S.U.; Monsur, K.A.; Rahman, M.A.; Latif, M.A.; et al. Clinical studies of the use of bacteriophage in the treatment of cholera. *Bull. World Health Organ.* **1971**, *45*, 77–83. [PubMed]
54. Goodridge, L.D. Bacteriophages for managing *Shigella* in various clinical and non-clinical settings. *Bacteriophage* **2013**, *3*, e25098. [CrossRef]
55. Zhvania, P.; Hoyle, N.; Nadareishvili, L.; Nizharadze, D.; Kutateladze, M. Phage Therapy in a 16-Year-Old boy with Netherton Syndrome. *Front. Med.* **2017**, *4*, 94. [CrossRef]
56. Jonczyk-Matysiak, E.; Weber-Dabrowska, B.; Zaczek, M.; Miedzybrodzki, R.; Letkiewicz, S.; Lusiak-Szelchowska, M.; Gorski, A. Prospects of phage application in the treatment of acne caused by *Propionibacterium acnes*. *Front Microbiol.* **2017**, *8*, 164. [CrossRef]
57. Crutchfield, E.D.; Stout, B.F. Treatment of staphylococcic infections of the skin by the bacteriophage. *Arch. Derm. Syphilol.* **1930**, *22*, 1010–1021. [CrossRef]
58. Morozova, V.V.; Kozlova, Y.N.; Ganichev, D.A.; Tikunova, N.V. Bacteriophage treatment of infected diabetic foot ulcers. In *Bacteriophage Therapy: From Lab to Clinical Practice*; Azeredo, J., Sillankorva, S., Eds.; Humana Press: Clifton, NJ, USA; Springer: New York, NY, USA, 2018; Chapter 13; pp. 151–158.
59. Fish, R.; Kutter, E.; Wheat, G.; Blasdel, B.; Kutateladze, M.; Kuhl, S. Bacteriophage treatment of intransigent diabetic toe ulcers: A case series. *J. Wound Care* **2016**, *25* (Suppl. 7), S27–S33. [CrossRef]
60. Rose, T.; Verbeken, G.; de Vos, D.; Merabishvili, M.; Vaneechoutte, M.; Lavigne, R.; Jennes, S.; Zizi, M.; Pirnay, J.-P.P. Experimental phage therapy of burn wound infection: Difficult first steps. *Int. J. Burns Trauma* **2014**, *4*, 66–73.
61. Jennes, S.; Merabishvili, M.; Soentjens, P.; Pang, K.; Rose, T.; Keersebilck, E.; Soete, O.; François, P.-M.; Teodorescu, S.; Verween, G.; et al. Use of bacteriophages in the treatment of colistin-only-sensitive *Pseudomonas aeruginosa* septicaemia in a patient with acute kidney injury-a case report. *Crit. Care* **2017**, *21*, 129. [CrossRef]
62. Duplessis, C. Refractory *Pseudomonas* bacteremia in a 2-Year-Old sterilized by bacteriophage therapy. *J. Pediatr. Infect. Dis. Soc.* **2018**, *7*, 253–256. Available online: https://academic.oup.com/jpids/article/7/3/253/4004747 (accessed on 14 November 2018). [CrossRef]
63. Grimont, P.A.; Grimont, F.; Lacut, J.Y.; Issanchou, A.M.; Aubertin, J. Traitement d'une endocardite à *Serratia* par les bactériophages. *Nouvelle Presse Médicale* **1978**, *7*, 2251.
64. MacNeal, W.J.; Frisbee, F.C.; Blevins, A. Bacteriophage therapy of staphylococcic septic obstruction of cavernous sinus: II. Report of cases. *Arch. Ophthalmol.* **1943**, *29*, 341–368. [CrossRef]
65. MacNeal, W.J. The use of bacteriophages in wound infections and in bacteremias. *Am. J. Med. Sci.* **1932**, *184*, 805. [CrossRef]

66. Raiga, A. Septicémie à staphylocoque guérie par une inoculation intra-veineuse de bactériophage. *Bulletin et Mémoire de la Société des Chirurgiens de Paris* **1931**, *23*, 441–447.
67. Stroj, L.; Weber-Dabrowska, B.; Partyka, K.; Mulczyk, M.; Wojcik, M. Successful treatment with bacteriophage in purulent cerebrospinal meningitis in a newborn. *Neurologia i Neurochirurgia Polska* **1999**, *33*, 693–698.
68. Merril, C.R.; Biswas, B.; Carlton, R.; Jensen, N.C.; Creed, G.J.; Zullo, S.; Adhya, S. Long-circulating bacteriophage as antibacterial agents. *Proc. Natl. Acad. Sci. USA* **1996**, *93*, 3188–3192. [CrossRef]
69. Schless, R.A. *Staphylococcus aureus* meningitis: Treatment with specific bacteriophage. *Am. J. Dis. Child.* **1932**, *44*, 813–822. [CrossRef]
70. MacNeal, W.J.; Frisbee, F.C.; Blevins, A. Recoveries of staphylococcic meningitis following bacteriophage therapy. *Arch. Otolaryngol.* **1943**, *37*, 507–525. [CrossRef]
71. Martin, P. Méningite posttraumatique à pyocyaniques traitée par un bactériophage adapté intrarachidien. *Acta Chir. Belg.* **1959**, *58*, 85–90. [PubMed]
72. Sedallian, P.; Bertoye, A.; Gauthier, J.; Muller, M.; Courtieu, A.L. Méningite purulente à colibacilles traitée par un bactériophage adapté intrarachidien. *Lyon Med.* **1958**, *66*, 509–512.
73. Beckerich, A.; Hauduroy, P. Le traitement des infections urinaires à colibacille par le bactériophage de d'Hérelle. *Bull. Med.* **1923**, *37*, 273.
74. Schultz, E.W. Bacteriophage as a therapeutic agent in genito-urinary infections: Part I. *Calif. West. Med.* **1932**, *36*, 33–37.
75. Schultz, E.W. Bacteriophage as a therapeutic agent in genito-urinary infections: Part II. *Calif. West. Med.* **1932**, *36*, 91–96.
76. Wehrbein, H.; Nerb, L. Bacteriophage in the treatment of urinary infections: With an appendix on the technique of phage preparation. *Am. J. Surg.* **1935**, *29*, 48–53. [CrossRef]
77. Ujmajuridze, A.; Jvania, G.; Chanishvili, N.; Goderdzishvili, M.; Sybesma, W.; Managadze, L.; Chkhotua, A.; Kessler, T. Phage therapy for the treatment for urinary tract infection: Results of in-vitro screenings and in-vivo application using commercially available bacteriophage cocktails. *Eur. Urol. Suppl.* **2016**, *15*, e265. [CrossRef]
78. Khawaldeh, A.; Morales, S.; Dillon, B.; Alavidze, Z.; Ginn, A.; Thomas, L.; Chapman, S.; Dublanchet, A.; Smithyman, A.; Iredell, J. Bacteriophage therapy for refractory *Pseudomonas aeruginosa* urinary tract infection. *J. Med. Microbiol.* **2011**, *60*, 1697–1700. [CrossRef]
79. Melo, L.D.; Veiga, P.; Cerca, N.; Kropinski, A.M.; Almeida, C.; Azeredo, J.; Sillankorva, S. Development of a phage cocktail to control *Proteus mirabilis* catheter-associated urinary tract infections. *Front. Microbiol.* **2016**, *7*, 1024. [CrossRef] [PubMed]
80. Nzakizwanayo, J.; Hanin, A.; Alves, D.R.; McCutcheon, B.; Dedi, C.; Salvage, J.; Knox, K.; Stewart, B.; Metcalfe, A.; Clark, J.; et al. Bacteriophage can prevent encrustation and blockage of urinary catheters by *Proteus mirabilis*. *Antimicrob. Agents Chemother.* **2015**, *60*, 1530–1536. [CrossRef] [PubMed]
81. Letkiewicz, S.; Miedzybrodzki, R.; Fortuna, W.; Weber-Dabrowska, B.; Górski, A. Eradication of *Enterococcus faecalis* by phage therapy in chronic bacterial prostatitis-case report. *Folia Microbiol.* **2009**, *54*, 457–461. [CrossRef] [PubMed]
82. Letkiewicz, S.; Międzybrodzki, R.; Kłak, M.; Jończyk, E.; Weber-Dąbrowska, B.; Górski, A. The perspectives of the application of phage therapy in chronic bacterial prostatitis. *FEMS Immunol. Med. Microbiol.* **2010**, *60*, 99–112. [CrossRef] [PubMed]
83. Furr, C.L.; Lehman, S.M.; Morales, S.P.; Rosas, F.X.; Gaidamaka, A.; Bilinsky, I.P.; Grint, P.C.; Schooley, R.T.; Aslam, S. Bacteriophage treatment of multidrug-resistant *Pseudomonas aeruginosa* pneumonia in a cystic fibrosis patient. In 41st European Cystic Fibrosis Conference. *J. Cystic Fibrosis* **2018**, *17* (Suppl. 3), S1–S150. [CrossRef]
84. Kvachadze, L.; Balarjishvili, N.; Meskhi, T.; Tevdoradze, E.; Skhirtladze, N.; Pataridze, T.; Adamia, R.; Topuria, T.; Kutter, E.; Rohde, C.; et al. Evaluation of lytic activity of staphylococcal bacteriophage Sb-1 against freshly isolated clinical pathogens. *Microb. Biotechnol.* **2011**, *4*, 643–650. [CrossRef]
85. Pherecydes Pneumophage. Available online: https://www.pherecydes-pharma.com/pneumophage.html (accessed on 14 November 2018).
86. Zhang, G.; Zhao, Y.; Paramasivan, S.; Richter, K.; Morales, S.; Wormald, P.; Vreugde, S. Bacteriophage effectively kills multidrug resistant *Staphylococcus aureus* clinical isolates from chronic rhinosinusitis patients. *Int. Forum Allergy Rhinol.* **2018**, *8*, 406–414. [CrossRef]

87. Fong, S.A.; Drilling, A.; Morales, S.; Cornet, M.E.; Woodworth, B.A.; Fokkens, W.J.; Psaltis, A.J.; Vreugde, S.; Wormald, P.-J. Activity of bacteriophages in removing biofilms of *Pseudomonas aeruginosa* isolates from chronic rhinosinusitis patients. *Front. Cell. Infect. Microbiol.* **2017**, *7*, 418. [CrossRef]
88. Drilling, A.J.; Ooi, M.L.; Miljkovic, D.; James, C.; Speck, P.; Vreugde, S.; Clark, J.; Wormald, P.J. Long-term safety of topical bacteriophage application to the frontal sinus region. *Front. Cell. Infect. Microbiol.* **2017**, *7*, 49. [CrossRef]
89. Drilling, A.; Morales, S.; Jardeleza, C.; Vreugde, S.; Speck, P.; Wormald, P.J. Bacteriophage reduces biofilm of *Staphylococcus aureus* ex vivo isolates from chronic rhinosinusitis patients. *Am. J. Rhinol. Allergy* **2014**, *28*, 3–11. [CrossRef]
90. Town, A.E.; Frisbee, F.C. Bacteriophage in ophthalmology. *Arch. Ophthalmol.* **1932**, *8*, 683–689. [CrossRef]
91. Fadlallah, A.; Chelala, E.; Legeais, J.-M.M. Corneal infection therapy with topical bacteriophage administration. *Open Ophthalmol. J.* **2015**, *9*, 167–168. [CrossRef] [PubMed]
92. Górski, A.; Targonska, M.; Borysowski, J.; Weber-Dabrowska, B. The potential of phage therapy in bacterial infections of the eye. *Ophthalmologica* **2009**, *223*, 162–165. [CrossRef] [PubMed]
93. Shlezinger, M.; Houri-Haddad, Y.; Coppenhagen-Glazer, S.; Resch, G.; Que, Y.A.; Beyth, S.; Dorfman, E.; Hazan, R.; Beyth, N. Phage therapy: A new horizon in the antibacterial treatment of oral pathogens. *Curr. Top. Med. Chem.* **2017**, *17*, 1199–1211. [CrossRef] [PubMed]
94. Khalifa, L.; Shlezinger, M.; Beyth, S.; Houri-Haddad, Y.; Coppenhagen-Glazer, S.; Beyth, N.; Hazan, R. Phage therapy against *Enterococcus faecalis* in dental root canals. *J. Oral Microbiol.* **2016**, *8*, 32157. [CrossRef] [PubMed]
95. Ly, M.; Abeles, S.R.; Boehm, T.K.; Robles-Sikisaka, R.; Naidu, M.; Santiago-Rodriguez, T.; Pride, D.T. Altered oral viral ecology in association with periodontal disease. *mBio* **2014**, *5*, e01133-14. [CrossRef] [PubMed]
96. Rossitto, M.; Fiscarelli, E.V.; Rosati, P. Challenges and promises for planning future clinical research into bacteriophage therapy against Pseudomonas aeruginosa in cystic fibrosis. An argumentative review. *Front. Microbiol.* **2018**, *9*, 775. [CrossRef]
97. Matsuzaki, S.; Uchiyama, J.; Takemura-Uchiyama, I.; Ujihara, T.; Daibata, M. Isolation of bacteriophages for fastidious bacteria. In *Bacteriophage Therapy: From Lab to Clinical Practice, Humana Press ed.*; Azeredo, J., Sillankorva, S., Eds.; Springer: New York, NY, USA, 2018; Chapter 1; pp. 3–10.
98. Wan, X.Q.; Li, H.M.; Bai, Y. Advances in phage therapy of Helicobacter pylori infection. *World Chin. J. Digestol.* **2009**, *17*, 3623–3626. [CrossRef]
99. Shan, J.; Teulieres, L.; Clockie, M. Is there a place for bacteriophages in diagnosis and treatment of Lyme Disease? In Proceedings of the Lymes Disease Action Conference, International Lyme And Associated Diseases Society (ILADS), Philadelphia, PA, USA, 3–6 November 2016.
100. Zakowska, D.; Bartoszcze, M.; Niemcewicz, M.; Bielawska-Drozd, A.; Knap, J.; Cieslik, P.; Chomiczewski, K.; Kocik, J. Bacillus anthracis infections—New possibilities of treatment. *Ann. Agric. Environ. Med. AAEM* **2015**, *22*, 202–207. [CrossRef]
101. Filippov, A.A.; Kirill, V.S.; Mikeljon, P.N. Bacteriophages against biothreat bacteria: Diagnostic, environmental and therapeutic applications. *J. Bioterrorism Biodefense* **2013**, *S3*, 010. [CrossRef]
102. Kremers, H.M.; Nwojo, M.E.; Ransom, J.E.; Wood-Wentz, C.M.; Melton, L.J., III; Huddleston, P.M., III. Trends in the epidemiology of osteomyelitis: A population-based study, 1969 to 2009. *J. Bone Jt. Surg.* **2015**, *97*, 837–845. [CrossRef] [PubMed]
103. Grammatico-Guillon, L.; Baron, S.; Gettner, S.; Lecuyer, A.-I.; Gaborit, C.; Rosset, P.; Rusch, E.; Bernard, L. Surveillance hospitalière des infections ostéo-articulaires en France: Analyse des données médico-administratives, PMSI 2008. *Bull. Epidémiol. Hosp.* **2013**, *4–5*, 39–44.
104. Albee, F.H. The treatment of osteomyelitis by bacteriophage. *J. Bone Jt. Surg.* **1933**, *15*, 58–66.
105. Kutateladze, M. Experience of the Eliava Institute in bacteriophage therapy. *Virol. Sin.* **2015**, *30*, 80–81. [CrossRef] [PubMed]
106. Slopek, S.; Weber Dabrowska, B.; Dabrowski, M.; Kucharewicz-Krukowska, A. Results of bacteriophage treatment of suppurative bacterial infections in the years 1981–1986. *Archivum Immunologiae et Therapiae Experimentalis* **1987**, *37*, 369–383.

107. Chanishvili, N.; Sharp, R. Bacteriophage therapy: Experience from the Eliva Institute, Georgia. *Microbiol. Aust.* **2008**, *20*, 96–101.
108. Raiga, A. Considérations Générales sur L'ostéomyélite Aiguë et son Traitement par le Bactériophage de d'Hérelle. In Proceedings of the 52ème Congrès Français de Chirurgie, Paris, France, 4 October 1949.
109. Lang, G.; Kher, P.; Mathevon, H.; Clavert, J.M.; Sejourne, P.; Pointu, J. Bactériophages et chirurgie orthopédique—A propos de sept cas. *Rev. Chir. Orthop. Reparatrice Appar. Mot.* **1979**, *65*, 33–37.
110. Chanishvili, N. Phage Therapy—History from Twort and d'Herelle through soviet experience to current approaches. *Adv. Virus Res.* **2012**, *82*, 3–40.
111. Ferry, T.; Boucher, F.; Fevre, C.; Perpoint, T.; Chateau, J.; Petitjean, C.; Josse, J.; Chidiac, C.; L'hostis, G.; Leboucher, G.; et al. Innovations for the treatment of a complex bone and joint infection due to XDR *Pseudomonas aeruginosa* including local application of a selected cocktail of bacteriophages. *J. Antimicrob. Chemother.* **2018**, *73*, 2901–2903. [CrossRef]
112. Yilmaz, C.; Colak, M.; Yilmaz, B.C.; Ersoz, G.; Kutateladze, M.; Gozlugol, M. Bacteriophage therapy in implant-related infections: An experimental study. *J. Bone Jt. Surg.* **2013**, *95*, 117–125. [CrossRef]
113. Kishor, C.; Mishra, R.R.; Saraf, S.K.; Kumar, M.; vastav, A.K.; Nath, G. Phage therapy of staphylococcal chronic osteomyelitis in experimental animal model. *Indian J. Med. Res.* **2016**, *143*, 87–94. [PubMed]
114. Kaur, S.; Harjai, K.; Chhibber, S. In vivo assessment of phage and linezolid based implant coatings for treatment of methicillin resistant *S. aureus* (MRSA) mediated orthopaedic device related infections. *PLoS ONE* **2016**, *11*, e0157626. [CrossRef] [PubMed]
115. Zhang, L.; Sun, L.; Wei, R.; Gao, Q.; He, T.; Xu, C.; Liu, X.; Wang, R. Study of intracellular *Staphylococcus aureus* control by virulent bacteriophage within MAC-T bovine mammary epithelial cells. *Antimicrob. Agents Chemother.* **2017**, *61*, e01990-16. [CrossRef] [PubMed]
116. Pherecydes Phosa. Available online: https://www.pherecydes-pharma.com/phosa-collaborative-project.html (accessed on 14 November 2018).
117. Vieu, J.-F.; Guillermet, F.; Minck, R.; Nicolle, P. Données actuelles sur les applications thérapeutiques des bactériophages. *Bull. Acad. Nat. Méd.* **1979**, *1*, 61–66.
118. Houssaye, C. Evaluation In vitro D'une Suspension de Bactériophages Anti-Staphylococcique à Usage Thérapeutique. Ph.D. Thesis, Université Pierre et Marie Curie, Paris, France, 2004.
119. Comeau, A.; Tétart, F.; Trojet, S.; Prere, M.; One, K.H. Phage-antibiotic synergy (PAS): β-lactam and quinolone antibiotics stimulate virulent phage growth. *PLoS ONE* **2007**, *2*, e799. [CrossRef] [PubMed]
120. Kamal, F.; Dennis, J.J. *Burkholderia cepacia* complex phage-antibiotic synergy (PAS): Antibiotics stimulate lytic phage activity. *Appl. Environ. Microbiol.* **2015**, *81*, 1132–1138. [CrossRef] [PubMed]
121. Oechslin, F.; Piccardi, P.; Mancini, S.; Gabard, J.; Moreillon, P.; Entenza, J.M.; Resch, G.; Que, Y.A. Synergistic interaction between phage therapy and antibiotics clears *Pseudomonas aeruginosa* infection in endocarditis and reduces virulence. *J. Infect. Dis.* **2017**, *215*, 703–712. [CrossRef]
122. Valério, N.; Oliveira, C.; Jesus, V.; Branco, T.; Pereira, C.; Moreirinha, C.; Almeida, A. Effects of single and combined use of bacteriophages and antibiotics to inactivate *Escherichia coli*. *Virus Res.* **2017**, *240*, 8–17. [CrossRef]
123. Knezevic, P.; Curcin, S.; Aleksic, V.; Petrusic, M.; Vlaski, L. Phage-antibiotic synergism: A possible approach to combatting *Pseudomonas aeruginosa*. *Res. Microbiol.* **2013**, *164*, 55–60. [CrossRef]
124. Kumaran, D.; Taha, M.; Yi, Q.; Ramirez-Arcos, S.; Diallo, J.-S.; Carli, A.; Abdelbary, H. Does treatment order matter? Investigating the ability of bacteriophage to augment antibiotic activity against *Staphylococcus aureus* biofilms. *Front. Microbiol.* **2018**, *9*, 127. [CrossRef]
125. Chan, B.K.; Abedon, S.T. Bacteriophages and their enzymes in biofilm control. *Curr. Pharm. Des.* **2015**, *21*, 85–99. [CrossRef] [PubMed]
126. Sanchez, C.J.; Ward, C.L.; Romano, D.R.; Hurtgen, B.J.; Hardy, S.K.; Woodbury, R.L.; Trevino, A.V.; Rathbone, C.R.; Wenke, J.C. *Staphylococcus aureus* biofilms decrease osteoblast viability, inhibits osteogenic differentiation, and increases bone resorption in vitro. *BMC Musculoskeletal Disord.* **2013**, *14*, 187–198. [CrossRef] [PubMed]
127. Tevdoradze, E.; Kvachadze, L.; Kutateladze, M.; Stewart, C.R. Bactericidal genes of staphylococcal bacteriophage Sb-1. *Curr. Microbiol.* **2014**, *68*, 204–210. [CrossRef] [PubMed]

128. Dąbrowska, K. Interaction of bacteriophages with the immune system: Induction of bacteriophage-specific antibodies. *Methods Mol. Biol.* **2018**, *1693*, 139–150. [PubMed]
129. Aragón, I.M.; Herrera-Imbroda, B.; Queipo-Ortuño, M.I.; Castillo, E.; Moral, J.S.; Gómez-Millán, J.; Yucel, G.; Lara, M.F. The urinary tract microbiome in health and disease. *Eur. Urol. Focus* **2018**, *4*, 128–138. [CrossRef] [PubMed]
130. Oh, J.; Byrd, A.L.; Park, M.; Program, N.; Kong, H.H.; Segre, J.A. Temporal Stability of the Human Skin Microbiome. *Cell* **2016**, *165*, 854–866. [CrossRef]
131. Miller-Ensminger, T.; Garretto, A.; Brenner, J.; Thomas-White, K.; Zambom, A.; Wolfe, A.J.; Putonti, C. Bacteriophages of the urinary microbiome. *J. Bacterial.* **2018**, *200*, JB-00738. [CrossRef]
132. Gilbert, J.A.; Blaser, M.J.; Caporaso, G.J.; Jansson, J.K.; Lynch, S.V.; Knight, R. Current understanding of the human microbiome. *Nat. Med.* **2018**, *24*, 392–400. [CrossRef]
133. Xian, P.; Xuedong, Z.; Xin, X.; Yuqing, L.; Yan, L.; Jiyao, L.; Xiaoquan, S.; Shi, H.; Jian, X.; Ga, L. The Oral Microbiome Bank of China. *Int. J. Oral Sci.* **2018**, *10*, 16. [CrossRef]
134. Kong, H.H. Skin microbiome: Genomics-based insights into the diversity and role of skin microbes. *Trends Mol. Med.* **2011**, *17*, 320–328. [CrossRef]
135. Chu, D.M.; Ma, J.; Prince, A.L.; Antony, K.M.; Seferovic, M.D.; Aagaard, K.M. Maturation of the infant microbiome community structure and function across multiple body sites and in relation to mode of delivery. *Nat. Med.* **2017**, *23*, 314–326. [CrossRef] [PubMed]
136. Ravel, J.; Brotman, R.M. Translating the vaginal microbiome: Gaps and challenges. *Genome Med.* **2016**, *8*, 35. [CrossRef] [PubMed]
137. Manrique, P.; Bolduc, B.; Walk, S.T.; van der Oost, J.; de Vos, W.M.; Young, M.J. Healthy human gut phageome. *Proc. Natl. Acad. Sci. USA* **2016**, *113*, 10400–10405. [CrossRef] [PubMed]
138. Zarate, S.; Taboada, B.; Yocupicio-Monroy, M.; Arias, C.F. Human virome. *Arch. Med. Res.* **2017**, *48*, 701–716. [CrossRef] [PubMed]
139. Microbiome: Phage community in the gut. *Nat. Rev. Microbiol.* **2016**, *14*, 605. [CrossRef] [PubMed]
140. Kashyap, P.C.; Chia, N.; Nelson, H.; Segal, E.; Elinav, E. Microbiome at the frontier of personalized medicine. *Mayo Clin. Proc.* **2017**, *92*, 1855–1864. [CrossRef] [PubMed]
141. Sunderland, K.S.; Yang, M.; Mao, C. Phage-enabled nanomedicine: From probes to therapeutics in precision medicine. *Angew. Chem. Int. Engl.* **2017**, *56*, 1964–1992. [CrossRef]
142. Palmela, C.; Chevarin, C.; Xu, Z.; Torres, J.; Sevrin, G.; Hirten, R.; Barnich, N.; Ng, S.C.; Colombel, J.-F.F. Adherent-invasive *Escherichia coli* in inflammatory bowel disease. *Gut* **2018**, *67*, 574–587. [CrossRef]
143. Mirzaei, M.K.; Maurice, C.F. Ménage à trois in the human gut: Interactions between host, bacteria and phages. *Nat. Rev. Microbiol.* **2017**, *15*, 397–408. [CrossRef]
144. Waldschmitt, N.; Metwaly, A.; Fischer, S.; Haller, D. Microbial signatures as a predictive tool in IBD-Pearls and pitfalls. *Inflamm. Bowel Dis.* **2018**, *24*, 1123–1132. [CrossRef]
145. Knights, D.; Parfrey, L.W.; Zaneveld, J.; Lozupone, C.; Knight, R. Human-associated microbial signatures: Examining their predictive value. *Cell Host Microbe* **2011**, *10*, 292–296. [CrossRef] [PubMed]
146. Carding, S.; Davis, N.; Hoyles, L. Review article: The human intestinal virome in health and disease. *Aliment. Pharmacol. Ther.* **2017**, *46*, 800–815. [CrossRef] [PubMed]
147. Galtier, M.; Sordi, L.; Sivignon, A.; de Vallée, A.; Maura, D.; Neut, C.; Rahmouni, O.; Wannerberger, K.; Darfeuille-Michaud, A.; Desreumaux, P.; et al. Bacteriophages targeting adherent invasive *Escherichia coli* strains as a promising new treatment for Crohn's disease. *J. Crohn's Colitis* **2017**, *11*, 840–847. [CrossRef] [PubMed]
148. López, R.; Burgos, M.J.; Gálvez, A.; Pulido, R. The human gastrointestinal tract and oral microbiota in inflammatory bowel disease: A state of the science review. *APMIS Acta Pathol. Microbiol. Immunol. Scand.* **2017**, *125*, 3–10. [CrossRef] [PubMed]
149. Nale, J.Y.; Spencer, J.; Hargreaves, K.R.; Buckley, A.M.; Trzepiński, P.; Douce, G.R.; Clokie, M.R. Bacteriophage Combinations Significantly Reduce *Clostridium dificile* Growth In vitro and Proliferation In vivo. *Antimicrob. Agents Chemother.* **2016**, *60*, 968–981. [CrossRef] [PubMed]
150. Rea, M.C.; Alemayehu, D.; Ross, R.; Hill, C. Gut solutions to a gut problem: Bacteriocins, probiotics and bacteriophage for control of *Clostridium difficile* infection. *J. Med. Microbiol.* **2013**, *62*, 1369–1378. [CrossRef] [PubMed]

151. Thanki, A.M.; Taylor-Joyce, G.; Dowah, A.; Nale, J.Y.; Malik, D.; Clokie, M.R.J. Unravelling the links between phage adsorption and successful infection in *Clostridium difficile*. *Viruses* **2018**, *10*, 411. [CrossRef]
152. Shan, J.; Ramachandran, A.; Thanki, A.M.; Vukusic, F.B.; Barylski, J.; Clokie, M.R. Bacteriophages are more virulent to bacteria with human cells than they are in bacterial culture; insights from HT-29 cells. *Sci. Rep.* **2018**, *8*, 5091. [CrossRef]
153. Ott, S.J.; Waetzig, G.H.; Rehman, A.; Moltzau-Anderson, J.; Bharti, R.; Grasis, J.A.; Cassidy, L.; Tholey, A.; Fickenscher, H.; Seegert, D.; et al. Efficacy of sterile fecal filtrate transfer for treating patients with *Clostridium difficile* infection. *Gastroenterology* **2017**, *152*, 799–811. [CrossRef]
154. WHO. *Global Action Plan on Antimicrobial Resistance*; World Health Organization: Geneva, Switzerland, 2015; Available online: http://www.who.int/antimicrobial-resistance/global-action-plan/en/ (accessed on 14 November 2018).

13

Enterococcus faecalis Countermeasures Defeat a Virulent *Picovirinae* Bacteriophage

Julien Lossouarn [1,*], Arnaud Briet [1], Elisabeth Moncaut [1], Sylviane Furlan [1], Astrid Bouteau [1], Olivier Son [1], Magali Leroy [2], Michael S. DuBow [2], François Lecointe [1], Pascale Serror [1] and Marie-Agnès Petit [1]

1 Micalis Institute, INRA, AgroParisTech, Université Paris-Saclay, 78350 Jouy-en-Josas, France; Arnaud.Briet@ANSES.FR (Ar.B.); elisabeth.moncaut@inra.fr (E.M.); sylviane.furlan@inra.fr (S.F.); astridbouteau@gmail.com (As.B.); olivier.son@inra.fr (O.S.); françois.lecointe@inra.fr (F.L.); pascale.serror@inra.fr (P.S.); marie-agnes.petit@inra.fr (M.-A.P.)

2 Institute for Integrative Biology of the Cell (I2BC), CEA, CNRS, Université Paris-Sud, Université Paris-Saclay, 91198 Gif-sur-Yvette, France; magali.o.leroy@gmail.com (M.L.); micheal.dubow@igmors.u-psud.fr (M.S.D.)

* Correspondence: julien.lossouarn@inra.fr

Abstract: *Enterococcus faecalis* is an opportunistic pathogen that has emerged as a major cause of nosocomial infections worldwide. Many clinical strains are indeed resistant to last resort antibiotics and there is consequently a reawakening of interest in exploiting virulent phages to combat them. However, little is still known about phage receptors and phage resistance mechanisms in enterococci. We made use of a prophageless derivative of the well-known clinical strain *E. faecalis* V583 to isolate a virulent phage belonging to the *Picovirinae* subfamily and to the P68 genus that we named Idefix. Interestingly, most isolates of *E. faecalis* tested—including V583—were resistant to this phage and we investigated more deeply into phage resistance mechanisms. We found that *E. faecalis* V583 prophage 6 was particularly efficient in resisting Idefix infection thanks to a new abortive infection (Abi) mechanism, which we designated Abiα. It corresponded to the Pfam domain family with unknown function DUF4393 and conferred a typical Abi phenotype by causing a premature lysis of infected *E. faecalis*. The *abiα* gene is widespread among prophages of enterococci and other Gram-positive bacteria. Furthermore, we identified two genes involved in the synthesis of the side chains of the surface rhamnopolysaccharide that are important for Idefix adsorption. Interestingly, mutants in these genes arose at a frequency of ~10^{-4} resistant mutants per generation, conferring a supplemental bacterial line of defense against Idefix.

Keywords: abortive infection; prophage; adsorption; *Enterococcus*; rhamnopolysaccharide

---

1. Introduction

Enterococci are ubiquitous Gram-positive facultative anaerobic bacteria that colonize the mammalian gastrointestinal tract [1]. In particular, the two species *Enterococcus faecalis* and *Enterococcus faecium* are part of the normal human gut microbiota and generally have no adverse effects on healthy individuals. However, they also represent opportunistic pathogens that have emerged as a leading source of nosocomial infections, particularly in immunocompromised patients [2]. *E. faecalis* and *E. faecium* mostly cause urinary tract infections, peritonitis, bacteraemia, and endocarditis [2]. The clinical importance of these bacterial species is directly related to their antibiotic resistance. The rapid spread of clinical isolates resistant to last resort antibiotics such as vancomycin and daptomycin has been of particular concern and associated hospital acquired infections have become a growing problem [3].

Virulent bacteriophages, i.e., viruses that infect and obligatorily lyse bacteria, have long held promise to treat bacterial infections and combat multi-drug resistant (MDR) bacteria [4]. In the recent years, the complete genome and phage cycle characteristics of a dozen virulent *E. faecalis* and *E. faecium* phages have been reported, emphasizing the growing interest for phage therapy in the future [5–15]. However, similar to the phenomenon of antibiotic resistance, bacterial resistance to phage is also taking place. For instance, mutations in the cell wall protein PIP_{EF} were recently found to provide resistance to two siphophages by limiting phage DNA entry in *E. faecalis* [16]. Apart from this, the modes of defence of enterococci against phages largely remain a *terra incognita*.

Keeping in mind that, in most ecosystems, bacteria co evolve with a plethora of bacteriophages, which imperatively depend on them for their reproduction, it is no surprise that bacteria invest efforts in fighting against them. They deploy for this goal different functions that have been studied for decades (reviewed in [17,18]), and still led to new discoveries [19–23]. The *E. faecalis* species, however, seems to have few acquired and innate immune systems. The only common clustered regularly interspaced short palindromic repeat (CRISPR)-CRISPR associated (Cas) locus found in *E. faecalis* isolates has lost its *cas* genes, and two complete type II CRISPR-Cas systems occur variably across the species [24–26]. Furthermore, no restriction-modification (R-M) system is commonly found within the species, and to date only a single type II R-M system has been described in three *E. faecalis* chromosomes [27,28]. Finally, no complete defense island system associated with restriction-modification was detected in *E. faecalis* to date [22]. The relative scarcity of R-M and CRISPR-Cas systems in MDR strains may facilitate plasmid-encoded antibiotic resistance genes acquisition [29,30].

Although less studied, phages themselves compete for their hosts on the bacterial battlefield [31]. Phage genes involved in anti-phage mechanisms are mainly found in temperate or defective prophages, rather than in virulent phages. During the prophage state (where the temperate phage is stably associated with its host), in addition to repressor-dependent immunity against similar phages, some phage express genes conferring resistance to infection by more or less unrelated phages. These genes can encode generalist functions such as R-M systems [32] or CRISPR-Cas loci [33], or specific ones. For instance, the *Escherichia coli* temperate phage P2 has three genes, *fun*, *tin*, and *old*, preventing growth of T5, T-even, and lambda respectively [34]. Furthermore, the O-antigen acetylase of *Salmonella typhimurium* phage BTP1 is reported to prevent adsorption of other phages [35]. Other typical prophage-encoded superinfection exclusion (Sie) systems act to block phage DNA injection into *E. coli* [36], *Lactococcus lactis* [37], and *Streptococcus thermophilus* [38]. Similar systems have also been recently discovered in *Pseudomonas* [39] and *Mycobacterium* prophages [40].

Prophages can also encode abortive infection (Abi) mechanisms that cause an interruption of invasive phage development and a premature death of the infected bacteria. This leads to the release of few or no progeny particles and thus prevents the expansion of the infection to the neighboring bacteria [17,18]. Abi are very diverse; among those carried by prophages, some have been well characterized such as the two component Rex system preventing lambda-lysogenic *E. coli* strain infection by T4 phage [41] or the tyrosine kinase Stk of coliphage 933W that blocks the replication cycle of HK97 [41,42].

Our earlier work showed that the vancomycin-resistant *E. faecalis* V583 clinical isolate hosts seven prophage elements. One prophage is remnant and completely domesticated (prophage 2) while the six others have various degrees of autonomy and different levels of interference with each other [43]. Only three of them—prophages 1, 3, and 5—are fully active and grow as plaques on a V583 derivative cured of all six prophages. However, prophage 1 is parasitized during the induction of it lytic cycle by the satellite prophage 7 also named a phage inducible chromosomal island. Prophages 4 and 6 finally retain some phage-like behavior but no longer produce infective virions. They excise from the bacterial chromosome in a process controlled by the other prophages, and once excised, prophage 4 replicates, while prophage 6 cannot [43].

To investigate putative anti-phage roles played by V583 prophages, we performed a phage screening using the V583 derivative strain cured of all plasmids and the six active prophages. We isolated a virulent phage belonging to the *Picovirinae* subfamily and to the P68 genus that contains phages with small size genome (19–20 kb). This prompted us to name this phage Idefix, after the French name of the small dog from Asterix comics. The genome sequence of two phages similar to Idefix have been reported recently [13,44]. We showed that *E. faecalis* prophage 6, which apparently belongs to the *Siphoviridae* family, is especially efficient in resisting to Idefix infection due to a new abortive infection system that we call Abiα. This latter confers a typical Abi phenotype, by causing a premature lysis of infected *E. faecalis*. The *abiα* gene is notably widespread among prophages integrated in enterococci and other Gram-positive bacteria. Furthermore, the bacterium itself provides another line of defence against Idefix through efficient mutagenesis of the phage bacterial receptor encoded within the variable part of the *epa* locus responsible for the building up of the surface rhamnopolysaccharide of *E. faecalis*.

2. Materials and Methods

2.1. Sample for Bacteriophage Isolation, Bacterial Strains, Plasmids, and Growth Conditions

One raw sewage water sample from the Sèvres wastewater treatment plant (Paris area, France) was used as a source of phage. *E. faecalis* indicator strain (cured of active prophages (strain VE18590)) used for phage Idefix isolation, as well as strains and plasmids used for *E. faecalis* phage-resistance characterization are listed in Table S1 (with supplementary references [45–50]). *Enterococcus* strains tested to determine phage Idefix host range are detailed in Table S2 (with supplementary references [51,52]). *E. coli* was cultivated at 37 °C in LB medium with shaking. *L. lactis* was grown statically at 30 °C in M17 medium supplemented with glucose 0.5% (M17G). *Enterococcus* strains were cultivated statically at 37 °C either in BHI medium or in M17G medium. Following antibiotics were added when necessary: erythromycin, 10 $\mu g \cdot mL^{-1}$ for *E. faecalis* and 100 $\mu g \cdot mL^{-1}$ for *L. lactis* and *E. coli* strains; chloramphenicol, 20 $\mu g \cdot mL^{-1}$ and 10 $\mu g \cdot mL^{-1}$ for *E. coli* and *E. faecalis* strains, respectively; kanamycin, 50 $\mu g \cdot mL^{-1}$ for *E. coli* strains.

2.2. Phage Isolation

Phage Idefix was isolated using the standard double overlay plaque assay technique as previously described [44] with minor modifications. A standard Petri dish was filled with 20–30 mL of BHI medium containing agar 1.5% and $MgSO_4$ 10 mM. One hundred microliters of 0.45 μm filtered sewage was mixed with 500 μL of an overnight culture of the indicator strain, then added to 5 mL of BHI medium containing agarose 0.4% and $MgSO_4$ 10 mM, and poured onto the bottom agar. The double agar/agarose plate was incubated 24 h at 37 °C and screened for plaque appearance. Many different plaques were obtained, and among them, a large clear plaque was picked and streaked on an agar base before applying the second layer of BHI top agarose mixed with the overnight culture of the indicator strain. The plate was incubated 24 h at 37 °C and a large clear plaque was streaked again twice, to ensure phage purity.

2.3. Phage Concentration and Purification

Starting from a large clear plaque, virions were resuspended in 1 mL of SM buffer (Tris-HCl 10 mM pH 7.5, $MgSO_4$ 10 mM, NaCl 300 mM) and the suspension was centrifuged 10 min at 7500× *g* and room temperature. Phage titer in the supernatant was determined by preparing serial dilutions in SM buffer and using the double overlay method. High-titer phage stock was obtained as previously described [53] with slight modifications. Five hundred to one thousand phages were plated using the double overlay method, which led to a confluent lysis after 12 h at 37 °C. The plate was then flooded with 5 mL of SM buffer and incubated 2 h at 4 °C. The overlay was carefully collected and centrifuged 20 min at 7500× *g* at room temperature and the phages-containing supernatant was passed through a 0.45 μm filter. Phage stocks were titrated (~10^{11} $PFU \cdot mL^{-1}$) and stored at 4 °C for further experiments. Ten milliliters of filtered phage stock was incubated 12 h at 4 °C under stirring in the presence of NaCl 1M and PEG 8000 10%. Precipitated phages were then centrifuged 20 min at 10,000× *g* and 4 °C and slowly resuspended in 1 mL of SM buffer for 1 h at 4 °C prior to be purified by centrifugation in a CsCl buoyant gradient. The purified phage-containing fraction was then recovered (density 1.4), titrated and stored at 4 °C for further experiments.

2.4. Phage Examination in Transmission Electron Microscopy

Ten microliters of purified phage Idefix fraction were directly spotted onto a Formwar carbon coated copper grid. Phages were allowed to adsorb to the carbon layer for 5 min and excess of liquid was removed. Ten microliters of a staining uranyl acetate solution (1%) was then spotted to the grid for 10 s and excess of liquid was removed again. The grid was imaged at 80 kV in a Hitachi HT7700 transmission electron microscope.

2.5. Phage Genomic Nucleic Acid Extraction, Whole Genome Sequencing, and Bioinformatic Analysis

Total DNA was extracted as described in [54,55]. Prior to DNA extraction, 10 mL of the phage stock (10^{11} PFU·mL^{-1}) was treated with 40 μL of nuclease mix (50% glycerol, 0.25 mg·mL^{-1} RNAse A, 0.25 mg·mL^{-1} Dnase I, 150 mM NaCl), for 15 min at 37 °C. Particles were then precipitated by adding PEG 8000 (10%, *w/v*) and NaCl to 1 M, and let sit overnight at 4 °C once PEG was solubilized. Phages were centrifuged 10 min at 10,000× *g* and room temperature, and resuspended into 500 μL of SM buffer. Insoluble particles were removed by centrifugation (20 s at 12,000× *g*), and the clarified supernatant was used for DNA extraction. The PROMEGA Wizard DNA Clean up kit (ref A7280) was then used, following essentially the manufacturer instructions. Prior to DNA elution from the column, a washing step with 5.4 M guanidium thiocyanate (resin solution) was applied. DNA was sent to a 454-sequencing platform, and reads were assembled with Newbler [56]. The phage genome was annotated using RAST [57], followed by manual inspection. The genome sequence is available under the accession number LT630001.1. All genomic figures, including Idefix genome comparison, were generated using Easyfig [58].

2.6. Determination of Phage Burst Size

The one-step growth kinetic curve of phage Idefix was measured using a standard method [59] with minor modifications. One milliliter of a log-phase culture of indicator strain was centrifuged 5 min at 10,000× *g* and room temperature, and resuspended in 100 μL of prewarmed BHI medium with $MgSO_4$ (10 mM). Phage from the high-titer phage stock was added at a MOI of 0.001 and allowed to adsorb for 5 min at 37 °C. The phage/bacteria mix was centrifuged 2 min at 10,000× *g* and room temperature. The supernatant was titrated to count unadsorbed phage particles, whereas the bacterial pellet was washed in 100 μL of prewarmed BHI medium with $MgSO_4$ (10 mM) and recentrifuged. The pellet was suspended and diluted in 10 mL of prewarmed BHI medium with $MgSO_4$ (10 mM) and cultured at 37 °C. Samples were taken at regular intervals and plated at the correct dilution for phage titration. A second set of samples from a synchronized 100-fold diluted culture was taken at same intervals and titrated. The values indicate the means and standard deviations of three independent experiments.

2.7. Determination of Phage Host Range

Ten microliters of serially diluted high-titer phage stock were spotted (10 μL) on top of agarose overlays containing overnight culture of enterococci, as described above (Table S2). Plates were incubated at 37 °C and examined for plaque appearance 6, 12, and 24 h after spotting.

2.8. Determination of Phage Efficiency of Plaquing

Efficiency of plaquing (EOP) was determined for *E. faecalis* derivative strains (Table S1). One hundred phages were plated using the double overlay plaque assay technique. EOP were calculated as ((phage titer on tested strain) × (phage titer on the indicator strain)$^{-1}$) × 100. These experiments were independently performed three times and average values are reported with standard deviations.

2.9. *Phage Adsorption Assay*

Adsorption of phage to *E. faecalis* derivative strains were determined as reported previously [60] with minor modifications. One milliliter of log-phase cultures was harvested and resuspended in 100 μL of BHI medium with $MgSO_4$ (10 mM), and then phage from the high-titer phage stock was added at a MOI of 0.001. Following incubation for 10 min at 37 °C, the phage/bacteria mixtures were centrifuged 2 min at 10,000× *g* and room temperature. Supernatants were plated at the correct dilution and titrated for phage. Percentages of adsorption were calculated as ((control titer - residual titer) × (control titer)$^{-1}$) × 100. These experiments were independently conducted three times and average values are given with standard deviations.

2.10. *Determination of Phage Efficiency of Center of Infection*

Efficiency of center of infection (ECOI) was determined for *E. faecalis* derivative strains as detailed by [61] with minor modifications. One milliliter of log-phase cultures was harvested and resuspended as previously, and then phage from the high-titer phage stock was added at a MOI of 0.001. Following incubation for 5 min at 37 °C, the phage/bacteria mixtures were centrifuged 1 min at 10,000× *g* and 4 °C, washed twice, diluted, and assayed for infective centers. An *E. faecalis* strain which does not adsorb Idefix was used as control to monitor the effectiveness of phage removal during washing. Percentages of ECOI were calculated as ((number of centers on indicator strain) × (number of centers on tested strain)$^{-1}$) × 100. These experiments were independently performed three times and average values are reported with standard deviations.

2.11. *Bacterial Survival Assay*

E. faecalis derivative strains survival was assayed as essentially described in [62] with slight modifications. Briefly, one milliliter of log-phase bacterial cultures was harvested and resuspended as previously described, and then phage from the high-titer phage stock was added at both MOI of 1 and 10. Following incubation for 20 min at 37 °C, bacterial suspensions were plated at the correct dilution on agar plates and surviving bacteria were enumerated as CFU. Percentages of bacterial death were calculated as ((CFU·mL^{-1} in cultures without phage − CFU·mL^{-1} in cultures with phage) × (CFU·mL^{-1} in cultures without phage)$^{-1}$) × 100. These experiments were independently conducted three times and average values are shown with standard deviations.

2.12. *Lysis Curve Experiments*

One milliliter of log-phase bacterial cultures was harvested and resuspended as previously described, and then phage from the high-titer phage stock was added at an MOI of 10. Following incubation for 10 min at 37 °C, the phage/bacteria mixtures were centrifuged 2 min at 10,000× *g* and room temperature. Pellets were resuspended in 200 μL of BHI medium with $MgSO_4$ (10 mM) and the suspensions were transferred in wells of a 96-wells plate. Empty wells are filled with BHI medium or uninfected bacterial suspensions to have negative and positive growth control respectively. Bacterial growths were then monitored during 30–50 min at 37 °C using a Tecan plate reader (OD 600 nm, measurements at 2 min intervals after shakings). During the experiment, each sample was prepared and monitored in triplicates. Kinetics shown are representative of three independent experiments.

2.13. *Luria–Delbrück Fluctuation Tests*

An exponentially growing *E. faecalis* strain cured of prophage 6 (strain VE18306) culture supplemented with 10 mM $MgSO_4$ was distributed in a 96-wells plate (180 μL, corresponding to ~2 × 10^4 CFU, in 93 wells), and infected with phage Idefix (20 μL, corresponding to ~2 × 10^9 PFU, which are dispensed before bacteria, in 90 of the 96 wells). Remaining wells contained either BHI medium or uninfected VE18306 cultures. Following static incubation of the plates for 12 h at 37 °C, bacterial growth was evaluated using a Tecan plate reader, after a 1 min shaking step (OD 600 nm). If mutations occur at random in the bacterial population, the number of mutational events per well follows a Poisson distribution [63], and the proportion of wells in which no mutant resisting to Idefix was present at the time of infection P_0, is related to h, the expectation of this law, by the formula $P_0 = e^{-h}$. Knowing the average number of bacteria per well at infection, N, mutation frequency $f = h/N$, so $f = -\ln P_0/N$. These experiments were independently performed three times giving a similar value of f.

2.14. General Molecular Biology Methods

All PCR reactions to clone or sequence *IDF_13, IDF_15, ef2833, ef2847, ef2850, ef2169,* and *ef2170* genes were performed in a Mastercycler Eppendorf with Phusion high-fidelity DNA polymerase (NEB) and according to manufacturer's instructions. PCR products and DNA restriction fragments were purified with QIAquick kits (QIAGEN, Hilden, Germany) when necessary. Electro-transformation of *E. coli, L. lactis,* and *E. faecalis* were carried out as previously described [64,65] using a Gene Pulser apparatus (Bio-Rad Laboratories, Inc., Hercules, CA, USA). Transformations of chemically competent *E. coli* ER2566 were carried out by a heat shock procedure.

2.15. Cloning of IDF_13 and IDF_15, Expression and Preparation of Extracts of E. coli, and Spot Assay of the Extracts on the Indicator Strain

PCR amplification of *IDF_13* and *IDF_15* were performed using primer pairs OFL264/OFL265 and OFL266/267 respectively, with Idefix genomic DNA as template. PCR products were purified and digested by *NdeI* and *BamHI* restriction enzymes. Digested products were purified and cloned between the *NdeI* and *BamHI* sites of a linearized pJ411 derivative (Table S1). JM105 transformants were selected on LB plates supplemented with kanamycin. The resulting plasmids, pAB1and pAB2, contained the corresponding ORF fused in 5′ to a sequence coding for a His6-tag, placed under the control of a T7 promoter. His6-tagged IDF_13 and IDF_15 were produced in *E. coli* ER2566 transformed with pAB1 and pAB2 respectively. Cells were grown in 50 mL of LB supplemented with kanamycin at 37 °C. At $OD_{600} = 0.6$, production of the phage proteins was induced by addition of IPTG (0.5 mM final concentration) to the culture for 2.5 h. Cells were then harvested by centrifugation at 5200× *g* for 7 min at 4 °C and resuspended in 1 mL of lysis buffer (Tris-HCl 50 mM pH 8, NaCl 150 mM). Cells suspensions were stored at −20 °C until preparation of crude extracts. After thawing, bacteria were lyzed by sonication on ice. The lysates were centrifuged at 4 °C for 20 min at 20,000× *g* and the supernatants were stored at −20 °C. Production and solubility of IDF_13 and IDF_15 were verified by SDS-PAGE. Lysis activity of IDF_13 and IDF_15 was assessed by spotting 5 μL of the supernatants alone or a mix of both fractions on an indicator strain bacterial lawn as previously described.

2.16. Construction of E. faecalis VE18306 ef2833-, ef2847- and ef2850-Complemented Strains and E. faecalis VE18590 ef2833- Complemented Strain

Complementations of the prophage 6 genes *ef2833, ef2847,* and *ef2850* were done using the pJIM2246 vector (Table S1). The three genes were amplified including their constitutive promoters and ribosome binding sites from DNA of *E. faecalis* strain containing all prophages (strain VE14089) with primer pairs JL12/JL13, JL10/JL11, and JL8/JL9 respectively (Table S1). The three purified products were separately cloned into pJIM2246 yielding plasmids pJL1, pJL2, and pJL3 after respective transformation into *E. coli* JM105 and chloramphenicol selection. pJL1, pJL2, and pJL3 were then separately electroporated into *E. faecalis* cured of prophage 6 (strain VE18306). The *ef2833-, ef2847-,* and *ef2850*-complemented strains were respectively selected on chloramphenicol. The nucleotide sequences of cloned PCR products were systematically confirmed by sequencing using primer pairs OEF879/1233 (Table S1). pJL3 and pJIM2246 were also separately electroporated into the indicator strain and selected as previously described.

2.17. *PCR Amplification in epaX Region*

epaX region was amplified from total DNA of nine Idefix spontaneous resisting mutants using primer pairs OEF394/OEF397 and OEF527/OEF397 (Table S1). PCR analysis was extended for the three mutants for which no IS insertion was discovered with larger amplifications downstream and upstream *epaX* region using primer pairs OEF857/OEF527 and OEF885/OEF858; and OEF528/OEF856 and OEF859/OEF823 (Table S1) respectively.

2.18. *Construction of E. faecalis VE18306ΔepaX Strain*

A deletion of *epaX* in the VE18306 background was constructed by double homologous recombination using pVE14283 plasmid (Table S1). pVE14283 was electroporated into strain VE18306, and the *epaX* deletion (strain VE18393, Table S1) was selected as described in [49,66].

2.19. *Construction of E. faecalis VE18393 epaX—Complemented Strain*

A complementation of *epaX* was constructed using pVE14297 plasmid (Table S1). This latter, containing *epaX* under the control of the constitutive promoter P_{aphA3}, was electroporated into the VE18306 Δ*epaX* strain (strain VE18393) and the complementation (strain VE18945, Table S1) was selected as described in [49]. A control strain, harboring pVE14176 vector devoid of *epaX*, was also obtained (strain VE18944, Table S1).

3. Results

3.1. *Characterization of the Enterococcus Phage Idefix*

3.1.1. Isolation, Morphological Characterization, and Phage–Host Relationship

One municipal sewage water sample from Sèvres (Paris area, Ile de France region) was screened by direct plating without enrichment for phages forming plaques on the indicator strain. This latter, VE18590 (here below pp$^-$, complete names of all strains used are listed in Table S1), corresponds to an *E. faecalis* V583 derivative deleted from its endogenous plasmids and six active prophages [43]. A phage making particularly large and clear plaques was isolated with the double-layer technique. After purification and amplification, transmission electron microscopy revealed a virion with an icosahedral head ~40 nm in diameter and a very short non-contractile tail (Figure 1A). This phage, Idefix, therefore belongs to the *Caudovirales* order and the *Podoviridae* family. A one-step growth kinetic indicated that Idefix has a latent period of 15 min and a burst size ~50 PFUs per infected pp$^-$ bacterium (Figure 1B).

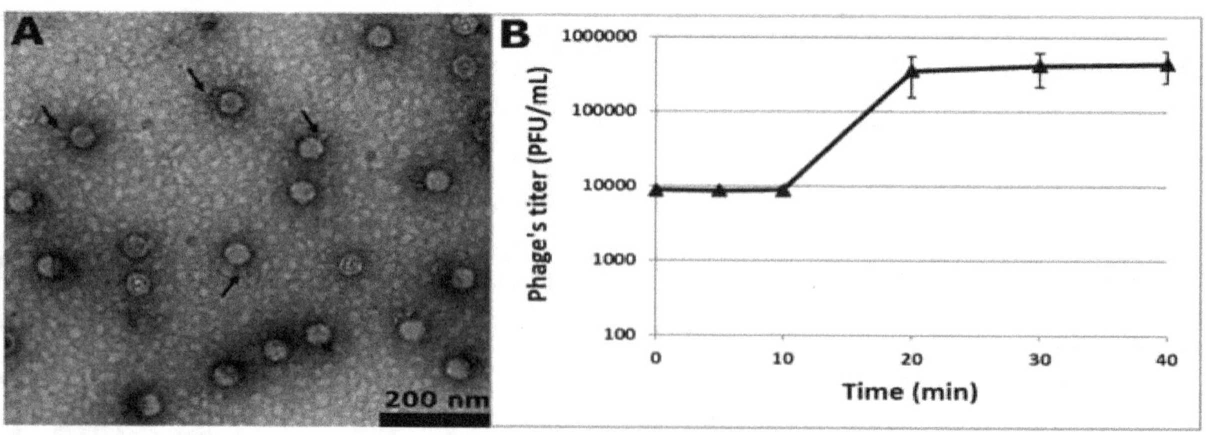

Figure 1. Characterization of the virulent phage Idefix. (**A**) Electron micrograph of Idefix particles negatively stained with 2% uranyl acetate (some Idefix tails are shown by arrows). (**B**) One step growth kinetic of phage Idefix determined in its host strain *E. faecalis* pp$^-$. The values indicate the means and standard deviations of three independent experiments.

3.1.2. Genomic Characterization

The genome of phage Idefix is a double stranded linear DNA, consisting of 18,168 bp with inverted terminal repeats 61 bp long and an average GC content of 33.2%. It is highly homologous to *Enterococcus* phages vB_EfaP_IME195 (95% coverage and 92% nt identity) and vB_Efae230P-4 (75% coverage and 85% identity) (Figure 2). These genomes belong to virulent podophages, which were isolated from sewage samples in China and Poland, respectively [13,44]. A close relative phage, vB_EfaP_IME199, infecting an *E. faecium* strain has also been described [14]. Genbank accession numbers of these genomes are listed in Table S3.

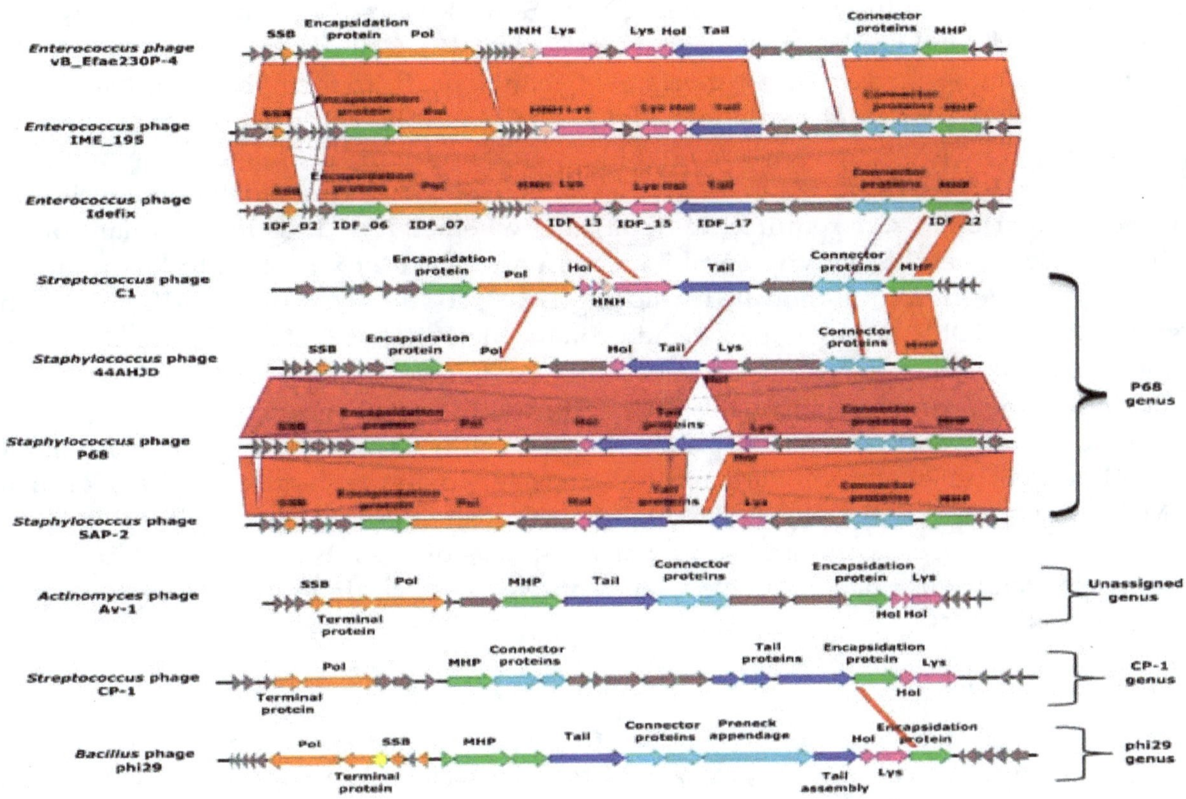

Figure 2. Annotation and comparison of the phage Idefix genome. *Enterococcus* phage genomes from vB_Efae230P-4, vB_EfaP_IME195, and Idefix compared to *Streptococcus* phage C1, *Staphylococcus* phages 44AHJD, P68, SAP-2, 66, *Actinomyces* phage Av-1, *Streptococcus* phage CP-1 and *Bacillus* phage phi29 all belonging to the *Picovirinae* subfamily. Gene functions are color-coded and detailed (yellow: transcriptional regulation, orange: DNA metabolism, green: DNA packaging and head, light blue: head to tail, dark blue: tail, pink: HNH endonuclease, fuchsia: lysis, grey: hypothetical proteins).

The Idefix genome encodes 25 ORFs, 12 of which were assigned a function (Figure 2 and Table S4). The replication module contains a single strand DNA binding protein (SSB, IDF_02) and a DNA polymerase belonging to the B type superfamily (Pol, IDF_07). This polymerase presents all the conserved motifs typical of phage phi29 polymerase, including the specific regions of the "protein priming" subfamily [67–71] (Figure S1).We next searched for the gene coding the terminal protein used to initiate the replication at both ends of *Picovirinae* linear genomes. Such genes are generally located near the polymerase gene but very poorly conserved. Terminal proteins share features like a small size and a high isoelectric point [72,73]. Based on these criteria, *IDF_05* appears the best candidate (Table S4) but additional investigations are needed to confirm this hypothesis. A gene encoding an encapsidation protein (IDF_06) separates this putative terminal gene and the polymerase gene. The lysis module is composed of a holin (Hol, IDF_16) and two different putative endolysins (Lys): IDF_15 and IDF_13. IDF_15 displays homology with *N*-acetylmuramoyl-L-alanine amidases (Figure S2A,B). To test whether this gene expresses an active endolysin, *IDF_15* was cloned in an expression vector based on a T7 promoter (plasmid pAB2) and expressed in *E. coli* ER2566 (Figure S4A). Spotting of a soluble cell extract (containing IDF_15, Figure S4A) on a pp- bacterial lawn revealed a lysis zone (Figure S4B). This result tends to show that IDF_15 has an endolysin activity. IDF_13 displays homology with PlyCA [74–76], a subunit of the PlyC endolysin synthetized by the *Streptococcus* podophage C1 (Figure S3A). Indeed *IDF_13*, like *plyCA*, encodes a protein with two catalytic domains. A putative glycosidase domain (homologous to the one of PlyCA) and a putative "CHAP" domain (more divergent compared with the one found in PlyCA) are respectively located in the N and the C terminus of the protein (Figure S3B,C). In contrast to IDF_15, a soluble cell extract of an *E. coli* strain expressing the *IDF_13* (via plasmid pAB1) did not lead to a bacterial lysis (Figure S4A,B). Moreover, a mix of extracts containing IDF_13 and IDF_15 did not produce increased lysis (Figure S4B). C1 is the only reported phage whose endolysin PlyC is synthesized from two genes: *plyCA* and *plyCB*. To form the complete enzyme, the catalytic subunit PlyCA and eight subunits PlyCB harboring the cell wall binding domain (CBD) are associated [75,77]. However, we were not able to find an Idefix ORF displaying any significant similarity with PlyCB. We concluded that *IDF_15* seems to encode a canonical monomeric endolysin, and that more experiments are required to determine whether *IDF_13* is just remnant of a former endolysin module, or retains activity combined with another Idefix protein to form a multimeric endolysin. Finally, the structural module includes genes encoding a tail protein (IDF_17), connector proteins (IDF_20 and IDF_21) and a major head protein (MHP, IDF_22) (Table S4).

Comparative genomic analyses clearly show that Idefix and the other homologous *Enterococcus* phages belong to the *Picovirinae* subfamily [78] composed of small virulent podophages infecting Gram-positive bacteria and encoding a phi29-like DNA polymerase. The *Picovirinae* subfamily is subdivided into P68, phi29, Cp-1 genera and one unassigned genus (Figure 2). The overall synteny and the MHP similarities [14] both lead to assign Idefix and all other *Enterococcus Picovirinae* to the P68 genus, including one *Streptococcus* and some *Staphylococcus* phages (Figure 2). Within this genus, a hallmark of all *Enterococcus* phages is the presence of two genes coding putative endolysins (IDF_13 and IDF_15 in Idefix).

3.1.3. Phage Host Range

Plaque assays of Idefix were performed on fifty-nine *Enterococcus* strains, belonging to the *E. faecalis* (47) and to the *E. faecium* (12) species. *E. faecalis* strains had sewage, clinical, commensal, or food origins and represented a range of different clonal complexes and capsule types, whereas *faecium* strains essentially belonged to different sequence types from the most prevalent clinical clonal complex (Table S2). Idefix did not propagate on any of them, including the wild type strain V583 (wt), from which our indicator sensitive strain pp^- is derived (Figure 3A,B).

3.2. Characterization of E. faecalis V583 Resistance to Idefix

3.2.1. Novel Abi System Encoded by V583 Prophage 6

To investigate the mechanism by which *E. faecalis* V583 resists Idefix infection, we made use of our collection of V583 derivatives deleted for either plasmids or prophages [43]. The plasmids hosted by V583 were not responsible for the resistance to Idefix, as the use of the plasmidless V583 derivative strain VE14089 (pp^+, Table S1), did not permit Idefix growth (Figure 3C). Plaque assays were next performed on V583 plasmidless derivatives where only one of the prophages remains. Idefix grew on all derivatives (Figure 3D–H) but one, VE18581 ($pp6^+$) in which prophage 6 is present (Figure 3I). We concluded that prophage 6 is necessary to confer resistance to Idefix. Plaque assays on the V583 derivative VE18306 ($pp6^-$) in which only prophage 6 is deleted, led to clear plaque appearance (Figure 3J) with efficiency of plaquing (EOP) similar to pp^- (Table 1). We concluded that prophage 6, which structural genes are notably related to the siphophage HK97, is sufficient for Idefix resistance. Interestingly, we noticed that plaque size was reduced (~three times smaller) whenever prophage 3 was present (Figure 3G,H,J) (Table 1), suggesting that prophage 3 slightly interferes during Idefix infection.

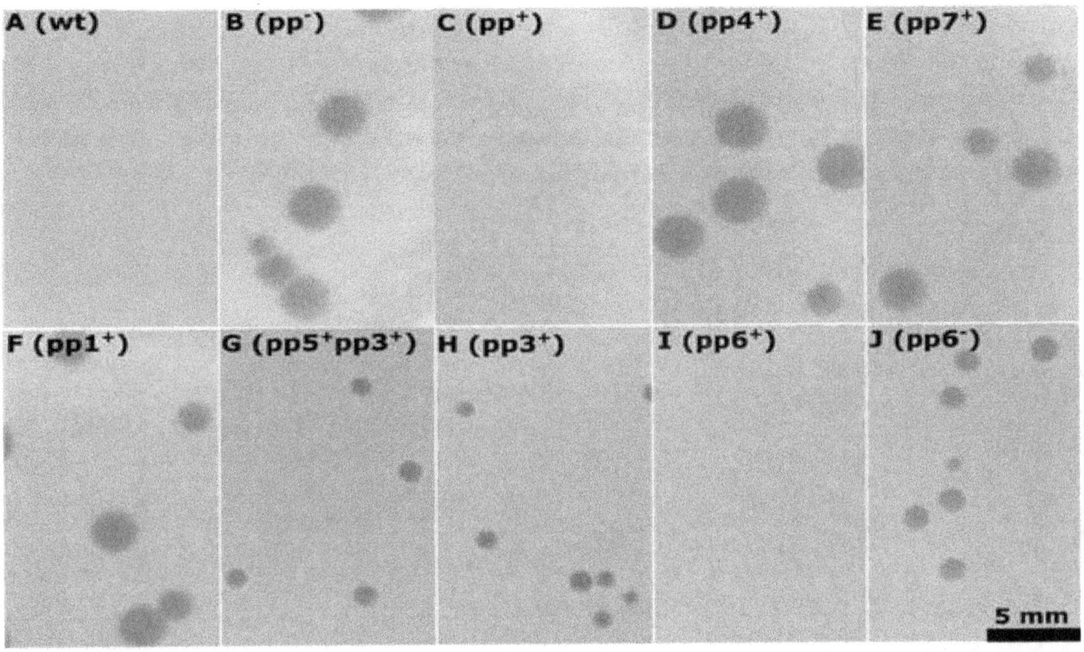

Figure 3. V583 endogenous prophages (pps) interference with Idefix infection, plaque assays performed on strains: A. wt (VE14002), V583 clinical isolate. B. pp- (VE18590), a V583 derivative deleted for all its plasmids and prophages. C. pp^+ (VE14089), a V583 derivative only deleted from all its plasmids. D. $pp4^+$ (VE18582), a VE14089 derivative deleted for all its pps but pp4. E. $pp7^+$ (VE18589), a VE14089 derivative deleted for all its pps but pp7. F. $pp1^+$ (VE18562), a VE14089 derivative deleted for all its pps but pp1. G. $pp3^+pp5^+$ (VE18583), a VE14089 derivative deleted for all its pps but pp3 and pp5. H. $pp3^+$ (VE18584), a VE14089 derivative deleted for all its pps but pp3. I. $pp6^+$ (VE18581), a VE14089 derivative deleted for all its pps but pp6. J. $pp6^-$ (VE18306), a VE14089 derivative only deleted from pp6.

Table 1. Efficiency of plaquing (EOP) of phage Idefix on *E. faecalis* V583 derivatives deleted from different prophages.

Strain (Genotype)	Average EOP of Idefix (sd)	Plaque (Diameter)
VE18590 (pp^-)	1	Big clear plaque (3–4 mm)
VE18562 ($pp1^+$)	1.1 (0.17)	Big clear plaque (3–4 mm)
VE18582 ($pp4^+$)	0.92 (0.14)	Big clear plaque (3–4 mm)
VE18589 ($pp7^+$)	1.03 (0.16)	Big clear plaque (3–4 mm)
VE18583 (pp3+, $pp5^+$)	0.97 (0.16)	Reduction in size (1 mm)
VE18584 ($pp3^+$)	0.92 (0.17)	Reduction in size (1 mm)
VE18581 ($pp6^+$)	0 *	No plaque visible
VE18306 ($pp6^-$)	1 (0.13)	Reduction in size (1 mm)

* Below the detectable limit of the assay, at least $< 1.2 \times 10^{-8}$.

To characterize the resistance conferred by prophage 6, adsorption assays were first performed on a panel of strains differing for the presence or absence of this prophage. Idefix adsorption was always efficient, regardless of the presence of prophage 6 (Table 2), showing therefore that prophage 6 does not prevent Idefix adsorption. We next assayed efficiency of center of infection (ECOI) by Idefix on the same panel of strains, which can detect infective events, regardless of phage burst size. It was reduced to 39% upon infection of strain $pp6^+$. This reduction was even more drastic when the strain pp^+, carrying all prophages, was tested, with only 15% of the infections leading to phage production. This suggests again that some other prophage gene(s) impede Idefix growth. However, infection of strain pp6$^-$ permitted to recover plaques for nearly 70% of all infecting particles, suggesting that prophage 6 contribution to interference is major (Table 2). We finally tested whether prophage 6 affected cell survival upon Idefix infection. Cell survival following exposure to Idefix was similar irrespective of the presence of prophage 6: even in the Idefix resistant strains, percentage of cell death was around 50–70% at MOI of 1, and around 100% at MOI of 10, like in Idefix sensitive strains (Table 2). We concluded that prophage 6 encodes a typical Abi mechanism affecting the production of virions while leading simultaneously to host cell death upon Idefix infection.

Table 2. Parameters of phage Idefix proliferation on *E. faecalis* strains differing by the presence or absence of prophage 6 or prophage 6-encoded *ef2833*.

Strain (Genotype)	% EOP (Plaques Diameter)	% Adsorption (sd)	% ECOI (sd)	% Bacterial Death at MOI 1 (sd) and MOI 10 (sd)
Indicator strain VE18590 (pp$^-$)	100 (3–4 mm)	96.5 (1.63)	100	69.0 (0.39) and 99.2 (0.78)
VE18306 (pp6$^-$)	100 (1 mm)	97.1 (1.35)	69.3 (3.10)	52.8 (3.00) and 98.2 (0.98)
VE18581 (pp6$^+$)	0 None plaques visible	97.5 (0.92)	39.5 (3.94)	66.8 (2.78) and 98.2 (1.32)
VE14089 (pp$^+$)	0 None plaques visible	98.1 (2.36)	15.9 (4.01)	60.2 (3.46) and 98.9 (0.19)
VEJL3 (pp6$^-$, *ef2833*$^+$)	0 None plaques visible	98.4 (0.68)	9.46 (2.68)	67.7 (1.65) and 98.6 (0.46)
VEJL5 (pp$^-$, *ef2833*$^+$)	0 None plaques visible	98.5 (1.33)	13.8 (0.58)	63.2 (1.98) and 96.6 (1.36)

To search for prophage 6 candidate genes involved in this Abi mechanism, we analyzed transcriptomic data of strain pp$^+$ [48]. Eight of the prophage 6 encoded genes are expressed constitutively during normal growth conditions, in contrast to the generally low expression level of the remaining 50 genes carried by the prophage (Figure 4A). Two of these genes, *ef2855* and *ef2852*, encode the integrase and repressor proteins, which are implicated in the lysogenic control of the prophage. Between these two genes, and probably forming an operon with them, genes *ef2854* and *ef2853* encode a putative membrane protein and a putative metallo-peptidase, respectively. A similar gene pair, placed between an integrase and a repressor, is found in several Sie prophage-encoded phage resistance systems within the *Lactococcus* genus [37,79]. These systems block the phage DNA injection step, due to the membrane protein. The nearby metallo-peptidase is dispensable, but sometimes enhances the resistance efficiency [37,79]. Given that Sie systems do not affect bacterial survival, we did not consider the gene pair *ef2853* and *ef2854* as responsible for the observed resistance to Idefix infection. Among the four last candidate genes, *ef2801* is disrupted by a transposable element invalidating a putative glycosyltransferase, so that our investigation was restricted to the three remaining genes *ef2833*, *ef2847*, and *ef2850*.

All of them are preceded by a promoter region including an experimentally mapped transcription-starting site [80] and encode proteins with unknown function. We thus cloned these three genes individually with their own promoters on pJIM2246 vector (Table S1), and performed Idefix infections in pp6$^-$ transformed by each of the plasmids. Plaque assays revealed that Idefix was able to infect all strains (Figure 4B(a,b) but the one hosting plasmid pJL3, in which *ef2833* is expressed (Figure 4B(c)). We additionally tested plasmid pJL3 in the pp$^-$ background and found that this strain was also resistant to Idefix (Figure 4B(d)) whereas the phage grew on the isogenic strain hosting the empty vector (Figure 4B(e)) as well as on pp$^-$ (Figure 4B(f)).

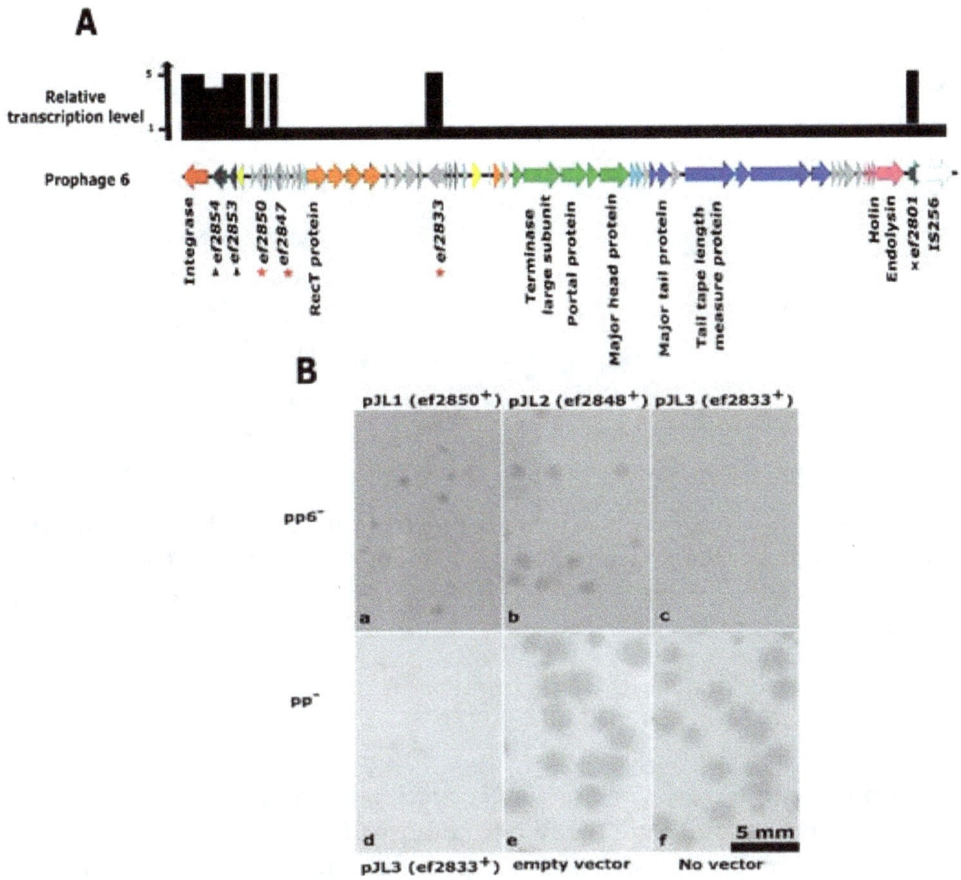

Figure 4. Identification of the V583 endogenous prophage 6 (pp6) gene responsible for Idefix resistance. (**A**) Genomic organization of pp6 and relative transcription level of each gene. The genomic organization of pp6 is modified from [43]. Gene functions are color-coded and detailed wherever possible (red: integrase, yellow: transcriptional regulation, orange: DNA metabolism, green: DNA packaging and head, light blue: head to tail, dark blue: tail, fuchsia: lysis, grey: hypothetical proteins, white: transposable element). Relative transcriptional level of each gene is indicated in black and designed from a previously published transcriptomic study [48]. Eight pp6 genes are constitutively expressed during V583 normal growth conditions. Among those not involved in pp6 lysogenic decision: a membrane protein and putative metallo-peptidase genes are indicated with triangles, a putative glycosyltransferase gene disrupted by a transposable element is indicated with a cross and the three other genes tested as *abi* candidates are indicated with red stars. (**B**) Interference with Idefix infection following the expression of the three pp6 *abi* candidates, plaque assays performed on strain pp6$^-$ (A to C) or pp$^-$ (D to F) transformed by: **a.** pJL1. **b.** pJL2. **c.** pJL3. **d.** pJL3. **e.** the pJIM2246 empty vector. **f.** no vector.

We then checked the other proliferation parameters of Idefix on the two strains hosting the pJL3 plasmid. The phage adsorbed as efficiently on these strains, its ECOI was reduced to ~10% and the percentage of cell death were around 60–70% at MOI 1 and around 100% at MOI 10 in both cases (Table 2). These results confirmed that *ef2833* is responsible for the abortive mechanism. As letters from *abiA* to *abiZ* have been used once to designate over 20 *L. lactis* Abi systems [18,81], we renamed *ef2833* as "*abiα*". The corresponding encoded protein contains 272 residues, and does not exhibit similarity with any domain or protein of known function. Abiα nevertheless constitutes a PFAM domain referred to as DUF4393 (158 sequences, 140 species, both Gram$^+$ and Gram$^-$), suggesting already its broad distribution (see below). Abiα also shares similarity with Pfam entry PF10987 and PDB entry 3H35 without providing any substantial information about Abiα function.

To characterize the Abiα mode of action, lysis curves were conducted and indicated that strain pp$^-$ containing plasmid pJL3 lyses ~10 min earlier than its isogenic strain devoid of *abiα* after infection by Idefix (MOI 10) (Figure 5A). The same results were obtained when comparing lysis curves of the prophage positive and prophageless strains pp6$^+$ and pp$^-$, respectively (Figure 5B). We concluded that Abiα provokes a lysis asynchrony.

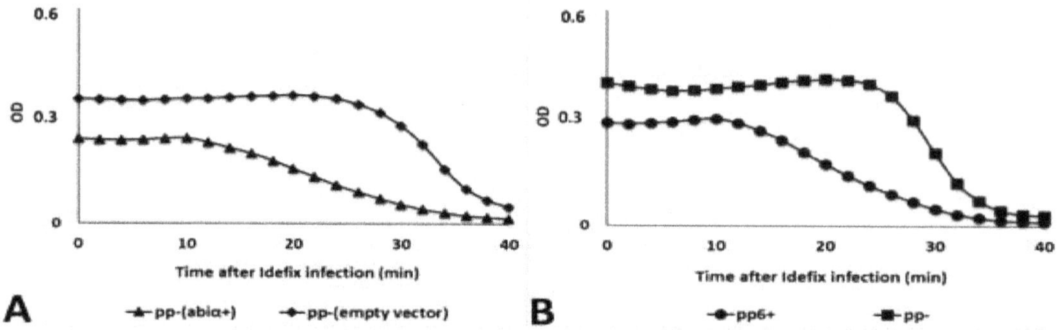

Figure 5. Lysis curves after Idefix infection at MOI 10. (**A**) Comparison between pp$^-$pJIM2246*abiα*$^+$ (VEJL5) and pp$^-$ pJIM2246 (VEJL4) in triangles and diamonds, respectively. (**B**) Comparison between pp6$^+$ and pp$^-$ in circles and squares, respectively. The results shown are representative of three biological replicates (see Figure S5).

To evaluate the prevalence of *abiα* and its genetic context, the protein sequence was searched in the JGI database with the IMG interface ([82]; BLASTP, E-value < 3.10^{-8}, Identity $\geq$ 25%). Homologs of Abiα were found mostly on prophages, with some of them shown in Figure S6: the closer relatives (61–59% sequence identity) came from various enterococci, such as *E. faecium* and *Enterococcus villorum* isolates, and subsequent analyses with the NCBI nt database also revealed a homolog in an *Enterococcus hirae* prophage (not shown in Figure S6). Other Abiα were found in about 50 *Lactobacillus* strains (27–42% sequence identity). Roughly, half of these genes are encoded on prophages (as in *L. johnsonii*, *L. salivarius* or *L. plantarum* isolates) whereas the other half are located on the chromosomes (as in *L. lindneri* and *L. helveticus* isolates). Interestingly, in *L. helveticus*, and in two *Oenococcus* species (*O. kitaharae* and *O. oeni*), the *abiα* gene is close to other putative Abi systems, and may belong to a phage resistance island. Sporadic occurrences (31–37% sequence identity) were also found in three *Streptococcus* species (*S. suis*, *S. bovis*, and *S. parasanguinis*), and one *Carnobacterium* isolate. A prophage context was detectable in this latter and in *S. parasanguinis*. Additional prophage-encoded genes with 25–27% sequence identity with *abiα* were located in one *Lactococcus lactis* ssp. *lactis* (not shown in Figure S6), *Bacillus velezensis*, *Staphylococcus epidermidis*, *Staphylococcus scuiri* and *Staphylococcus aureus*. We conclude that Abiα is widely distributed, and hypothesize it has a phage origin.

3.2.2. Mutagenesis in V583 *epa* Variable Region as Potential Additional Line of Defense

During this work, we regularly observed phage-resistant colonies growing within lysis zones of the pp6$^-$ strain. Fluctuation tests of Luria-Delbrück allowed estimating that the frequency of mutations resulting in resistance of the strain was 1.56 ($\pm$ 0.54) $\times$ 10^{-4} per cellular division. We conclude that spontaneous resistance to Idefix arises at high frequency in *E. faecalis* strain devoid of *abiα*.

To gain further insights into the bacterial mechanisms of resistance to Idefix, we tested nine spontaneous Idefix resistant mutants randomly isolated from fluctuation tests. Idefix adsorption was reduced for all mutants: three of them had a 2-to-4-fold reduced adsorption efficiency and the remaining six, rather a 10-fold defect (Table S5). We conclude that bacterial resistance to Idefix is due to an adsorption defect.

More than 10 years ago, a study of the podophage C1 distantly related to Idefix (see Figure 2) had proposed that the *N*-acetylgalactosamine (GalNac) composing the side chains of the group C streptococci surface rhamnopolysaccharide should be a crucial element of the bacterial receptor [83]. Enterococci, like group C streptococci, harbor a surface rhamnopolysaccharide or Epa (Enterococcal polysaccharide antigen), which is synthesized by more than thirty proteins encoded within a single cluster of genes. The upstream part of this gene cluster is shared among *E. faecalis* strains, while the immediately downstream region is variable between strains [84]. Within this *epa* variable region, *epaX* encodes a glycosyltransferase involved in the incorporation of galactose and/or GalNac proposed to form the side chains of the rhamnopolysaccharide in *E. faecalis* [49]. We therefore started by examining the *epaX* region in the nine mutants. PCR amplification of *epaX* led to a DNA product of increased size in six out of nine mutants (~4000 instead of ~2500 bp). Sequencing revealed that *epaX* gene was disrupted by an IS256 insertion sequence, positioned in either direction, and at six different locations, all of them in the very distal 3′ region of *epaX* (Figure 6 and Table S5).

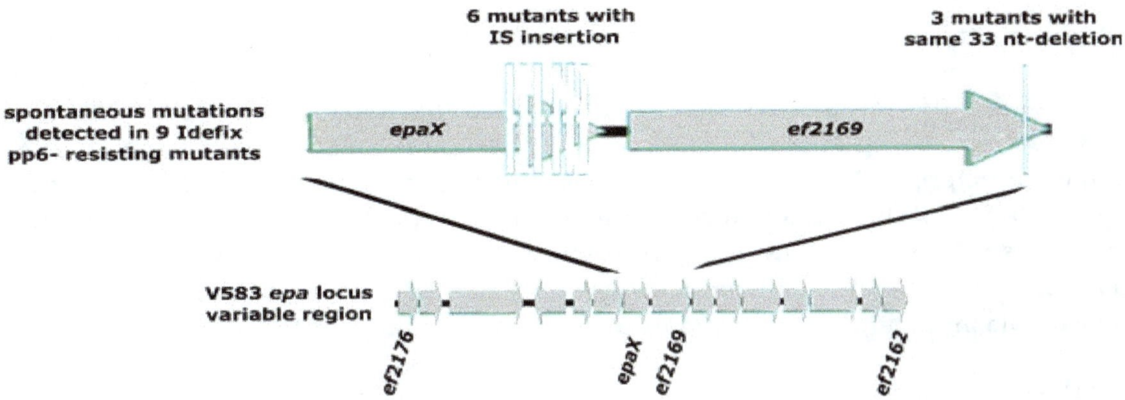

Figure 6. Genomic organization of V583 variable *epa* locus and focus on spontaneous mutations found in *epaX* region for nine Idefix pp6$^-$ resisting mutants.

We next reconstructed a deletion of *epaX* in the pp6$^-$ background. Again, Idefix was almost unable to adsorb to the resulting strain (VE18393, Table S1) with only 5% (± 8) of adsorption, nor to lyse it (Figure 7A). Complementation of this *epaX* mutant with plasmid pVE14176 expressing constitutively *epaX* under a strong promoter (strain VE18945, Table S1) restored Idefix adsorption, which reached 96% (± 2), as well as the capacity of plaquing (Figure 7B). Results on the isogenic strain (VE18944, Table S1) hosting the empty vector were 5% (± 6) of phage adsorption and no plaque formation (Figure 7C). We concluded that *epaX* is required for Idefix adsorption.

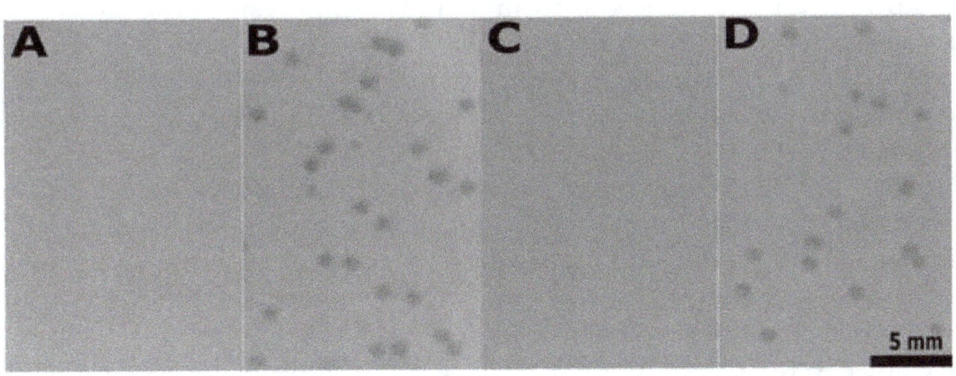

Figure 7. *epaX* gene expression is required for Idefix infection of pp6$^-$. Plaque assays performed on strains: (**A**) pp6$^-$*epaX*$^-$ (VE18393), a VE18306 derivative deleted from *epaX*. (**B**) pp6$^-$*epaX*$^-$pVE14176*epaX*$^+$ (VE18945), a VE18393 derivative complemented with *epaX*. (**C**) pp6$^-$*epaX*$^-$pVE14176 (VE18944), a VE18393 derivative carrying the empty vector. (**D**) pp6$^-$ (VE18306), a V583 derivative deleted from its plasmids and pp6.

To characterize the three remaining Idefix-resistant mutants, in which no IS was detected in the *epaX* region by PCR, we sequenced the genome of one of them, and mapped the reads against the pp6$^-$ reference genome. We identified a 33 nt-long deletion, flanked by 11 nt-long direct repeats, within ORF *ef2169* encoding a predicted O antigen polymerase, and located immediately downstream of *epaX*.

PCR amplification and sequencing of *ef2169* gene in the two last mutants allowed to detect the same 33 nt deletion in both of them (Figure 6 and Table S5). The observed deletion results in an in-frame 11 amino acids deletion in the C-terminal region of the putative O antigen polymerase. Additional single nucleotide polymorphisms (introducing amino acid substitution and a premature stop codon, respectively) were also observed in these two last *ef2169* mutants (Table S5). Complementation of the *ef2169* mutation could not be checked, due to our failure to clone the *ef2169* gene on a plasmid, despite repeated attempts in *E coli*, *L. lactis*, and *E. faecalis*.

4. Discussion

Enterococci are particularly successful at rapidly acquiring resistance to virtually any antibiotic used in therapy, with vancomycin-resistant enterococci (VRE) being a major clinical problem. If phage therapy is consequently nowadays (re)considered as an alternative to combat VRE infections, we are still nowhere near using enterococci phages as therapeutic agents in routine. Before that, we need to better characterize (i) enterococci phage receptors that define phage strain specificity, and (ii) enterococci resistance mechanisms that constitute the major constraint of phage therapy [7,16].

The present study with the new virulent podophage, Idefix, fulfills these goals. The phage was isolated by using the reference vancomycin-resistant *E. faecalis* V583 clinical isolate, deleted from its endogenous plasmids and prophages, as a recipient for phage infections. Idefix belongs to the *Picovirinae* subfamily and P68 genus and is closely related to three phages recently isolated on *E. faecalis* [13,44] or *E. faecium* [14]. They encode a DNA polymerase from the B type superfamily, which is a hallmark of the *Picovirinae*. As an additional hallmark of these enterococci podophages, they all encode two types of predicted endolysins. Endolysin engineering has emerged as a suitable strategy for food safety, environment decontamination, and infections control [85]. Some of the characterized enterococci phage endolysins show potential to combat VRE in vivo [15,86] and could represent an alternative to resolve the VRE problem. Idefix both encodes endolysin IDF_15, a predicted N-acetylmuramoyl-L-alanine amidase for which we could presume activity by spot assays on bacterial lawns, and IDF_13, similar to the catalytic subunit of the endolysin PlyC encoded by *Streptococcus* phage C1, which was inactive in the same spot assay. PlyC is the unique example of multimeric endolysin and represents the more active peptidoglycan hydrolase reported to date [85]. We were unable to identify by similarity an Idefix gene that could encode the CBD of this complex, and allow the formation of a putative multimeric endolysin. CBD of endolysins bind to specific substrates on the bacterial surfaces, often giving rise to near-species-specific binding, so that endolysins of the same class often share very little sequence similarity in the binding region [85]. Identification of the CBD subunit homolog in Idefix and complete characterization of this intriguing endolysin requires further investigation.

Idefix was unable to lyse any of our fifty-nine strains of *E. faecalis* and *E. faecium*, suggesting it could originate from another enterococcal species. Plaques were obtained against the indicator strain used for its isolation, and not on the wild type isolate V583 from which the indicator strain is derived. This apparently narrow host range could be explained by the reported Abiα-sensitivity and perhaps more importantly by the receptor-specificity of Idefix.

In V583, resistance to the phage was mainly due to the gene *abiα* (formerly ef2833) encoded by prophage 6. Upon Idefix infection, cells are dying while the Idefix lytic cycle is perturbed (ECOI of ~40% and ~10% whenever *abiα* is expressed on prophage 6 or overexpressed on cloning vectors, respectively) so that its efficiency of plaquing is below 10^{-8} and the detectable limits of the assay for Idefix. To our knowledge, it is the first time that an Abi system is described within enterococci, and the first one targeting a *Picovirinae*. This new Abi protein is widely distributed, it corresponds to the PFAM DUF 4393, and we report here that it is mostly found in prophages, arguing that it is essentially a temperate phage weapon to fight against other phages. Abi are specific anti-phage defence mechanisms present in many bacterial species including *Shigella dysenteriae*, *Streptococcus pyogenes*, *Vibrio cholerae*, *Bacillus subtilis*, and *Bacillus licheniformis* [62,87–90]. They have been more extensively studied in *L. lactis* and *E. coli* [17,81]. Most *abi* genes are encoded by a single gene on mobile genetic elements (MGE), on prophages in *E. coli* [91], or plasmids in *L. lactis* [81]. The fact that most *abi* genes are plasmidic in *L. lactis* may result however from a bias of human selection for plasmid-encoded systems in the dairy industry. Abi actually include a large collection of diverse mechanisms acting at any stage of the phage development to decrease or completely block virion production and cause host cell death. All these mechanisms display little or no known evolutionary relationship, apart from a very similar phenotype [18,81,92].

Lysis curve experiments show that the expression of *abiα* triggers a premature lysis of Idefix-infected *E. faecalis*. A similar phenotype was described in *L. lactis*, in which lysis, upon infection by siphophages from the P335 group, occurs earlier in the presence of AbiZ [93]. AbiZ speeds up the lysis of *L. lactis* bacteria in which the phage holin and endolysin are expressed, and enhances membrane permeability of bacteria expressing the phage holin. Durmaz and Klaenhammer propose that AbiZ interacts with phage holin to accelerate the lysis clock and prevent normal phage multiplication [93]. Abiα and AbiZ do not share any sequence similarity. We were unable to obtain Idefix mutants that were resistant to Abiα, suggesting a very high efficiency of this Abi system. Based on our results, we can only speculate that Abiα interferes with lysis, possibly by preventing timely holin and consequently endolysin(s) actions, as described for AbiZ. Another possibility is that Abiα targets a putative Idefix holin inhibitor. The holin triggering, which is determinant for optimal burst size, is critically regulated by the expressed ratio between the holin and its inhibitor. This latter is encoded within the lambda holin gene, as a separate transcript initiated at a dual-start motif [94,95]. Unlike lambda (and phi29), the Idefix holin gene does not harbor a dual-start motif and its regulation may be mediated by the expression of another non-identified Idefix gene, as described in other phages [94,95]. Finally, premature triggering of lambda holin can also be induced by any poison that efficiently reduces the proton-motrice force (pmf) of the cytoplasmic membrane [94,95]. Thus, we cannot exclude Abiα causes a holin-independent reduction of the pmf underlying an early trigger of the holin and/or a permeabilization of the membrane leading to endolysin release. If this is the case, you might imagine that Abiαcould be active against a wider range of phages and not only Idefix or related phages. Further experiments will be needed to test these different hypotheses and complete the characterization of this defence mechanism.

Genomes of V583 and other MDR *E. faecalis* isolates have few generalist anti-MGE systems, which favor horizontal gene transfer and polylysogeny [29]. MDR enterococci may thus provide a suitable ground for bacteriophages confrontation. Whereas the spread of Idefix infection is thus limited by V583 prophage 6, it is interesting to note this latter is itself strictly controlled by V583 prophages 3 and 5 that block its excision [43]. This 'domestication' could be seen as a way for both prophages to sustain the specific line of defense conferred by prophage 6 and thus protect themselves and their host from an external phage 'attack'.

Beyond the intra-bacteriophage warfare, bacteria are also able to evolve resistance to phages. We observed that *E. faecalis* mutants resisting to Idefix infection arose at a high frequency of 1.5×10^{-4} per generation. The nine Idefix-resistant mutants analyzed had either acquired an IS256 or recombined between eleven base paires long direct repeats in the *epa* variable region, indicating that *E. faecalis* has a high potential for evolution by recombination. Mutants in glycosyltransferase gene *epaX* had a 10-fold defect in Idefix adsorption, whereas mutants in the next o-polymerase gene had a milder adsorption defect. The fact that all mutations cluster into two genes of the *epa* variable region underlines the role of the rhamnopolysaccharide for Idefix adsorption. Epa was recently confirmed as a receptor of *E. faecalis* virulent phage NPV1 [96,97], and we provide here the first evidence for a role of Epa decoration chains in phage/host recognition in enterococci. Rhamnose-rich cell wall polysaccharides (CWPS) and their structural diversity are important in phage adsorption within lactococci and streptococci [98,99]. In *L. lactis* as well, CWPS biosynthesis is encoded on a large chromosomal gene cluster also including a conserved and a variable region. Based on sequence similarity and difference in the variable region, *L. lactis* strains were divided into three groups, and one of them in several subtypes [100]. These latter are distinguished by their glycosyltransferase-encoding genes composition and consequent differences between CWPS structures are critical in determining phage sensitivity [100]. The use of unconserved sugar decorations of the saccharidic chains as a receptor combined with the presence of a prophage-encoded Abi system targeting Idefix may explain Idefix very low success in *E. faecalis*.

5. Conclusions

This study of the *Enterococcus* infecting *Picovirinae* Idefix permitted to unveil two resistance mechanisms against it, one bacterial and the other viral. Bacterial mutations suppressed the Epa decoration needed for phage adsorption, and the prophage-encoded product Abiα interfered with Idefix timing of lysis. However, the bacterial line of defence is likely to be counterselected in vivo as V583 *epaX* mutants have a defect in mouse gut colonization [49]. In fact, phage selective pressure might be one of the actors of the observed diversification of the *epa* locus in enterococci. The viral line of defence based on Abiα is likely to be more robust, given that no escape mutant could be isolated. Indeed, Abiα is widespread both in enterococci and in *Firmicutes* and it may allow to fight against *Picovirinae* or other ranges of phages. Somehow, the different families of phages infecting the same bacterial species are in competition, so that their host resembles a battlefield. It is especially true if bacteria are devoid of generalist defense systems, as MDR *E. faecalis* strains tend to be. In this context, it might be expected that Abi and other specific defensive systems pave prophage genomes, allowing temperate phages to align their strategy with their host, and fight against virulent phage invaders.

Figure S1: Structural and functional map of family of B phage DNA polymerases belonging to the "protein priming" subfamily. Figure S2: IDF_15 alignments. Figure S3: Alignments of IDF_13. Figure S4: Activities of *E. coli* extracts containing putative Idefix endolysins (IDF_15 and IDF_13). Figure S5: Biological replicates relative to lysis curves experiments after Idefix infection at MOI 10. Figure S6: Putative *abiα* homologs identified on several prophages of Gram-positive bacteria. Table S1: Bacterial strains, plasmids, and oligonucleotide primers used. Table S2: Description of *Enterococcus* isolates tested as potential Idefix hosts. Table S3: Respective genome accession numbers of the *Enterococcus Picovirinae* phages. Table S4: Features of Idefix ORFs and predicted functions of their products. Table S5: Spontaneous mutation in *epaX* (ef2170) or *ef2169* in pp6^{-} and resistance to Idefix infection.

Author Contributions: Conceptualization, J.L., F.L., P.S., and M.-A.P.; Investigation, J.L., Ar.B., E.M., S.F., As.B., O.S., M.L., M.D., and F.L.; Supervision, M.-A.P.; Writing—original draft, J.L., F.L., P.S., and M.-A.P.; Writing—review & editing, J.L.

Acknowledgments: We thank Marianne De Paepe and Lionel Rigottier-Gois for their help during this study; Christine Longin from the MIMA2 facilities (UMR 1313 GABI, INRA) for the TEM observations; Laurent Debarbieux and Sylwia Bloch, Alicja Węgrzyn as well as Vincent Cattoir who respectively provided sewage water samples and enterococci isolates.

References

1. Lebreton, F.; Willems, R.J.; Gilmore, M.S. *Enterococcus* diversity, origins in nature, and gut colonization. In *Enterococci from Commensals to Leading Causes of Drug Resistant Infection*; Gilmore, M.S., Clewell, D.B., Ike, Y., Shankar, N., Eds.; Massachusetts Eye and Ear Infirmary: Boston, MA, USA, 2014; pp. 3–46.
2. Higuita, N.I.A.; Huycke, M.M. Enterococcal disease, epidemiology, and implications for treatment. In *Enterococci from Commensals to Leading Causes of Drug Resistant Infection*; Gilmore, M.S., Clewell, D.B., Ike, Y., Shankar, N., Eds.; Massachusetts Eye and Ear Infirmary: Boston, MA, USA, 2014; pp. 47–72.
3. Kristich, C.J.; Rice, L.B.; Arias, C.A. Enterococcal infection—Treatment and antibiotic resistance. In *Enterococci from Commensals to Leading Causes of Drug Resistant Infection*; Gilmore, M.S., Clewell, D.B., Ike, Y., Shankar, N., Eds.; Massachusetts Eye and Ear Infirmary: Boston, MA, USA, 2014; pp. 89–134.
4. Sulakvelidze, A.; Alavidze, Z.; Morris, J.G. Bacteriophage therapy. *Antimicrob. Agents Chemother.* **2001**, *45*, 649–659. [CrossRef] [PubMed]
5. Cheng, M.; Liang, J.; Zhang, Y.; Hu, L.; Gong, P.; Cai, R.; Zhang, L.; Zhang, H.; Ge, J.; Ji, Y.; et al. The bacteriophage EF-P29 efficiently protects against lethal vancomycin-resistant *Enterococcus faecalis* and alleviates gut microbiota imbalance in a murine bacteremia model. *Front. Microbiol.* **2017**, *8*, 837. [CrossRef]

6. Cheng, S.; Xing, S.; Zhang, X.; Pei, G.; An, X.; Mi, Z.; Huang, Y.; Tong, Y. Complete genome sequence of a new *Enterococcus faecalis* bacteriophage, vB_EfaS_IME197. *Genome Announc.* **2016**, *4*, e00827-16. [CrossRef] [PubMed]
7. Duerkop, B.A.; Palmer, K.L.; Horsburgh, M.J. Enterococcal bacteriophages and genome defense. In *Enterococci from Commensals to Leading Causes of Drug Resistant Infection*; Gilmore, M.S., Clewell, D.B., Ike, Y., Shankar, N., Eds.; Massachusetts Eye and Ear Infirmary: Boston, MA, USA, 2014; pp. 309–336.
8. Gelman, D.; Beyth, S.; Lerer, V.; Adler, K.; Poradosu-Cohen, R.; Coppenhagen-Glazer, S.; Hazan, R. Combined bacteriophages and antibiotics as an efficient therapy against VRE *Enterococcus faecalis* in a mouse model. *Res. Microbiol.* **2018**, *169*, 531–539. [CrossRef]
9. Gong, P.; Cheng, M.; Li, X.; Jiang, H.; Yu, C.; Kahaer, N.; Li, J.; Zhang, L.; Xia, F.; Hu, L.; et al. Characterization of *Enterococcus faecium* bacteriophage IME-EFm5 and its endolysin LysEFm5. *Virology* **2016**, *492*, 11–20. [CrossRef]
10. Khalifa, L.; Brosh, Y.; Gelman, D.; Coppenhagen-Glazer, S.; Beyth, S.; Poraduso-Cohen, R.; Que, Y.-A.; Beyth, N.; Hazan, R. Targeting *Enterococcus faecalis* biofilm using phage therapy. *Appl. Environ. Microbiol.* **2015**, *81*, 2696–2705. [CrossRef] [PubMed]
11. Khalifa, L.; Gelman, D.; Shlezinger, M.; Dessal, A.L.; Coppenhagen-Glazer, S.; Beyth, N.; Hazan, R. Defeating antibiotic-and phage-resistant *Enterococcus faecalis* using a phage cocktail in vitro and in a clot model. *Front. Microbiol.* **2018**, *9*, 326. [CrossRef]
12. Rahmat Ullah, S.; Andleeb, S.; Raza, T.; Jamal, M.; Mehmood, K. Effectiveness of a lytic Phage SRG1 against vancomycin-resistant *Enterococcus faecalis* in compost and soil. *Biomed. Res. Int.* **2017**, *2017*. [CrossRef]
13. Wang, R.; Xing, S.; Zhao, F.; Li, P.; Mi, Z.; Shi, T.; Liu, H.; Tong, Y. Characterization and genome analysis of novel phage vB_EfaP_IME195 infecting *Enterococcus faecalis*. *Virus Genes* **2018**, *54*, 804–811. [CrossRef]
14. Xing, S.; Zhang, X.; Sun, Q.; Wang, J.; Mi, Z.; Pei, G.; Huang, Y.; An, X.; Fu, K.; Zhou, L.; et al. Complete genome sequence of a novel, virulent Ahjdlikevirus bacteriophage that infects *Enterococcus faecium*. *Arch.Virol.* **2017**, *162*, 3843–3847. [CrossRef]
15. Zhang, W.; Mi, Z.; Yin, X.; Fan, H.; An, X.; Zhang, Z.; Chen, J.; Tong, Y. Characterization of *Enterococcus faecalis* phage IME-EF1 and its endolysin. *PLoS ONE* **2013**, *8*, e80435. [CrossRef] [PubMed]
16. Duerkop, B.A.; Huo, W.; Bhardwaj, P.; Palmer, K.L.; Hooper, L.V. molecular basis for lytic bacteriophage resistance in enterococci. *MBio* **2016**, *7*. [CrossRef] [PubMed]
17. Labrie, S.J.; Samson, J.E.; Moineau, S. Bacteriophage resistance mechanisms. *Nat. Rev. Microbiol.* **2010**, *8*, 317–327. [CrossRef] [PubMed]
18. Seed, K.D. Battling Phages: How bacteria defend against viral attack. *PLoS Pathog.* **2015**, *11*, e1004847. [CrossRef] [PubMed]
19. Goldfarb, T.; Sberro, H.; Weinstock, E.; Cohen, O.; Doron, S.; Charpak-Amikam, Y.; Afik, S.; Ofir, G.; Sorek, R. BREX is a novel phage resistance system widespread in microbial genomes. *EMBO J.* **2014**, *34*, 169–183. [CrossRef]
20. Doron, S.; Melamed, S.; Ofir, G.; Leavitt, A.; Lopatina, A.; Keren, M.; Amitai, G.; Sorek, R. Systematic discovery of antiphage defense systems in the microbial pangenome. *Science* **2018**, *359*, eaar4120. [CrossRef]
21. Depardieu, F.; Didier, J.-P.; Bernheim, A.; Sherlock, A.; Molina, H.; Duclos, B.; Bikard, D. A eukaryotic-like serine/threonine kinase protects staphylococci against phages. *Cell Host Microbe* **2016**, *20*, 471–481. [CrossRef]
22. Ofir, G.; Melamed, S.; Sberro, H.; Mukamel, Z.; Silverman, S.; Yaakov, G.; Doron, S.; Sorek, R. DISARM is a widespread bacterial defence system with broad anti-phage activities. *Nat. Microbiol.* **2018**, *3*, 90–98. [CrossRef]
23. Kronheim, S.; Daniel-Ivad, M.; Duan, Z.; Hwang, S.; Wong, A.I.; Mantel, I.; Nodwell, J.R.; Maxwell, K.L. A chemical defence against phage infection. *Nature* **2018**, *564*, 283–286. [CrossRef]
24. Burley, K.M.; Sedgley, C.M. CRISPR-Cas, a prokaryotic adaptive immune system, in endodontic, oral, and multidrug-resistant hospital-acquired *Enterococcus faecalis*. *J. Endod.* **2012**, *38*, 1511–1515. [CrossRef]
25. Hullahalli, K.; Rodrigues, M.; Schmidt, B.D.; Li, X.; Bhardwaj, P.; Palmer, K.L. Comparative analysis of the orphan CRISPR2 locus in 242 *Enterococcus faecalis* strains. *PLoS ONE* **2015**, *10*, e0138890. [CrossRef] [PubMed]
26. Lindenstrauß, A.G.; Pavlovic, M.; Bringmann, A.; Behr, J.; Ehrmann, M.A.; Vogel, R.F. Comparison of genotypic and phenotypic cluster analyses of virulence determinants and possible role of CRISPR elements towards their incidence in *Enterococcus faecalis* and *Enterococcus faecium*. *Syst. Appl. Microbiol.* **2011**, *34*, 553–560. [CrossRef] [PubMed]

27. Price, V.J.; Huo, W.; Sharifi, A.; Palmer, K.L. CRISPR-cas and restriction-modification act additively against conjugative antibiotic resistance plasmid transfer in *Enterococcus faecalis*. *mSphere* **2016**, *1*. [CrossRef] [PubMed]
28. Huo, W.; Adams, H.M.; Zhang, M.Q.; Palmer, K.L. Genome modification in *Enterococcus faecalis* OG1RF assessed by bisulfite sequencing and single-molecule real-time sequencing. *J. Bacteriol.* **2015**, *197*, 1939–1951. [CrossRef] [PubMed]
29. Palmer, K.L.; Gilmore, M.S. Multidrug-resistant enterococci lack CRISPR-cas. *MBio* **2010**, *1*, e00227-10. [CrossRef] [PubMed]
30. Hullahalli, K.; Rodrigues, M.; Nguyen, U.T.; Palmer, K. An attenuated CRISPR-cas system in *Enterococcus faecalis* permits DNA acquisition. *MBio* **2018**, *9*, e00414-18. [CrossRef]
31. Villarreal, L.P. Viral ancestors of antiviral systems. *Viruses* **2011**, *3*, 1933–1958. [CrossRef]
32. Arber, W.; Dussoix, D. Host specificity of DNA produced by *Escherichia coli*. I. Host controlled modification of bacteriophage lambda. *J. Mol. Biol.* **1962**, *5*, 18–36. [CrossRef]
33. Seed, K.D.; Lazinski, D.W.; Calderwood, S.B.; Camilli, A. A bacteriophage encodes its own CRISPR/cas adaptive response to evade host innate immunity. *Nature* **2013**, *494*, 489–491. [CrossRef]
34. Nilsson, A.S.; Karlsson, J.L.; Haggård-Ljungquist, E. Site-specific recombination links the evolution of P2-like coliphages and pathogenic enterobacteria. *Mol. Biol. Evol.* **2004**, *21*, 1–13. [CrossRef]
35. Kintz, E.; Davies, M.R.; Hammarlöf, D.L.; Canals, R.; Hinton, J.C.D.; van der Woude, M.W. A BTP1 prophage gene present in invasive non-typhoidal *Salmonella* determines composition and length of the O-antigen of the lipopolysaccharide. *Mol. Microbiol.* **2015**, *96*, 263–275. [CrossRef] [PubMed]
36. Cumby, N.; Edwards, A.M.; Davidson, A.R.; Maxwell, K.L. The bacteriophage HK97 gp15 moron element encodes a novel superinfection exclusion protein. *J. Bacteriol.* **2012**, *194*, 5012–5019. [CrossRef] [PubMed]
37. Mahony, J.; McGrath, S.; Fitzgerald, G.F.; van Sinderen, D. Identification and characterization of lactococcal-prophage-carried superinfection exclusion genes. *Appl. Environ. Microbiol.* **2008**, *74*, 6206–6215. [CrossRef] [PubMed]
38. Bebeacua, C.; Lorenzo Fajardo, J.C.; Blangy, S.; Spinelli, S.; Bollmann, S.; Neve, H.; Cambillau, C.; Heller, K.J. X-ray structure of a superinfection exclusion lipoprotein from phage TP-J34 and identification of the tape measure protein as its target. *Mol. Microbiol.* **2013**, *89*, 152–165. [CrossRef] [PubMed]
39. Bondy-Denomy, J.; Qian, J.; Westra, E.R.; Buckling, A.; Guttman, D.S.; Davidson, A.R.; Maxwell, K.L. Prophages mediate defense against phage infection through diverse mechanisms. *ISME J.* **2016**, *10*, 2854–2866. [CrossRef] [PubMed]
40. Dedrick, R.M.; Jacobs-Sera, D.; Bustamante, C.A.G.; Garlena, R.A.; Mavrich, T.N.; Pope, W.H.; Reyes, J.C.C.; Russell, D.A.; Adair, T.; Alvey, R.; et al. Prophage-mediated defence against viral attack and viral counter-defence. *Nat. Microbiol.* **2017**, *2*, 16251. [CrossRef] [PubMed]
41. Parma, D.H.; Snyder, M.; Sobolevski, S.; Nawroz, M.; Brody, E.; Gold, L. The Rex system of bacteriophage lambda: Tolerance and altruistic cell death. *Genes Dev.* **1992**, *6*, 497–510. [CrossRef] [PubMed]
42. Friedman, D.I.; Mozola, C.C.; Beeri, K.; Ko, C.-C.; Reynolds, J.L. Activation of a prophage-encoded tyrosine kinase by a heterologous infecting phage results in a self-inflicted abortive infection. *Mol. Microbiol.* **2011**, *82*, 567–577. [CrossRef]
43. Matos, R.C.; Lapaque, N.; Rigottier-Gois, L.; Debarbieux, L.; Meylheuc, T.; Gonzalez-Zorn, B.; Repoila, F.; de Lopes, M.F.; Serror, P. *Enterococcus faecalis* prophage dynamics and contributions to pathogenic traits. *PLoS Genet.* **2013**, *9*, e1003539. [CrossRef]
44. Jurczak-Kurek, A.; Gąsior, T.; Nejman-Faleńczyk, B.; Bloch, S.; Dydecka, A.; Topka, G.; Necel, A.; Jakubowska-Deredas, M.; Narajczyk, M.; Richert, M.; et al. Biodiversity of bacteriophages: Morphological and biological properties of a large group of phages isolated from urban sewage. *Sci. Rep* **2016**, *6*, 34338. [CrossRef]
45. Dumoulin, R.; Cortes-Perez, N.; Gaubert, S.; Duhutrel, P.; Brinster, S.; Torelli, R.; Sanguinetti, M.; Posteraro, B.; Repoila, F.; Serror, P. Enterococcal Rgg-like regulator ElrR activates expression of the elrA operon. *J. Bacteriol.* **2013**, *195*, 3073–3083. [CrossRef]
46. Gasson, M.J. Plasmid complements of *Streptococcus lactis* NCDO 712 and other lactic streptococci after protoplast-induced curing. *J. Bacteriol.* **1983**, *154*, 1–9. [PubMed]
47. Renault, P.; Corthier, G.; Goupil, N.; Delorme, C.; Ehrlich, S.D. Plasmid vectors for gram-positive bacteria switching from high to low copy number. *Gene* **1996**, *183*, 175–182. [CrossRef]

48. Rigottier-Gois, L.; Alberti, A.; Houel, A.; Taly, J.-F.; Palcy, P.; Manson, J.; Pinto, D.; Matos, R.C.; Carrilero, L.; Montero, N.; et al. Large-scale screening of a targeted *Enterococcus faecalis* mutant library identifies envelope fitness factors. *PLoS ONE* **2011**, *6*, e29023. [CrossRef]
49. Rigottier-Gois, L.; Madec, C.; Navickas, A.; Matos, R.C.; Akary-Lepage, E.; Mistou, M.-Y.; Serror, P. The surface rhamnopolysaccharide Epa of *Enterococcus faecalis* is a key determinant of intestinal colonization. *J. Infect. Dis.* **2015**, *211*, 62–71. [CrossRef]
50. Sahm, D.F.; Marsilio, M.K.; Piazza, G. Antimicrobial resistance in key bloodstream bacterial isolates: Electronic surveillance with the Surveillance Network Database-USA. *Clin. Infect. Dis.* **1999**, *29*, 259–263. [CrossRef] [PubMed]
51. Fritzenwanker, M.; Kuenne, C.; Billion, A.; Hain, T.; Zimmermann, K.; Goesmann, A.; Chakraborty, T.; Domann, E. Complete Genome Sequence of the Probiotic *Enterococcus faecalis* Symbioflor 1 Clone DSM 16431. *Genome Announc.* **2013**, *1*, e00165-12. [CrossRef] [PubMed]
52. Jamet, E.; Akary, E.; Poisson, M.-A.; Chamba, J.-F.; Bertrand, X.; Serror, P. Prevalence and characterization of antibiotic resistant *Enterococcus faecalis* in French cheeses. *Food Microbiol.* **2012**, *31*, 191–198. [CrossRef]
53. Fortier, L.-C.; Moineau, S. Phage production and maintenance of stocks, including expected stock lifetimes. *Methods Mol. Biol.* **2009**, *501*, 203–219. [PubMed]
54. Pickard, D.J.J. Preparation of bacteriophage lysates and pure DNA. *Methods Mol. Biol.* **2009**, *502*, 3–9.
55. Summer, E.J. Preparation of a phage DNA fragment library for whole genome shotgun sequencing. *Methods Mol. Biol.* **2009**, *502*, 27–46. [PubMed]
56. Margulies, M.; Egholm, M.; Altman, W.E.; Attiya, S.; Bader, J.S.; Bemben, L.A.; Berka, J.; Braverman, M.S.; Chen, Y.-J.; Chen, Z.; et al. Genome sequencing in microfabricated high-density picolitre reactors. *Nature* **2005**, *437*, 376–380. [CrossRef] [PubMed]
57. Aziz, R.K.; Bartels, D.; Best, A.A.; DeJongh, M.; Disz, T.; Edwards, R.A.; Formsma, K.; Gerdes, S.; Glass, E.M.; Kubal, M.; et al. The RAST Server: Rapid annotations using subsystems technology. *BMC Genom.* **2008**, *9*, 75. [CrossRef] [PubMed]
58. Sullivan, M.J.; Petty, N.K.; Beatson, S.A. Easyfig: A genome comparison visualizer. *Bioinformatics* **2011**, *27*, 1009–1010. [CrossRef]
59. Hyman, P.; Abedon, S.T. Practical methods for determining phage growth parameters. *Methods Mol. Biol.* **2009**, *501*, 175–202.
60. Garvey, P.; Hill, C.; Fitzgerald, G.F. The lactococcal plasmid pNP40 encodes a third bacteriophage resistance mechanism, one which affects phage DNA penetration. *Appl. Environ. Microbiol.* **1996**, *62*, 676–679.
61. Sing, W.D.; Klahenhammer, T.R. Characteristics of phage abortion conferred in lactococci by the congugal plasmid pTR2030. *J. Mol. Biol.* **1990**, *136*, 1807–1815.
62. Behnke, D.; Malke, H. Bacteriophage interference in *Streptococcus pyogenes*. II. A25 mutants resistant to prophage-medicated interference. *Virology* **1978**, *85*, 129–136. [CrossRef]
63. Luria, S.E.; Delbrück, M. Mutations of bacteria from virus sensitivity to virus resistance. *Genetics* **1943**, *28*, 491–511.
64. Dower, W.J.; Miller, J.F.; Ragsdale, C.W. High efficiency transformation of *E. coli* by high voltage electroporation. *Nucleic Acids Res.* **1988**, *16*, 6127–6145. [CrossRef]
65. Dunny, G.M.; Lee, L.N.; LeBlanc, D.J. Improved electroporation and cloning vector system for gram-positive bacteria. *Appl. Environ. Microbiol.* **1991**, *57*, 1194–1201. [PubMed]
66. Brinster, S.; Furlan, S.; Serror, P. C-terminal WxL domain mediates cell wall binding in *Enterococcus faecalis* and other gram-positive bacteria. *J. Bacteriol.* **2007**, *189*, 1244–1253. [CrossRef] [PubMed]
67. Blanco, L.; Salas, M. Relating structure to function in phi29 DNA polymerase. *J. Biol. Chem.* **1996**, *271*, 8509–8512. [CrossRef] [PubMed]
68. Dufour, E.; Méndez, J.; Lázaro, J.M.; de Vega, M.; Blanco, L.; Salas, M. An aspartic acid residue in TPR-1, a specific region of protein-priming DNA polymerases, is required for the functional interaction with primer terminal protein1. *J. Mol. Biol.* **2000**, *304*, 289–300. [CrossRef] [PubMed]
69. Eisenbrandt, R.; Lázaro, J.M.; Salas, M.; Vega, M. de. Phi29 DNA polymerase residues Tyr59, His61 and Phe69 of the highly conserved ExoII motif are essential for interaction with the terminal protein. *Nucleic Acids Res.* **2002**, *30*, 1379–1386. [CrossRef]
70. Meijer, W.J.J.; Horcajadas, J.A.; Salas, M. φ29 Family of Phages. *Microbiol. Mol. Biol. Rev.* **2001**, *65*, 261–287. [CrossRef]

71. Rodríguez, I.; Lázaro, J.M.; Blanco, L.; Kamtekar, S.; Berman, A.J.; Wang, J.; Steitz, T.A.; Salas, M.; de Vega, M. A specific subdomain in phi29 DNA polymerase confers both processivity and strand-displacement capacity. *Proc. Natl. Acad. Sci. USA* **2005**, *102*, 6407–6412. [CrossRef]
72. Redrejo-Rodríguez, M.; Salas, M. Multiple roles of genome-attached bacteriophage terminal proteins. *Virology* **2014**, *468–470*, 322–329. [CrossRef]
73. Redrejo-Rodríguez, M.; Muñoz-Espín, D.; Holguera, I.; Mencía, M.; Salas, M. Nuclear and nucleoid localization are independently conserved functions in bacteriophage terminal proteins. *Mol. Microbiol.* **2013**, *90*, 858–868. [CrossRef] [PubMed]
74. Bateman, A.; Rawlings, N.D. The CHAP domain: A large family of amidases including GSP amidase and peptidoglycan hydrolases. *Trends Biochem. Sci.* **2003**, *28*, 234–237. [CrossRef]
75. McGowan, S.; Buckle, A.M.; Mitchell, M.S.; Hoopes, J.T.; Gallagher, D.T.; Heselpoth, R.D.; Shen, Y.; Reboul, C.F.; Law, R.H.P.; Fischetti, V.A.; et al. X-ray crystal structure of the streptococcal specific phage lysin PlyC. *Proc. Natl. Acad. Sci. USA* **2012**, *109*, 12752–12757. [CrossRef] [PubMed]
76. Rigden, D.J.; Jedrzejas, M.J.; Galperin, M.Y. Amidase domains from bacterial and phage autolysins define a family of gamma-D,L-glutamate-specific amidohydrolases. *Trends Biochem. Sci.* **2003**, *28*, 230–234. [CrossRef]
77. Nelson, D.; Schuch, R.; Chahales, P.; Zhu, S.; Fischetti, V.A. PlyC: A multimeric bacteriophage lysin. *Proc. Natl. Acad. Sci. USA* **2006**, *103*, 10765–10770. [CrossRef] [PubMed]
78. Lavigne, R.; Seto, D.; Mahadevan, P.; Ackermann, H.-W.; Kropinski, A.M. Unifying classical and molecular taxonomic classification: Analysis of the Podoviridae using BLASTP-based tools. *Res. Microbiol.* **2008**, *159*, 406–414. [CrossRef] [PubMed]
79. McGrath, S.; Fitzgerald, G.F.; van Sinderen, D. Identification and characterization of phage-resistance genes in temperate lactococcal bacteriophages. *Mol. Microbiol.* **2002**, *43*, 509–520. [CrossRef] [PubMed]
80. Innocenti, N.; Golumbeanu, M.; d' Hérouël, A.F.; Lacoux, C.; Bonnin, R.A.; Kennedy, S.P.; Wessner, F.; Serror, P.; Bouloc, P.; Repoila, F.; et al. Whole-genome mapping of 5′ RNA ends in bacteria by tagged sequencing: A comprehensive view in *Enterococcus faecalis*. *Rna* **2015**, *21*, 1018–1031. [CrossRef] [PubMed]
81. Chopin, M.-C.; Chopin, A.; Bidnenko, E. Phage abortive infection in lactococci: Variations on a theme. *Curr. Opin. Microbiol.* **2005**, *8*, 473–479. [CrossRef]
82. Paez-Espino, D.; Roux, S.; Chen, I.-M.A.; Palaniappan, K.; Ratner, A.; Chu, K.; Huntemann, M.; Reddy, T.B.K.; Pons, J.C.; Llabrés, M.; et al. IMG/VR v.2.0: An integrated data management and analysis system for cultivated and environmental viral genomes. *Nucleic Acids Res.* **2018**. [CrossRef]
83. Nelson, D.; Schuch, R.; Zhu, S.; Tscherne, D.M.; Fischetti, V.A. Genomic sequence of C1, the first streptococcal phage. *J. Bacteriol.* **2003**, *185*, 3325–3332. [CrossRef]
84. Palmer, K.L.; Godfrey, P.; Griggs, A.; Kos, V.N.; Zucker, J.; Desjardins, C.; Cerqueira, G.; Gevers, D.; Walker, S.; Wortman, J.; et al. Comparative genomics of enterococci: Variation in Enterococcus faecalis, clade structure in E. faecium, and defining characteristics of E. gallinarum and E. casseliflavus. *MBio* **2012**, *3*, e00318-11. [CrossRef]
85. Nelson, D.C.; Schmelcher, M.; Rodriguez-Rubio, L.; Klumpp, J.; Pritchard, D.G.; Dong, S.; Donovan, D.M. Endolysins as antimicrobials. *Adv. Virus Res.* **2012**, *83*, 299–365. [PubMed]
86. Cheng, M.; Zhang, Y.; Li, X.; Liang, J.; Hu, L.; Gong, P.; Zhang, L.; Cai, R.; Zhang, H.; Ge, J.; et al. Endolysin LysEF-P10 shows potential as an alternative treatment strategy for multidrug-resistant *Enterococcus faecalis* infections. *Sci. Rep.* **2017**, *7*, 10164. [CrossRef] [PubMed]
87. Chowdhury, R.; Biswas, S.K.; Das, J. Abortive replication of choleraphage phi 149 in *Vibrio cholerae* biotype el tor. *J. Virol.* **1989**, *63*, 392–397. [PubMed]
88. Rettenmier, C.W.; Hemphill, H.E. Abortive infection of lysogenic *Bacillus subtilis* 168(SPO2) by bacteriophage phi 1. *J. Virol.* **1974**, *13*, 870–880. [PubMed]
89. Smith, H.S.; Pizer, L.I.; Pylkas, L.; Lederberg, S. Abortive infection of *Shigella dysenteriae* P2 by T2 bacteriophage. *J. Virol.* **1969**, *4*, 162–168. [PubMed]
90. Tran, L.S.; Szabó, L.; Ponyi, T.; Orosz, L.; Sík, T.; Holczinger, A. Phage abortive infection of *Bacillus licheniformis* ATCC 9800; identification of the abiBL11 gene and localisation and sequencing of its promoter region. *Appl. Microbiol. Biotechnol.* **1999**, *52*, 845–852. [CrossRef] [PubMed]
91. Snyder, L. Phage-exclusion enzymes: A bonanza of biochemical and cell biology reagents? *Mol. Microbiol.* **1995**, *15*, 415–420. [CrossRef]

92. Stern, A.; Sorek, R. The phage-host arms race: Shaping the evolution of microbes. *Bioessays* **2011**, *33*, 43–51. [CrossRef]
93. Durmaz, E.; Klaenhammer, T.R. Abortive phage resistance mechanism AbiZ speeds the lysis clock to cause premature lysis of phage-infected Lactococcus lactis. *J. Bacteriol.* **2007**, *189*, 1417–1425. [CrossRef]
94. Young, R. Phage lysis: Three steps, three choices, one outcome. *J. Microbiol.* **2014**, *52*, 243–258. [CrossRef]
95. Wang, I.N.; Smith, D.L.; Young, R. Holins: The protein clocks of bacteriophage infections. *Annu. Rev. Microbiol.* **2000**, *54*, 799–825. [CrossRef] [PubMed]
96. Ho, K.; Huo, W.; Pas, S.; Dao, R.; Palmer, K.L. Loss-of-Function Mutations in epaR Confer Resistance to ϕNPV1 Infection in *Enterococcus faecalis* OG1RF. *Antimicrob. Agents Chemother.* **2018**, *62*. [CrossRef] [PubMed]
97. Teng, F.; Singh, K.V.; Bourgogne, A.; Zeng, J.; Murray, B.E. Further characterization of the *epa* gene cluster and Epa polysaccharides of *Enterococcus faecalis*. *Infect. Immun.* **2009**, *77*, 3759–3767. [CrossRef] [PubMed]
98. Chapot-Chartier, M.-P. Interactions of the cell-wall glycopolymers of lactic acid bacteria with their bacteriophages. *Front. Microbiol.* **2014**, *5*, 236. [CrossRef] [PubMed]
99. Mistou, M.-Y.; Sutcliffe, I.C.; van Sorge, N.M. Bacterial glycobiology: Rhamnose-containing cell wall polysaccharides in Gram-positive bacteria. *FEMS Microbiol. Rev.* **2016**, *40*, 464–479. [CrossRef]
100. Ainsworth, S.; Sadovskaya, I.; Vinogradov, E.; Courtin, P.; Guerardel, Y.; Mahony, J.; Grard, T.; Cambillau, C.; Chapot-Chartier, M.-P.; van Sinderen, D. Differences in lactococcal cell wall polysaccharide structure are major determining factors in bacteriophage sensitivity. *MBio* **2014**, *5*, e00880-14. [CrossRef]

14

Evaluation of Phage Therapy in the Context of *Enterococcus faecalis* and its Associated Diseases

Andrei S. Bolocan [1,2,†], Aditya Upadrasta [1,2,†], Pedro H. de Almeida Bettio [1,2], Adam G. Clooney [1,2], Lorraine A. Draper [1,2], R. Paul Ross [1,2,3] and Colin Hill [1,2,*]

1 APC Microbiome Ireland, University College Cork, Cork T12 YT20, Ireland; andrei.s.bolocan@gmail.com (A.S.B.); aupadrasta@gmail.com (A.U.); pedro.almeida.bettio@gmail.com (P.H.d.A.B.); adam.clooney@ucc.ie (A.G.C.); L.Draper@ucc.ie (L.A.D.); p.ross@ucc.ie (R.P.R.)

2 School of Microbiology, University College Cork, Cork T12 YN60, Ireland

3 Teagasc Food Research Centre, Moorepark, Fermoy, Cork P61 C996, Ireland

* Correspondence: c.hill@ucc.ie

† These authors contributed equally to this work.

Abstract: Bacteriophages (phages) or bacterial viruses have been proposed as natural antimicrobial agents to fight against antibiotic-resistant bacteria associated with human infections. *Enterococcus faecalis* is a gut commensal, which is occasionally found in the mouth and vaginal tract, and does not usually cause clinical problems. However, it can spread to other areas of the body and cause life-threatening infections, such as septicemia, endocarditis, or meningitis, in immunocompromised hosts. Although *E. faecalis* phage cocktails are not commercially available within the EU or USA, there is an accumulated evidence from in vitro and in vivo studies that have shown phage efficacy, which supports the idea of applying phage therapy to overcome infections associated with *E. faecalis*. In this review, we discuss the potency of bacteriophages in controlling *E. faecalis*, in both in vitro and in vivo scenarios. *E. faecalis* associated bacteriophages were compared at the genome level and an attempt was made to categorize phages with respect to their suitability for therapeutic application, using orthocluster analysis. In addition, *E. faecalis* phages have been examined for the presence of antibiotic-resistant genes, to ensure their safe use in clinical conditions. Finally, the domain architecture of *E. faecalis* phage-encoded endolysins are discussed.

Keywords: phage therapy; *E. faecalis*; OrthoMCL

---

1. Introduction

Enterococcus is a genus of gram-positive non-spore-forming bacteria that typically inhabit the gastrointestinal tract (GIT), which currently contains thirty five well-recognized species [1], including *Enterococcus faecalis*. The enterococci possess a remarkable ability to adapt to different environments and have a propensity to acquire antibiotic resistance, which has led to the emergence of multi-drug resistant variants, across the genus [1]. *E. faecalis* is mainly described as a core commensal member of the human gut, but it can also act as an opportunistic pathogen and translocate across the mucosal barrier to cause systemic infections [2,3]. More than 90% of the bacterial isolates frequently recovered from clinical specimens (blood, and other infectious site samples) are *E. faecalis* and *E. faecium* [4,5]. Life-threatening infections generally linked to *E. faecalis* include endocarditis, bacteremia, urinary tract infections, meningitis, and root canal infections. In contrast, *E. faecalis* Symbioflor 1 strain (Symbiopharm, Herborn, Germany) has been demonstrated to be a safe and effective probiotic and a few other enterococcal strains have been used as starter cultures in the cheese industry [6]. However, the genus *Enterococcus* is not listed in the Qualified Presumption of Safety (QPS) of the European Food

Safety Authority, nor does it have a generally regarded as safe (GRAS) status [6]. Hence the continued use of enterococci in traditional fermented foods and as probiotics, is controversial, because of their association with human infections [7].

Antimicrobial resistance (AMR) causes 700,000 global deaths each year, and it is estimated that it will rise to 10 million deaths by 2050 [7,8]. The high prevalence of Multi-Drug Resistant (MDR) bacteria and inefficiency of available antibiotics to overcome infectious diseases, has inspired a search for viable alternatives. Bacteriophages, also known as phages, and their associated cell wall lysing enzymes (endolysins), have the potential to be useful tools to combat MDR pathogens [9–11].

Phages are prokaryotic viruses that have the ability to infect and replicate within their host bacterial cell, and to subsequently lyse the cell, to release their progeny. Based on their replication strategy, phages can undergo two different life cycles; the lytic (virulent) and the lysogenic (temperate). Naturally virulent phages are suitable candidates for phage therapy, but temperate phages are not as useful. However, genome engineering strategies can be applied to convert temperate phages to virulent, for their effective use in phage therapy [12]. Phage therapy is described as the application of phages to treat bacterial infections [13,14]. There are some indications that phages could be suitable alternatives to combat *Enterococcus*-associated infections [2,15–18]. In this review, we focus on (i) phage therapy to treat *E. faecalis* infections using in vitro and in vivo models; (ii) the genetic relationships between currently isolated *E. faecalis* bacteriophages; (iii) identification of candidates suitable for phage therapy; (iv) *E. faecalis* phages endolysins as alternative to phage therapy; and (v) conclusions and recommendations for further development of *E. faecalis* phage therapy.

2. The Necessity of *E. faecalis* Phage Therapy

E. faecalis is one of the first colonizers of the human GIT and it plays a role in intestinal immune development at the very early stages of life [19]. *E. faecalis* is a ubiquitous microorganism that possesses the ability to survive and persist in a broad range of environments. In susceptible hosts, *E. faecalis* can act as an opportunistic pathogen, causing severe infections, including urinary tract infections (UTIs), endocarditis, bacteremia, catheter-related infections, wound infections, and intra-abdominal and pelvic infections [1].

An important question is, what makes this bacterium an opportunistic pathogen and under what circumstances? The key factors linked to the pathogenic role of *E. faecalis* in the GIT is its ability to generate reactive oxygen species (ROS) and extracellular superoxide, which can cause genomic instability and damage to the colonic DNA [20]. Opportunistic infection has been associated with the production of virulence factors, adherence to Caco-2 and HEP-2 cells, capacity for biofilm formation and resistance to antimicrobials [21–23]. Numerous virulence factors have been identified that are associated with a wide range of *E. faecalis* infections; namely, aggregation substance (AS), adhesion to collagen of *E. faecalis* (Ace), cell wall glycopeptides, gelatinase (GelE) and biofilm-associated Pili (Ebp), Enterococcal fibronectin-binding protein A (EfbA), membrane metalloprotease (Eep), and biofilm formation. AS is a pheromone-inducible plasmid-encoded cell surface protein, involved in bacterial aggregation during conjugation, via binding to the enterococcal binding substance (EBS) [22–26]. There are three AS proteins (Asa1, Asc10, and Asp1), which belong to a family of surface adhesions and are highly similar to each other. These factors are responsible for the initial adherence and biofilm formation at infected sites [25,27]. Other important cell wall-associated virulence factors are pili and fimbriae, which are anchored to the outer cell surface of the bacterium and aid the bacterium to adhere to host cells. In *E. faecalis*, these are encoded by a three-gene locus (ebpABC), with an associated enzyme sortase, srtC. This ebpABC locus has also been shown to encode proteins involved in biofilm formation [24,28].

Other virulence factors such as Ace, a cell-wall anchored adhesion, plays a pivotal role in in vitro adherence [27,29]. Similarly, EfbA, located on the outer cell membrane, confers adhesion to the host glycoprotein fibronectin [30]. One more critical virulence factor is GelE, an extracellular zinc-metallo protease that contributes to the degradation of various host proteins, such as collagen, fibrinogen, fibrin, and immune complement components C3 and C3a. Many of these factors associated with virulence are also known to promote biofilm formation in *E. faecalis*, suggesting that biofilms are crucial to development of severe infections [31].

In addition, *E. faecalis* is intrinsically resistant to numerous antibiotics, such as penicillin, ampicillin, piperacillin, imipenem, and vancomycin—which have only bacteriostatic rather than bactericidal effects [32]. Over the last decade vancomycin-resistant *E. faecalis* (VREF), together with the other vancomycin-resistant enterococci (VRE), have generated much concern. In the context of a cumulative mortality rate of 20–40% for infective endocarditis, generated by *E. faecalis* and *E. faecium*, *E. faecalis* accounts for approximately 97% of cases [33]. In contrast to that, in leukemia patients, the VR *E. faecium* is more prevalent, accounting for 84%, followed by *E. faecalis* accounting for 6% and the rest 10% was occupied by all other *Enterococcus* sp. [34] and these percentages slightly varied in different studies [35]. In addition, it has been reported that VR *E. faecium* was the leading cause of early infection-related mortality in older (≥60 years) acute leukemia patients, who were receiving induction chemotherapy [36]. Moreover, enterococcal bloodstream infections occurs frequently in patients with acute leukemia, and causes significant morbidity and mortality (87% due to *E. faecium*, while only 13% due to *E. faecalis*) [37]. However, the role of *E. faecalis* and *E. faecium* in colorectal cancer and other diseases such as inflammatory bowel disease (IBD), remains unclear, and their involvement in colorectal cancer is still under investigation [38]. It is presumed that it is the inefficient activity of β-lactams, as well as the biofilm-forming ability of *E. faecalis* which makes these infections difficult to treat. Often, combinations of antibiotic therapies are required for treatment of severe infections associated with *E. faecalis*. However, even these antibiotic treatment options are limited, considering that 50% of isolates exhibit a high-level of aminoglycoside resistance, mediated by aminoglycoside-modifying enzymes, which eliminate the synergistic bactericidal effect, usually seen when a cell wall-active agent is combined with an aminoglycoside [33,39].

3. Strategies for Obtaining *E. faecalis* Phages for Phage Therapy

There are several advantages associated with bacteriophages over antibiotics to treat bacterial infections. For example, unlike antibiotics, bacteriophages are highly specific to their corresponding target and, thus, do not perturb indigenous microbial communities [13,40–42]. Phages targeting *Enterococcus* spp. have been isolated from various sources, like sewage, animal yard effluents, human feces, urogenital secretions or by inducing chromosomally integrated prophages [17,43–46].

In general, plaque and spot assays are the methods applied by researchers to isolate phages, using bacterial hosts of interest. In an attempt to increase the recovery of phages from environments where they are scarce, a pre-enrichment step has been widely used, prior to plaque/spot assay. In the case of *E. faecalis*, typically, vancomycin-resistant strains or other clinical isolates have been used for screening, in order to realize the potential of phages as novel therapeutics [38,41].

Many factors can affect the process of phage isolation. For example, poor or invisible plaque morphology, difficulty in obtaining confluency of bacterial lawns, poor enrichment of samples containing very low numbers of phages, or sample availability [47]. Furthermore, bacterial host strains might adapt to routine laboratory culturing practices resulting in changes to their cell physiology. Such genotypic and phenotypic changes which occur during sub-culturing, can reduce the chances for the discovery new phages. To overcome such hurdles, Purnell et al. [37], suggest the isolation of target bacterial hosts, and their cognate bacteriophages, from the same sample, to achieve a higher success rate. Therefore, it is advisable to obtain a fresh culture from the glycerol stock and avoid multiple sub-culturing and serial broth-to-broth transfers, prior to phage isolation. In addition, bacteria can rapidly evolve to overcome phage infection by means of spontaneous mutation, or by acquiring CRISPR-*cas* mediated adaptive immunity, resulting in bacteriophage-insensitive mutants (BIMs) [48–50]. In addition, since multiple bacterial strains can be involved in diseases, the application of phage cocktails are deemed to be more appropriate over single-phage preparations, in therapeutic interventions [16].

4. Orthocluster Analysis of *E. faecalis* Phages

On the 30 December 2018, fifty-four *Enterococcus* phage genome sequences were available (http://millardlab.org/bioinformatics/bacteriophage-genomes/), of which 89% had *E. faecalis* and 11% had *E. faecium* as a target (Table S1). Usually, these phages infect both species at varying efficiencies [16,17,51–54].

To determine the gene content relationship between these bacteriophages, a cluster analysis was performed on the basis of the percentage of shared orthologous genes. For the orthocluster analysis, the phage genomes were downloaded from the NCBI database, and potential Open Reading Frames (ORFs) were predicted by Prodigal [55]. Identification of the bacteriophage protein Orthologous Groups (OG, cluster of proteins from at least two phages) was performed, using orthoMCL [56]. OrthoMCL phage clusters identified from this analysis were defined as "orthoclusters". This analysis allowed the identification of ten distinct and well-supported (100% bootstrap support) clusters of *Enterococcus* phage genomes. Of the fifty-four *Enterococcus* phage genomes, fifty-two fell into one of the ten distinct clusters, designated as orthoclusters I–V, VII, IX–X, as depicted in Figure 1. The remaining two phages used in this analysis, did not cluster with any other phages. Therefore, we hypothesize that the phages EF62phi and phiFL4, formed two different orthoclusters, V and VII, respectively. The distinct orthoclusters, typically contain phages of the same family, with similar genome size, GC content and morphology. The clustering was in good agreement with classical taxonomical phage families, as determined by the morphology and genome analysis—virulent *Myoviridae* family—orthocluster II, virulent *Siphoviridae* family—orthoclusters I, III, V, VII, IX, and X, temperate *Siphoviridae* family—orthoclusters IV and VIII, and temperate *Podoviridae* family—orthocluster V, and virulent *Podoviridae* family—orthocluster VI.

With respect to phage therapy, orthoclusters comprising native virulent phages, are of immense interest. Of the *Enterococcus* phages characterized to date, 77% are known to be virulent, and belong to the orthoclusters I, II, III, IV, VI, IX, and X. Although temperate phages have less obvious usefulness with respect to phage therapy, molecular mechanisms of phage conversion from temperate to virulent, might make this possible.

Orthocluster I, which is supported by a bootstrap value of 1000, contains 19 phages belonging to the *Siphoviridae* family. This orthocluster is particularly interesting as the phages differ significantly from each other, in terms of their genome length and mean GC content, features which are conserved among the other orthoclusters. The genome sizes range from ~17 kb to ~42 kb, and the mean GC content varies from 17.35% to 36.7%. The suitability of these phages for phage therapy is questionable, as the orthologous group 32, which belongs to orthocluster I, contains the putative metallo-beta-lactamase gene, a gene related to antibiotic resistance (Figure 2) [57,58]. All phages harbor this gene, except for EFRM31 and EFAP_1, within the orthocluster I. However, the functionality of this gene is currently unknown. Further studies are warranted to evaluate these phages and their involvement in antibiotic gene dissemination in the gut. In addition, gene editing tools could be applied to either delete or inactivate the metallo-beta-lactamase gene, before considering therapeutic applications. A study by Nezhad Fard et al. [59], demonstrated that the phage EFRM31 was efficient at transducing gentamicin resistance to multiple enterococcal species. In fact, this was the first example of inter-species host range generalized transduction, and thus, it did not support a role for such phages in therapeutic applications.

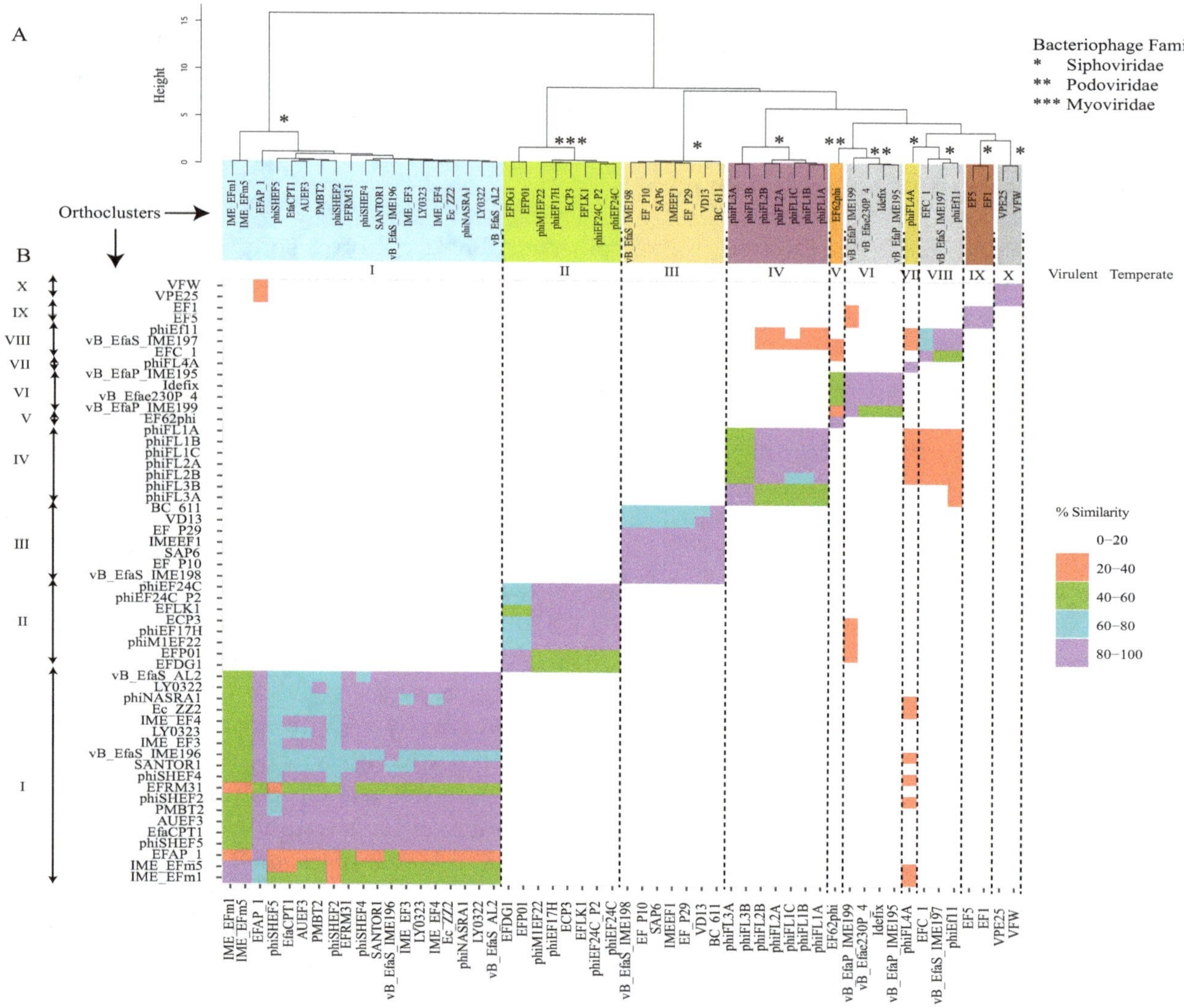

Figure 1. Genomic comparison of *Enterococcus* phages. (**A**) Neighbor-joining tree based on the percentage of shared orthologous genes (1000 bootstrap replicates); squares indicate the 10 phage putative orthoclusters. (**B**) Dot plot comparison of amino acids identity among the 10 orthoclusters; genes that share more than 40% homology were considered as being part of the same orthologous group. The vertical axis shows phage clusters and phage IDs.

Interestingly, Orthocluster II incorporates all the *Myoviridae* phages described so far, which infect *E. faecalis*. These phages can infect and proliferate in multiple strains of *E. faecalis* and *E. faecium* strains. The size of the genomes ranged between ~130 kb to ~150 kb, and the mean GC content was estimated to be 35.3% to 37.2%. These phages were related to SPO1-like viruses, such as the *Staphylococcus* phage K, *Listeria* phage P100, and *Lactobacillus* phage LP65. Interestingly, no *E. faecalis* temperate phages belonging to the *Myoviridae* family have ever been described [16,60].

Orthocluster III contains the most studied *E. faecalis* virulent phages from the *Siphoviridae* family (genus *Sap6virus*). The size of the genomes ranged between ~53 kb to ~59 kb, and the mean GC content was estimated to be 39% to 40%. These phages exhibited a broad host range and a high level of efficiency in in vitro and in vivo studies, which have been discussed in more detail, later on. Genome analysis did not reveal any putative virulence factors or antibiotic-resistant genes, and to date no transduction potential has been described. Members of this orthocluster should, therefore, be considered and studied with respect to their therapeutic potential [61,62].

The phages from Orthocluster IV were induced using norfloxacin and UV from bacteremia isolates of the *Enterococcus* sp. These temperate phages belonged to the *Siphoviridae* family, with a genome size of 30–40 kb, and a mean GC content of 30%–40%. Currently, only virulent phages have been considered as suitable candidates for phage therapy, but there is a possibility to convert these lysogenic phages to virulent entities, which would allow us to investigate these phages in the context of phage therapy. However, the use of genetically-modified phages, is not acceptable, for now [12]. Further inspection of the orthocluster IV harboring temperate phages, revealed their ability to pack its bacterial host DNA, a generalized transduction potential event observed in some other temperate phages, as well. As a result, these phages are not suitable for phage therapy. It is unfortunate that on rare occasions generalized transduction events have also been observed in some virulent phages [43].

The *Podoviridae* phage, EF62phi (~30 kb, mean GC content 32.7%) which forms the putative orthocluster V, is a pseudotemperate linear bacteriophage identified in the genome of *E. faecalis* strain 62, isolated from a healthy Norwegian infant. EF62ph is the only pseudotemperate enterococcal phage described to date. EF62ph is maintained in the bacterial genome by means of RepB and a toxin–antitoxin system [63]. There have been no studies, so far, on pseudotemperate enterococcal phages and their involvement in phage therapy.

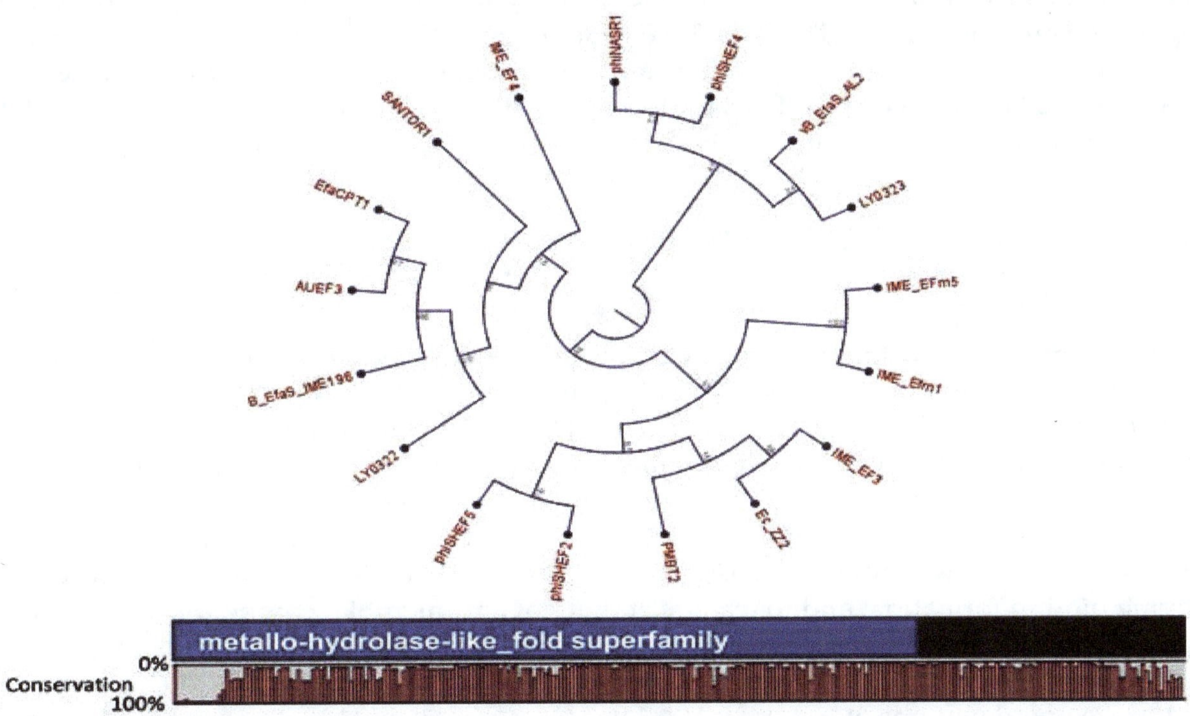

Figure 2. Maximum likelihood phylogenetic analysis sequence relatedness of the *Enterococcus faecalis* phage putative metallo-beta-lactamase gene (orthologous group 32); tree node labels represent bootstrap values.

Orthocluster VI is comprised of the *Podoviridae* phages, of the genus *Ahjdlikevirus*. These phages have been isolated from sewage, and infect both *E. faecalis* and *E. faecium* strains. The size of the genomes range from ~17 kb to ~18 kb, and have a mean GC content of 33.2% to 34.6%. With no evidence of antibiotic-resistance-associated genes or transduction potential, these phages should be explored further for potential therapeutic applications [17,54,64].

The phage phiFL4A, which forms the putative orthocluster VII (*Siphoviridae* family, *Phifelvirus* genus, 37 kb, mean GC content 37.8%) was induced from bacteremia isolates, using mitomycin C, in the same study as that of the phages of orthocluster IV. This phage is also temperate and has the ability of generalized transduction and, therefore, is not eligible for phage therapy [43].

Orhocluster VIII contains three temperate prophages and is part of the *Siphoviridae* family. phiEf11 was induced with mitomycin C from the root isolate *E. faecalis* TUSoD11 [65], EFC1 was induced with mitomycin C from the raw milk isolate *E. faecalis* KBL101 [66] and vB_EfaS_IME197 was isolated from sewage. The size of the genomes range from ~40 kb to ~42 kb and the mean GC content from 34% to 35%. This group is particularly interesting from the point of view of phage therapy, as Ef11 phage have been converted from temperate to virulent, followed by successful testing against *E. faecalis*. Therefore, the temperate phages from this orthocluster opens the direction for a new type of *E. faecalis* phage therapy, based on genetically engineered phages [67–69]

The phages that form orthocluster IX, EF1, and EF5, were previously annotated as part of the *Myoviridae* family. However, our genome annotation using RASTtk and BLAST suggest that these two virulent phages are part of the *Siphoviridae* family. By comparison with the other *Siphoviridae* virulent *E. faecalis* phages, these two phages have a large genome of 141.996 kb, with a mean content GC of 31.9%. Larger genomes are typical for *Myoviridae* family, which may be the reason for their previous attribution in the database. No therapeutic studies have been performed using these phages and, therefore, their potential role in phage therapy could not be predicted. Despite this, our genome analysis did not reveal any genes that would hinder further research of these phages for therapeutic potential.

Phages VPE25 and VFW formed orthocluster X. They were isolated from sewage and shared 95% homology at the nucleotide level. The size of the genomes of both phages was ~86 kb, with a mean GC of 33.2%. VPE25 and VFW were obligate lytic and their isolation, using VR *E. faecalis* V583 as a host, suggested them to be putative candidates for therapy [70].

Phages from each of the described orthocluster are now discussed in more details, with respect to the published in vitro and in vivo phage therapy studies.

5. *E. faecalis* Phage Therapy in In Vitro Models

5.1. *Biofilm Eradication*

Various studies describe the ability of single phage or phage cocktails in the treatment of bacterial biofilms. For example, biofilms formed by pathogenic bacteria *Streptococcus mutants* [71], *E. coli* [72], *Pseudomonas aeruginosa* [73], *Staphylococcus aureus* [74], and *E. faecalis* [75], can be disrupted by phages. Phage treatment is more efficient against biofilms, compared to conventional antibiotics, since, as the phages infect the bacteria from the upper layer, upon replication they release a new virion progeny, which subsequently attacks the bottom layer(s). As a result of this layer-by-layer mode of action, the biofilms are effectively eradicated [75,76]. Microtiter plates are the most commonly used method for studying biofilm formation, and to test the activity of antimicrobial compounds. More advanced techniques like confocal microscopy can also be applied for the visualization of biofilm matrices, before and after phage treatment [77]. Using this method, the efficiency of phage EFDG1 (orthocluster II) to reduce two-week-old biofilms of *E. faecalis* V583 has been described [18]. The genetically-engineered orthocluster VIII phage phiEf11 (phiEf11/phiFL1C(Δ36)PnisA [67]), reduced the static biofilm of *E. faecalis* strains JH2-2 (pMSP3535 nisR/K) and V583 (pMSP3535nisR/K), which had formed on coverslips. After 24 and 48 h of incubation, a 10–100-fold decrease in viable cells (CFU/biofilm) was observed [69].

5.2. *Human Root Canal Model (In Vitro/Ex Vivo)*

E. faecalis has been found, over time, to be more prevalent (24% to 77% of cases) in asymptomatic and persistent endodontic infections [78,79]. The extreme survival ability and highly adaptive nature of *E. faecalis* in harsh environments, allows the bacterium to cause persistent infections in root canals. Furthermore, it can resist nutritional deprivation and invade dental tubules to form endodontic biofilms. In this scenario, treatment with 2% chlorhexidine, combined with sodium hypochlorite, is generally effective. However, a number of failures have been recorded in endodontic treatment, due to technical difficulties associated with dental practices [78,80]. Therefore, the development of alternative strategies are necessary to prevent such situations. In this regard, the efficacy of phage treatment has been evaluated using an ex vivo two chamber bacterial leakage model of human teeth [18]. No turbidity was observed in the obturated root canals, which were subjected to 10^8 PFU/mL of EFDG1 phage (orthocluster II) irrigation and the results also indicated a 7-log reduction of bacterial leakage, from the root apex, when compared to the control. In a similar study, Paisano et al. [81] showed that a phage lysate of 2×10^8 PFU/mL was able to significantly inhibit *E. faecalis* in human dental roots inoculated for 6 days with a suspension of *E. faecalis* ATCC 29212 at the three different multiplicities of infection; 0.1, 1.0, and 10.0. Moreover, in the study of Tinoco et al [12]. extracted human dentin root segments were cemented into a sealable double-chamber and inoculated for 7 days, with an overnight suspension of either VR *E. faecalis* V583, or *E. faecalis* JH2-2, which is vancomycin sensitive, but resistant to fusidic acid and rifampin. The treatment with genetically-engineered phage, phiEf11/phiFL1C (Δ36)PnisA, generated a reduction of 18% for the JH2-2-infected models, and by 99% for the V583-infected models. These examples certainly strengthen the efficacy of phage therapy in the treatment of *E. faecalis* root canal infections.

5.3. Fibrin Clot Model

Clots are gel-like clumps of blood that occurs when thrombin converts fibrinogen to fibrin, a structural protein that assembles into a polymer [82]. An in vitro fibrin clot model has been successfully used to test the role of antibiotics in the treatment of bacterial endocarditis [83], demonstrating the in vitro clotting ability of bacterial strains *Bacillus cereus* [84], *Staphylococcus aureus* [85], *E. faecalis* [86], and *E. faecium* [83,84]. Recently, the in vitro fibrin clot model has been used to demonstrate the efficacy of individual phages and phage cocktails [16]. The authors spiked the plasma with vancomycin-resistant and sensitive *E. faecalis* strains, and triggered the plasma coagulation with the addition of bovine thrombin and $CaCl_2$. The resultant clots were subjected to a 10^8 PFU/mL bacteriophage treatment. Bacterial counts were significantly reduced by 3–6 logs, after treatment with phage(s) EFDG1 and EFLK1 (orthocluster II).

5.4. *E. faecalis* Phages as Biocontrol Agents

Bacteriophages have long been recognized as effective biological entities in the control of undesired foodborne bacteria. In 2007, a *Listeria*-specific bacteriophage preparation, Listex P100, obtained U.S. FDA approval for use as a biopreservative, in ready-to-eat meat products (U.S. Food and Drug Administration, 2007). In a recent study, phage Q69 has been shown to be effective against *E. faecalis*, in a cheese model system. This phage significantly reduced *E. faecalis* numbers and subsequently eliminated the accumulation of toxic biogenic amine tyramine, during cheese ripening [87].

6. *E. faecalis* Phage Therapy in In Vivo Models

To date, we are only aware of a single human study describing the phage treatment *of E. faecalis* associated chronic prostatitis (Table 1). Three subjects were selected for phage therapy who had failed to respond to antibiotic, auto-vaccine, and laser bio-stimulation treatments. During phage treatment, 10 mL of bacterial phage lysate was rectally applied, twice daily, for 30 days. In all three cases, the pathogen was eradicated, clinical symptoms abated, and early disease recurrence was not observed [88].

Table 1. Target infections, phage dosage, and outcomes in *Enterococcus faecalis* phage therapy in vivo models.

Disease (Target Strain)	No (n) and Type of Subjects	Form and Dosage	Application Route and Clinical Outcome	Reference
Chronic bacterial prostatitis	$n = 3$ human male	Phage lysate ~10^7–10^9 PFU/mL	Rectal Pathogen eradication, Abatement of clinical symptoms Lack of early disease recurrence	[88]
Infection (EF14 VRE2)	$n = 20$; BALB/c mice female 6 to 8 week old	CsCl; 1×10^{12} PFU/mL;	Intraperitoneal; Significantly effective, Efficiently rescued mice;	[89]
Bacteremia (VAN)	$n = 5$ BALB/c mice 1 month old	CsCl 3×10^8 PFU/mL	Intraperitoneal 100% survival 45 min after bacterial challenge 50% of moribund mice rescued after delayed phage administration	[90]
Sepsis 002	$n = 8$ 7 different dosage groups BALB/c female mice 6 to 8 weeks old	PEG 3.9×10^9 PFU/mL or 0.2 mg endolysin	Intraperitoneal 60% survival at 30 min post bacterial inoculation 40% survival at 4 h post bacterial administration	[52]
E. faecalis challenge	$n = 10$ 5 different dosage groups BALB/c F 6 to 8 weeks old	CsCl 4×10^3, 4×10^4, 4×10^5, 4×10^6, 4×10^7 PFU/mouse	Intraperitoneal Mice were protected from the infection	[91]
Septic peritonitis	$n = 15$ 4 groups ICR(CD-1C)	Dialyzed phage lysate 2×10^8	Intraperitoneal 100% survival No harmful effect on the microbiome	[60]
E. faecalis challenge (VAN)	$n = 5$ 4 different groups BALB/c n female mice 6 to 8 weeks old	LysEF-P10 endolysin 1 µg, 5 µg, 10 µg	Intraperitoneal Reduced *E. faecalis* colonization Alleviated the gut microbiota imbalance caused by VRE	[92]

VAN- experiment performed using vancomycin resistant *E. faecalis*; CsCl- Cesium chloride gradient purified phages; PEG- phage prepared by PEG precipitation.

Other positive results obtained on treating infectious disease unresponsive to antibiotics, caused by other bacteria, such as *S. aureus*, *E. coli*, *Klebsiella*, *Proteus*, *Pseudomonas*, and *Enterobacter*, support the idea of using phage therapy against antibiotic-resistant *E. faecalis* [93]. All highlight the efficiency of phages in disease resolution, and as future options for treating multi-drug-resistant bacterial infections. Another example describes a life-threatening multi-drug-resistant pathogen *Acinetobacter baumannii* infection, which was treated with an intravenous bacteriophage cocktail. This reversed the patient's clinical trajectory, cleared the *A. baumannii* infection, and restored the individual from a state of coma to complete health [94]. More clinical scenarios like these will undoubtedly open new avenues for phages or phage-derived enzybiotics as biotherapeutics, to combat situations where antibiotic treatments are no longer viable.

6.1. Vertebrate Models

Meanwhile, some studies have shown the efficacy of phages, in vivo, against *E. faecalis*, using mouse models (Table 1). An intraperitoneal application of phages, significantly rescued mice, when deliberately challenged with the *E. faecalis* EF14 and *E. faecalis* VRE2 strains [95]. Similarly, another study has showed that mice treated with different phage doses were protected from the VREF systemic infection, and alleviated the gut microbial imbalance that occurred as a result of infection [91]. In another study, a single dose of the lytic phage cocktail was effective in completely reversing a 100% mortality in a septic peritonitis mouse model caused by VREF, and without causing any collateral damage to the gut microbiome [60]. Furthermore, phage therapy has proven to be safe and effective in treating *E. faecalis*-induced bacteremia [90] and sepsis [52], in mouse models.

6.2. Invertebrate Models

The larvae of wax moth *Galleria mellonella* has been used as a model system to examine pathogenesis of many bacteria, such as *S. aureus*, *P. aeruginosa*, *L. monocytogenes*, *Klebsiella pneumoniae*, *E. faecalis*, and *E. faecium*, and the fungi *Candida albicans* and *Aspergillus fumigatus* [96–100]. This model involves monitoring *G. mellonella* caterpillars infected with bacterial culture, followed by the administration of a test drug or saline solution as a negative control. A number of *E. faecalis* virulence gene factors have been associated with larval mortality [101]. This method has been demonstrated as a suitable model for studying *E. faecalis*-drug interaction, for example, studies have used distamycin, linezolid, rifampicin, and extracts of *Zingiber officinale* [101–103]. The most significant advantage of this model is that it allows a precise measurement of the inoculum and the quantity of the administrated drug, over time. Not only are promising results obtained using this larval model, but it involves simple methodological approaches. To date, there are no reports of phages treatment of *E. faecalis* in *G. mellonella*. However, Yasmin et al. [43] infected *G. mellonella* with *E. faecalis* JH2-2 lysogenized by phiFL3A and phiFL3B (orthocluster IV), and found that it increased the mortality of caterpillars. Conversely, some of the other lysogens obtained in the same study, but with different phages, such as phiFL1B and phiFL2B (orthocluster IV), and phiFL4A (putative orthocluster VII), did not show any death in the caterpillars, when compared to the JH2-2 generic strain group. This *G. mellonella* model could be a valuable tool to pre-screen the ability of phages in an in vivo scenario, before performing large scale animal trials. In fact, the *Galleria* larval model has been used to examine the therapeutic potential of bacteriophages against other bacterial pathogens, such as *C. difficile* [104], *Burkholderia cepacia* [105], *Pseudomonas aeruginosa* [106], *Escherichia coli*, *K. pneumoniae*, *Enterobacter cloacae* [100], and *Cronobacter sakazakii* [107].

7. *E. faecalis* Phage Endolysins as Viable Alternatives for Phage Therapy

Endolysins, also termed phage lysins, have the ability to degrade the peptidoglycan layer of bacterial cell walls, leading to cell death. These phage-derived enzymes allow the release of nascent virions, following intracellular replication [108]. Endolysins possess a wide degree of killing activity, which also makes them potential therapeutic agents. Considering the bottlenecks associated with the production and purification of phages, to ensure the removal of host-derived endotoxins for therapeutic use, endolysin manufacture is a less arduous process, with a potentially similar outcome. Moreover, with the advent of mass sequencing technologies and the availability of curated gene functional databases, it is now possible to access the genomes of uncultured phages and their enigmatic gene content, to develop potential lytic enzymes, without the necessity for phage isolation. In fact, an in silico examination of uncultured phage genomes, revealed enormous diversity among endolysins [109]. With a varied host specificity and domain architecture, the development of robust novel antimicrobials for future application are within our reach.

7.1. *Domain Architecture of E. faecalis Phage Endolysins*

Based on their muralytic activity, four types of phage endolysins have already been identified; type I (lysozymes) and type II (transglycosidases); both of which act on the glycosidic bond linking the amino sugars in the cell wall. Type III (amidases) and type IV (endopeptidases), both act on the amide and peptide bonds of the oligopeptide cross-linking stems [110]. Endolysins typically consist of an N-terminal catalytic domain targeting the peptidoglycan network, and a C-terminal cell wall binding domain (termed as carbohydrate binding domain, CBD), which initializes the binding for corresponding enzymatic action, against the specific substrate (Loessner, 2005). A comprehensive in silico analysis on endolysin classes revealed that most (more than 74%) of the *E. faecalis* phage endolysins have an LysM module as a part of their Cell Binding Domain (CBD), whereas the Enzyme Catalytic Domain (ECD) consists of a glycosidase hydrolase (GH) module GH25 (the predominant one 50–74%) and cysteine, and hsitidine-dependent amidohydrolase/peptidase (CHAP) (accounting for less than 25%) (Oliveira et al. [111]). We identified a total of 54 putative and reference endolysin sequences in *E. faecalis* phages (Figure 3). They were clustered into orthologous groups (OGs) using OrthoMCL with default settings (Li et al. [57]). All but one (an endolysin associated with the phage EF62phi) clustered into one of the four distinct orthologous groups (OG 22, OG 28, OG 78, and OG 236), which mirrored the orthologous groups of their parental phages (Figures 2 and 3).

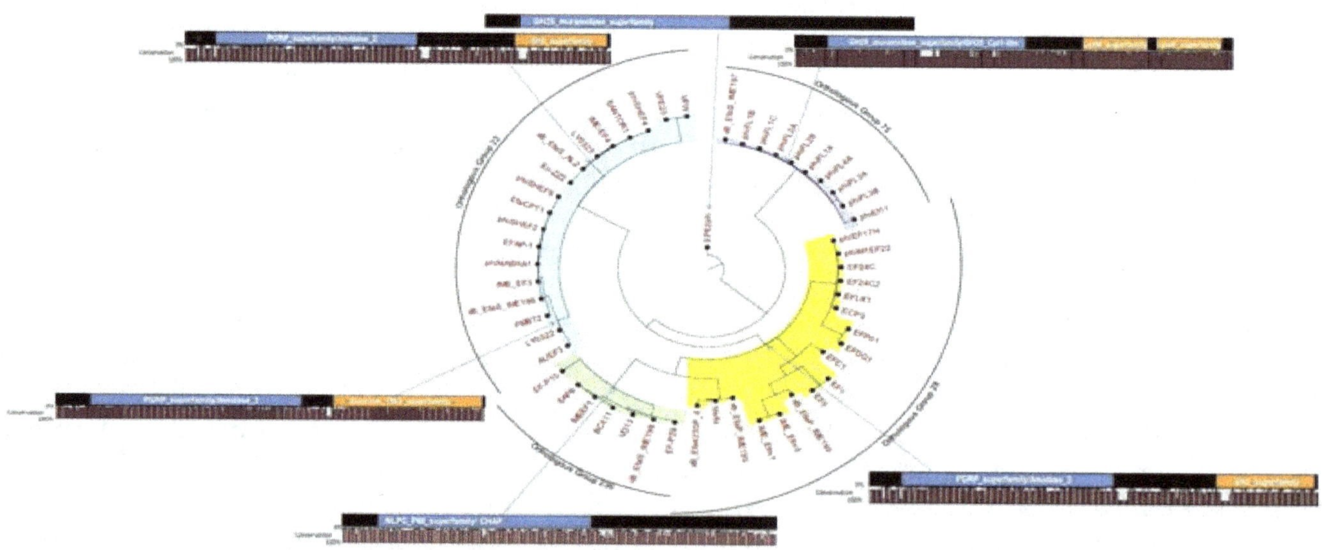

Figure 3. Maximum likelihood phylogenetic analysis sequence relatedness of *E. faecalis* phage endolysin functional domains; tree node labels represent the bootstrap values; the sequence similarity between functional domains is evidenced by using identical filling patterns; in blue—active domain; in orange—biding in domain; each of the four orthologous group is represented by a different color; Ef62phi could not be associated to any orthologous group.

One representative sequence was selected from each OG and subjected to HHMER [112] or HHPRED [113] analysis, to determine the protein domain architecture. Proteins assigned to the same OG often displayed the identical domain architectures, although a few exceptions were observed.

In the case of ECD, three major domains—GH25, Amidase_2, and CHAP—were observed across the four OGs, whereas in CBD, three domains—LysM, SH3, and PET-M23 (ZoocinA)—were identified (Figure 3). This observation was consistent with the findings of Oliveira et al. [114].

7.2. *Applications of E. faecalis Phage Endolysins*

Of note, endolysins could also be used in combination with traditional antibiotics to treat polyantibiotic-resistant bacterial pathogens. Many studies have shown the successful application of phage endolysins, in treating multi-drug resistant bacterial infections caused by *A. baumannii*, *S. aureus*, Methicillin resistance *S. aureus* (MRSA), *E. coli*, *Proteus mirabilis*, *Klebsiella*, *Pseudomonas*, *Morganella*, *Enterobacter*, *Enterococcus*, and *Salmonella* [111]. A small number of studies have demonstrated the in vivo efficacy of *E. faecalis* specific endolysins. One recent study evaluated endolysin LysEF-P10 to treat multi-drug resistant *E. faecalis* in a mouse model [92]. Here, a single intraperitoneal dose of 5 μg LysEF-P10 endolysin, was sufficient to eliminate the vancomycin resistant strain from the gut, without causing any collateral damage to the gut communities. Another study described the use of the endolysin IME-EF1, which protected 80% of mice challenged with a lethal dose of *E. faecalis* 002, and significantly reduced bacterial proliferation in the blood [52]. Several studies have described the in vitro antimicrobial action of *E. faecalis* endolysins. Heterologous expression of two endolysins Lys168 and Lys170 derived from *E. faecalis*, displayed a promising activity against clinical isolates of exponentially growing vancomycin-resistant and sensitive *E. faecalis* cultures, but failed to display a similar activity against log phase cultures [62]. Lys170 contains a catalytic domain of the amidase-2 family, which has an N-acetlymuramoyl-L-alanine amidase activity, while Lys168 was identified as being unique among the enterococcal phage endolysins, and highly similar to the endolysin of *S. aureus* phage SAP6, therefore, distantly related to all CHAP domain containing enterococcal endolysins [62]. In a follow-up study, these authors used a domain shuffling approach, by fusing a peptidase M23 catalytic domain to a cell-wall-binding domain of the native endolysin Lys170, to generate a bacteriolysin-like chimera, designated as EC300, to improve its anti- *E. faecalis* activity [115]. A recent study highlighted the advantage of using the phage endolysin IME-EFm5, over a narrow host range *E. faecalis* phage. Interestingly, the endolysin of phage IME-EFm5, displayed lytic activity against almost all tested strains [15]. Similarly, an expanded lytic activity of the *E. faecalis* bacteriophage ϕEF24C endolysin, ORF9 has been observed when heterologously expressed in *E. coli*. Further analysis has revealed that ORF9 belongs to the family of N-acetlymuramoyl-L-alanine amidases [44,116].

Antibacterial activity of a thermostable endolysin VD13 with an N-terminal CHAP domain has been demonstrated in vitro, against *E. faecalis*, with no activity observed against *E. faecium* or any other non-enterococcal strains tested [51]. In general, phage endolysins display a wider spectrum of activity than their parental phage counterparts.

8. Conclusions

We conclude that phages could provide a viable alternative therapy to antibiotics in the fight against *E. faecalis* infections. To date, only one clinical study has demonstrated the efficiency of *E. faecalis* phages in a clinical setting. However, there are increased chances of developing a successful phage therapy approach to an *E. faecalis* control, based on the in vitro and in vivo studies described in this review. As far as we are aware, no current phage clinical trials are focused on *E. faecalis*, but the outcomes of trials targeting other pathogens might be useful for the design of future *E. faecalis* phage therapy.

One of the issues of phage therapy is the narrow host range of the phages. In the case of *E. faecalis*, the diversity of phages showed in this review, based on the orthocluster identification, support the idea of expanding the phage host range by creating phage cocktails with a broader host range. It is unlikely that resistance will simultaneously occur for all virulent phages.

If this approach fails, there is the possibility of engineering temperate phages, as was done successfully for the *E. faecalis* phage phiEf11. Moreover, even if phages fail in providing a therapy for *E. faecalis*, their endolysins might prove to be a suitable alternative in the fight against *E. faecalis*-associated disease.

Author Contributions: Bioinformatics, writing, and editing, A.S.B.; writing and editing, A.U.; P.H.d.A.B.; writing, bioinformatics, and editing A.G.C.; writing and editing, L.A.D.; supervision and editing R.P.R. and C.H.

References

1. Arias, C.A.; Contreras, G.A.; Murray, B.E. Management of multidrug-resistant enterococcal infections. *Clin. Microbiol. Infect.* **2010**, *16*, 555–562. [CrossRef] [PubMed]
2. Sava, I.G.; Heikens, E.; Huebner, J. Pathogenesis and immunity in enterococcal infections. *Clin. Microbiol. Infect.* **2010**, *16*, 533–540. [CrossRef]
3. Berg, R.D. The indigenous gastrointestinal microflora. *Trends Microbiol.* **1996**, *4*, 430–435. [CrossRef]
4. Facklam, R.R.; da Carvalho, M.G.S.; Teixeira, L.M. History, Taxonomy, Biochemical Characteristics, and Antibiotic Susceptibility Testing of Enterococci. In *The Enterococci*; American Society of Microbiology: Washington, DC, USA, 2002; pp. 1–54.
5. Simonsen, G.S.; Småbrekke, L.; Monnet, D.L.; Sørensen, T.L.; Møller, J.K.; Kristinsson, K.G.; Lagerqvist-Widh, A.; Torell, E.; Digranes, A.; Harthug, S.; et al. Prevalence of resistance to ampicillin, gentamicin and vancomycin in Enterococcus faecalis and Enterococcus faecium isolates from clinical specimens and use of antimicrobials in five Nordic hospitals. *J. Antimicrob. Chemother.* **2003**, *51*, 323–331. [CrossRef] [PubMed]
6. Hanchi, H.; Mottawea, W.; Sebei, K.; Hammami, R. The Genus Enterococcus: Between Probiotic Potential and Safety Concerns—An Update. *Front. Microbiol.* **2018**, *9*, 1791. [CrossRef] [PubMed]
7. O'Neill, J. AMR Review Paper-Tackling a Crisis for the Health and Wealth of Nations. Available online: http://www.jpiamr.eu/wp-content/uploads/2014/12/AMR-Review-Paper-Tackling-a-crisis-for-the-health-and-wealth-of-nations_1-2.pdf (accessed on 19 April 2019).
8. Tagliabue, A.; Rappuoli, R. Changing Priorities in Vaccinology: Antibiotic Resistance Moving to the Top. *Front. Immunol.* **2018**, *9*, 1068. [CrossRef] [PubMed]
9. Bolocan, A.S.; Callanan, J.; Forde, A.; Ross, P.; Hill, C. Phage therapy targeting Escherichia coli-a story with no end? *FEMS Microbiol. Lett.* **2016**, *363*. [CrossRef] [PubMed]
10. Kortright, K.E.; Chan, B.K.; Koff, J.L.; Turner, P.E. Phage Therapy: A Renewed Approach to Combat Antibiotic-Resistant Bacteria. *Cell Host Microbe* **2019**, *25*, 219–232. [CrossRef] [PubMed]
11. Brüssow, H. Phage therapy: The Escherichia coli experience. *Microbiology* **2005**, *151*, 2133–2140. [CrossRef]
12. Pires, D.P.; Cleto, S.; Sillankorva, S.; Azeredo, J.; Lu, T.K. Genetically Engineered Phages: A Review of Advances over the Last Decade. *Microbiol. Mol. Biol. Rev.* **2016**, *80*, 523–543.
13. Moelling, K.; Broecker, F.; Willy, C. A Wake-Up Call: We Need Phage Therapy Now. *Viruses* **2018**, *10*, 688. [CrossRef] [PubMed]
14. Patey, O.; McCallin, S.; Mazure, H.; Liddle, M.; Smithyman, A.; Dublanchet, A. Clinical Indications and Compassionate Use of Phage Therapy: Personal Experience and Literature Review with a Focus on Osteoarticular Infections. *Viruses* **2018**, *11*, 18. [CrossRef] [PubMed]
15. Gong, P.; Cheng, M.; Li, X.; Jiang, H.; Yu, C.; Kahaer, N.; Li, J.; Zhang, L.; Xia, F.; Hu, L.; et al. Characterization of Enterococcus faecium bacteriophage IME-EFm5 and its endolysin LysEFm5. *Virology* **2016**, *492*, 11–20. [CrossRef]
16. Khalifa, L.; Gelman, D.; Shlezinger, M.; Dessal, A.L.; Coppenhagen-Glazer, S.; Beyth, N.; Hazan, R. Defeating Antibiotic- and Phage-Resistant Enterococcus faecalis Using a Phage Cocktail in Vitro and in a Clot Model. *Front. Microbiol.* **2018**, *9*, 326. [CrossRef]
17. Lossouarn, J.; Briet, A.; Moncaut, E.; Furlan, S.; Bouteau, A.; Son, O.; Leroy, M.; DuBow, M.; Lecointe, F.; Serror, P.; et al. Enterococcus faecalis Countermeasures Defeat a Virulent Picovirinae Bacteriophage. *Viruses* **2019**, *11*, 48. [CrossRef] [PubMed]
18. Khalifa, L.; Brosh, Y.; Gelman, D.; Coppenhagen-Glazer, S.; Beyth, S.; Poradosu-Cohen, R.; Que, Y.A.; Beyth, N.; Hazan, R. Targeting Enterococcus faecalis biofilms with phage therapy. *Appl. Environ. Microbiol.* **2015**, *81*, 2696–2705. [CrossRef] [PubMed]

19. Fanaro, S.; Chierici, R.; Guerrini, P.; Vigi, V. Intestinal microflora in early infancy: Composition and development. *Acta Paediatr.* **2007**, *92*, 48–55. [CrossRef]
20. Huycke, M.M.; Abrams, V.; Moore, D.R. Enterococcus faecalis produces extracellular superoxide and hydrogen peroxide that damages colonic epithelial cell DNA. *Carcinogenesis* **2002**, *23*, 529–536. [CrossRef]
21. Bhatty, M.; Cruz, M.R.; Frank, K.L.; Laverde Gomez, J.A.; Andrade, F.; Garsin, D.A.; Dunny, G.M.; Kaplan, H.B.; Christie, P.J. *Enterococcus faecalis* pCF10-encoded surface proteins PrgA, PrgB (aggregation substance) and PrgC contribute to plasmid transfer, biofilm formation and virulence. *Mol. Microbiol.* **2015**, *95*, 660–677. [CrossRef] [PubMed]
22. Kayaoglu, G.; Ørstavik, D. Virulence factors of Enterococcus faecalis: Relationship to endodontic disease. *Crit. Rev. Oral Biol. Med.* **2004**, *15*, 308–320. [CrossRef] [PubMed]
23. Upadhyaya, P.; Ravikumar, K.; Umapathy, B. Review of virulence factors of enterococcus: An emerging nosocomial pathogen. *Indian J. Med. Microbiol.* **2009**, *27*, 301. [CrossRef]
24. Singh, K.V.; Nallapareddy, S.R.; Murray, B.E. Importance of the *ebp* (Endocarditis- and Biofilm-Associated Pilus) Locus in the Pathogenesis of *Enterococcus faecalis* Ascending Urinary Tract Infection. *J. Infect. Dis.* **2007**, *195*, 1671–1677. [CrossRef]
25. Singh, K.V.; Nallapareddy, S.R.; Sillanpää, J.; Murray, B.E. Importance of the Collagen Adhesin Ace in Pathogenesis and Protection against Enterococcus faecalis Experimental Endocarditis. *PLoS Pathol.* **2010**, *6*, e1000716. [CrossRef]
26. Toledo-Arana, A.; Valle, J.; Solano, C.; Arrizubieta, M.J.; Cucarella, C.; Lamata, M.; Amorena, B.; Leiva, J.; Penadés, J.R.; Lasa, I. The enterococcal surface protein, Esp, is involved in Enterococcus faecalis biofilm formation. *Appl. Environ. Microbiol.* **2001**, *67*, 4538–4545. [CrossRef] [PubMed]
27. Nallapareddy, S.R.; Singh, K.V.; Duh, R.W.; Weinstock, G.M.; Murray, B.E. Diversity of ace, a gene encoding a microbial surface component recognizing adhesive matrix molecules, from different strains of Enterococcus faecalis and evidence for production of ace during human infections. *Infect. Immun.* **2000**, *68*, 5210–5217. [CrossRef] [PubMed]
28. Montealegre, M.C.; La Rosa, S.L.; Roh, J.H.; Harvey, B.R.; Murray, B.E. The Enterococcus faecalis EbpA Pilus Protein: Attenuation of Expression, Biofilm Formation, and Adherence to Fibrinogen Start with the Rare Initiation Codon ATT. *MBio* **2015**, *6*, e00467-15. [CrossRef] [PubMed]
29. Hubble, T.S.; Hatton, J.F.; Nallapareddy, S.R.; Murray, B.E.; Gillespie, M.J. Influence of Enterococcus faecalis proteases and the collagen-binding protein, Ace, on adhesion to dentin. *Oral Microbiol. Immunol.* **2003**, *18*, 121–126. [CrossRef] [PubMed]
30. Singh, K.V.; La Rosa, S.L.; Somarajan, S.R.; Roh, J.H.; Murray, B.E. The fibronectin-binding protein EfbA contributes to pathogenesis and protects against infective endocarditis caused by Enterococcus faecalis. *Infect. Immun.* **2015**, *83*, 4487–4494. [CrossRef] [PubMed]
31. Nallapareddy, S.R.; Qin, X.; Weinstock, G.M.; Höök, M.; Murray, B.E. Enterococcus faecalis adhesin, ace, mediates attachment to extracellular matrix proteins collagen type IV and laminin as well as collagen type I. *Infect. Immun.* **2000**, *68*, 5218–5224. [CrossRef]
32. Kristich, C.J.; Rice, L.B.; Arias, C.A. *Enterococcal Infection—Treatment and Antibiotic Resistance*; Massachusetts Eye and Ear Infirmary: Boston, MA, USA, 2014.
33. Beganovic, M.; Luther, M.K.; Rice, L.B.; Arias, C.A.; Rybak, M.J.; Laplante, K.L. A Review of Combination Antimicrobial Therapy for Enterococcus Faecalis Bloodstream Infections and Infective Endocarditis Citation/Publisher Attribution. *Clin. Infect. Dis.* **2018**, *2*, 303–309. [CrossRef]
34. Matar, M.J.; Safdar, A.; Rolston, K.V.I. Relationship of colonization with vancomycin-resistant enterococci and risk of systemic infection in patients with cancer. *Clin. Infect. Dis.* **2006**, *42*, 1506–1507. [CrossRef] [PubMed]
35. Gedik, H.; Şimşek, F.; Kantürk, A.; Yıldırmak, T.; Arıca, D.; Aydın, D.; Yokuş, O.; Demirel, N. Vancomycin-resistant enterococci colonization in patients with hematological malignancies: Screening and its cost-effectiveness. *Afr. Health Sci.* **2014**, *14*, 899. [PubMed]
36. Hicks, K.L.; Breto, L.; Halbur, L. *Vancomycin Resistant Enterococcus as a Leading Cause of Early Infection-Related Mortality in Older (≥60 Years) AML Patients Admitted to a Community Hospital for Standard Induction Chemotherapy*; American Society of Hematology: Washington, DC, USA, 2006.

37. Messina, J.A.; Sung, A.D.; Chao, N.J.; Alexander, B.D. *The Timing and Epidemiology of Enterococcus Faecium and E. Faecalis Bloodstream Infections (BSI) in Patients with Acute Leukemia Receiving Chemotherapy*; American Society of Hematology: Washington, DC, USA, 2017.
38. De Almeida, C.V.; Taddei, A.; Amedei, A. The controversial role of *Enterococcus faecalis* in colorectal cancer. *Ther. Adv. Gastroenterol.* **2018**, *11*, 175628481878360. [CrossRef] [PubMed]
39. Koehler, P.; Jung, N.; Cornely, O.A.; Rybniker, J.; Fätkenheuer, G. Combination Antimicrobial Therapy for *Enterococcus faecalis* Infective Endocarditis. *Clin. Infect. Dis.* **2019**. [CrossRef] [PubMed]
40. Abdelkader, K.; Gerstmans, H.; Saafan, A.; Dishisha, T.; Briers, Y. The Preclinical and Clinical Progress of Bacteriophages and Their Lytic Enzymes: The Parts are Easier than the Whole. *Viruses* **2019**, *11*, 96. [CrossRef]
41. Elbreki, M.; Ross, R.P.; Hill, C.; O'Mahony, J.; McAuliffe, O.; Coffey, A. Bacteriophages and Their Derivatives as Biotherapeutic Agents in Disease Prevention and Treatment. *J. Viruses* **2014**, *2014*, 1–20. [CrossRef]
42. Purnell, S.E.; Ebdon, J.E.; Taylor, H.D. Bacteriophage lysis of enterococcus host strains: A tool for microbial source tracking? *Environ. Sci. Technol.* **2011**, *45*, 10699–10705. [CrossRef] [PubMed]
43. Yasmin, A.; Kenny, J.G.; Shankar, J.; Darby, A.C.; Hall, N.; Edwards, C.; Horsburgh, M.J. Comparative genomics and transduction potential of Enterococcus faecalis temperate bacteriophages. *J. Bacteriol.* **2010**, *192*, 1122–1130. [CrossRef]
44. Uchiyama, J.; Rashel, M.; Maeda, Y.; Takemura, I.; Sugihara, S.; Akechi, K.; Muraoka, A.; Wakiguchi, H.; Matsuzaki, S. Isolation and characterization of a novel Enterococcus faecalis bacteriophage ϕEF24C as a therapeutic candidate. *FEMS Microbiol. Lett.* **2008**, *278*, 200–206. [CrossRef] [PubMed]
45. Santiago-Rodriguez, T.M.; De vila, C.; Gonzalez, J.; Bonilla, N.; Marcos, P.; Urdaneta, M.; Cadete, M.; Monteiro, S.; Santos, R.; Domingo, J.S.; et al. Characterization of Enterococcus faecalis-infecting phages (enterophages) as markers of human fecal pollution in recreational waters. *Water Res.* **2010**, *44*, 4716–4725. [CrossRef] [PubMed]
46. Bonilla, N.; Santiago, T.; Marcos, P.; Urdaneta, M.; Santo Domingo, J.; Toranzos, G.A. Enterophages, a group of phages infecting Enterococcus faecalis, and their potential as alternate indicators of human faecal contamination. *Water Sci. Technol.* **2010**, *61*, 293–300. [CrossRef] [PubMed]
47. Mullan, M. Factors Affecting Plaque Formation by Bacteriophages. *Dairy Sci.* **2002**, *5*, 1–12.
48. Örmälä, A.-M.; Jalasvuori, M. Phage therapy. *Bacteriophage* **2013**, *3*, e24219. [CrossRef]
49. Rostøl, J.T.; Marraffini, L. (Ph)ighting Phages: How Bacteria Resist Their Parasites. *Cell Host Microbe* **2019**, *25*, 184–194. [CrossRef] [PubMed]
50. Duerkop, B.A.; Palmer, K.L.; Horsburgh, M.J. Enterococcal Bacteriophages and Genome Defense. In *Enterococci: From Commensals to Leading Causes of Drug Resistant Infection*; Eye and Ear Infirmary: Boston, MA, USA, 2014.
51. Swift, S.M.; Rowley, D.T.; Young, C.; Franks, A.; Hyman, P.; Donovan, D.M. The endolysin from the *Enterococcus faecalis* bacteriophage VD13 and conditions stimulating its lytic activity. *FEMS Microbiol. Lett.* **2016**, *363*, fnw216. [CrossRef]
52. Zhang, W.; Mi, Z.; Yin, X.; Fan, H.; An, X.; Zhang, Z.; Chen, J.; Tong, Y. Characterization of Enterococcus faecalis phage IME-EF1 and its endolysin. *PLoS ONE* **2013**, *8*, e80435. [CrossRef] [PubMed]
53. Wang, Y.; Wang, W.; Lv, Y.; Zheng, W.; Mi, Z.; Pei, G.; An, X.; Xu, X.; Han, C.; Liu, J.; et al. Characterization and complete genome sequence analysis of novel bacteriophage IME-EFm1 infecting Enterococcus faecium. *J. Gen. Virol.* **2014**, *95*, 2565–2575. [CrossRef] [PubMed]
54. Wang, R.; Xing, S.; Zhao, F.; Li, P.; Mi, Z.; Shi, T.; Liu, H.; Tong, Y. Characterization and genome analysis of novel phage vB_EfaP_IME195 infecting Enterococcus faecalis. *Virus Genes* **2018**, *54*, 804–811. [CrossRef]
55. Hyatt, D.; Chen, G.-L.; LoCascio, P.F.; Land, M.L.; Larimer, F.W.; Hauser, L.J. Prodigal: Prokaryotic gene recognition and translation initiation site identification. *BMC Bioinform.* **2010**, *11*, 119. [CrossRef]
56. Li, L.; Stoeckert, C.J.; Roos, D.S.; Roos, D.S. OrthoMCL: Identification of ortholog groups for eukaryotic genomes. *Genome Res.* **2003**, *13*, 2178–2189. [CrossRef] [PubMed]
57. Li, X.; Ding, P.; Han, C.; Fan, H.; Wang, Y.; Mi, Z.; Feng, F.; Tong, Y. Genome analysis of Enterococcus faecalis bacteriophage IME-EF3 harboring a putative metallo-beta-lactamase gene. *Virus Genes* **2014**, *49*, 145–151. [CrossRef]
58. Son, J.S.; Jun, S.Y.; Kim, E.B.; Park, J.E.; Paik, H.R.; Yoon, S.J.; Kang, S.H.; Choi, Y.-J. Complete genome sequence of a newly isolated lytic bacteriophage, EFAP-1 of *Enterococcus faecalis*, and antibacterial activity of its endolysin EFAL-1. *J. Appl. Microbiol.* **2010**, *108*, 1769–1779. [CrossRef] [PubMed]

59. Mazaheri Nezhad Fard, R.; Barton, M.D.; Heuzenroeder, M.W. Bacteriophage-mediated transduction of antibiotic resistance in enterococci. *Lett. Appl. Microbiol.* **2011**, *52*, 559–564. [CrossRef]
60. Gelman, D.; Beyth, S.; Lerer, V.; Adler, K.; Poradosu-Cohen, R.; Coppenhagen-Glazer, S.; Hazan, R. Combined bacteriophages and antibiotics as an efficient therapy against VRE Enterococcus faecalis in a mouse model. *Res. Microbiol.* **2018**, *169*, 531–539. [CrossRef] [PubMed]
61. Lee, Y.-D.; Park, J.-H. Complete genome sequence of enterococcal bacteriophage SAP6. *J. Virol.* **2012**, *86*, 5402–5403. [CrossRef]
62. São-José, C.; Proença, D.; Leandro, C.; Fernandes, S.; Pimentel, M.; Mato, R.; Lopes, F.; Santos, S.; Cavaco-Silva, P.; Silva, F.A. Phage Endolysins with Broad Antimicrobial Activity Against Enterococcus faecalis Clinical Strains. *Microb. Drug Resist.* **2012**, *18*, 322–332.
63. Brede, D.A.; Snipen, L.G.; Ussery, D.W.; Nederbragt, A.J.; Nes, I.F. Complete genome sequence of the commensal Enterococcus faecalis 62, isolated from a healthy Norwegian infant. *J. Bacteriol.* **2011**, *193*, 2377–2378. [CrossRef] [PubMed]
64. Xing, S.; Zhang, X.; Sun, Q.; Wang, J.; Mi, Z.; Pei, G.; Huang, Y.; An, X.; Fu, K.; Zhou, L.; et al. Complete genome sequence of a novel, virulent Ahjdlikevirus bacteriophage that infects Enterococcus faecium. *Arch. Virol.* **2017**, *162*, 3843–3847. [CrossRef] [PubMed]
65. Stevens, R.H.; Porras, O.D.; Delisle, A.L. Bacteriophages induced from lysogenic root canal isolates of *Enterococcus faecalis*. *Oral Microbiol. Immunol.* **2009**, *24*, 278–284. [CrossRef] [PubMed]
66. Yoon, B.H.; Chang, H.-I. Genomic annotation for the temperate phage EFC-1, isolated from Enterococcus faecalis KBL101. *Arch. Virol.* **2015**, *160*, 601–604. [CrossRef]
67. Zhang, H.; Fouts, D.E.; DePew, J.; Stevens, R.H. Genetic modifications to temperate Enterococcus faecalis phage Ef11 that abolish the establishment of lysogeny and sensitivity to repressor, and increase host range and productivity of lytic infection. *Microbiology* **2013**, *159*, 1023–1035. [CrossRef] [PubMed]
68. Stevens, R.H.; Zhang, H.; Hsiao, C.; Kachlany, S.; Tinoco, E.M.B.; Depew, J.; Fouts, D.E.; Roy, F.; Stevens, H. Structural proteins of Enterococcus faecalis bacteriophage ϕEf11. *Bacteriophage* **2016**, *6*, e1251381. [CrossRef] [PubMed]
69. Tinoco, J.M.; Buttaro, B.; Zhang, H.; Liss, N.; Sassone, L.; Stevens, R. Effect of a genetically engineered bacteriophage on Enterococcus faecalis biofilms. *Arch. Oral Biol.* **2016**, *71*, 80–86. [CrossRef]
70. Duerkop, C.A.; Huo, B.A.; Bhardwaj, W.; Palmer, P.L.; Hooper, K.L. Molecular basis for lytic bacteriophage resistance in enterococci. *MBio* **2016**, *7*, 1304–1320. [CrossRef] [PubMed]
71. Dalmasso, M.; de Haas, E.; Neve, H.; Strain, R.; Cousin, F.J.; Stockdale, S.R.; Ross, R.P.; Hill, C. Isolation of a Novel Phage with Activity against Streptococcus mutans Biofilms. *PLoS ONE* **2015**, *10*, e0138651. [CrossRef]
72. Nazareth, N.; Magro, F.; Machado, E.; Ribeiro, T.G.; Martinho, A.; Rodrigues, P.; Alves, R.; Macedo, G.N.; Gracio, D.; Coelho, R.; et al. Prevalence of Mycobacterium avium subsp. paratuberculosis and Escherichia coli in blood samples from patients with inflammatory bowel disease. *Med. Microbiol. Immunol.* **2015**, *204*, 681–692. [CrossRef]
73. Fong, S.A.; Drilling, A.; Morales, S.; Cornet, M.E.; Woodworth, B.A.; Fokkens, W.J.; Psaltis, A.J.; Vreugde, S.; Wormald, P.-J. Activity of Bacteriophages in Removing Biofilms of Pseudomonas aeruginosa Isolates from Chronic Rhinosinusitis Patients. *Front. Cell. Infect. Microbiol.* **2017**, *7*, 418. [CrossRef]
74. Abdulamir, A.S.; Jassim, S.A.A.; Hafidh, R.R.; Bakar, F.A. The potential of bacteriophage cocktail in eliminating Methicillin-resistant Staphylococcus aureus biofilms in terms of different extracellular matrices expressed by PIA, ciaA-D and FnBPA genes. *Ann. Clin. Microbiol. Antimicrob.* **2015**, *14*, 49. [CrossRef]
75. Khalifa, L.; Shlezinger, M.; Beyth, S.; Houri-Haddad, Y.; Coppenhagen-Glazer, S.; Beyth, N.; Hazan, R. Phage therapy against Enterococcus faecalis in dental root canals. *J. Oral Microbiol.* **2016**, *8*, 32157. [CrossRef] [PubMed]
76. Szafrański, S.P.; Winkel, A.; Stiesch, M. The use of bacteriophages to biocontrol oral biofilms. *J. Biotechnol.* **2017**, *250*, 29–44. [CrossRef] [PubMed]
77. Sutherland, I.W.; Hughes, K.A.; Skillman, L.C.; Tait, K. The interaction of phage and biofilms. *FEMS Microbiol. Lett.* **2004**, *232*, 1–6. [CrossRef]
78. Stuart, C.H.; Schwartz, S.A.; Beeson, T.J.; Owatz, C.B. Enterococcus faecalis: Its role in root canal treatment failure and current concepts in retreatment. *J. Endod.* **2006** *32*, 93–98. [CrossRef] [PubMed]

79. Wang, Q.Q.; Zhang, C.F.; Chu, C.H.; Zhu, X.F. Prevalence of Enterococcus faecalis in saliva and filled root canals of teeth associated with apical periodontitis. *Int. J. Oral Sci.* **2012**, *4*, 19–23. [CrossRef]
80. Sundqvist, G.; Figdor, D.; Persson, S.; Sjögren, U. Microbiologic analysis of teeth with failed endodontic treatment and the outcome of conservative re-treatment. *Oral Surg. Oral Med. Oral Pathol. Oral Radiol. Endodontol.* **1998**, *85*, 86–93. [CrossRef]
81. Paisano, A.F.; Spira, B.; Cai, S.; Bombana, A.C. In vitro antimicrobial effect of bacteriophages on human dentin infected with Enterococcus faecalis ATCC 29212. *Oral Microbiol. Immunol.* **2004**, *19*, 327–330. [CrossRef] [PubMed]
82. Furie, B.; Furie, B.C. The molecular basis of blood coagulation. *Cell* **1988**, *53*, 505–518. [CrossRef]
83. Hershberger, E.; Coyle, E.A.; Kaatz, G.W.; Zervos, M.J.; Rybak, M.J. Comparison of a Rabbit Model of Bacterial Endocarditis and an In Vitro Infection Model with Simulated Endocardial Vegetations. *Antimicrob. Agents Chemother.* **2000**, *44*, 1921–1924. [CrossRef]
84. Kastrup, C.J.; Boedicker, J.Q.; Pomerantsev, A.P.; Moayeri, M.; Bian, Y.; Pompano, R.R.; Kline, T.R.; Sylvestre, P.; Shen, F.; Leppla, S.H.; et al. Spatial localization of bacteria controls coagulation of human blood by "quorum acting". *Nat. Chem. Biol.* **2008**, *4*, 742–750. [CrossRef]
85. McGrath, B.J.; Kang, S.L.; Kaatz, G.W.; Rybak, M.J. Bactericidal activities of teicoplanin, vancomycin, and gentamicin alone and in combination against Staphylococcus aureus in an in vitro pharmacodynamic model of endocarditis. *Antimicrob. Agents Chemother.* **1994**, *38*, 2034–2040. [CrossRef] [PubMed]
86. Houlihan, H.H.; Stokes, D.P.; Rybak, M.J. Pharmacodynamics of vancomycin and ampicillin alone and in combination with gentamicin once daily or thrice daily against Enterococcus faecalis in an in vitro infection model. *J. Antimicrob. Chemother.* **2000**, *46*, 79–86. [CrossRef]
87. Ladero, V.; Gómez-Sordo, C.; Sánchez-Llana, E.; del Rio, B.; Redruello, B.; Fernández, M.; Martín, M.C.; Alvarez, M.A. Q69 (an E. faecalis-Infecting Bacteriophage) As a Biocontrol Agent for Reducing Tyramine in Dairy Products. *Front. Microbiol.* **2016**, *7*, 445. [CrossRef]
88. Letkiewicz, S.; Międzybrodzki, R.; Fortuna, W.; Weber-Dąbrowska, B.; Górski, A. Eradication of Enterococcus faecalis by phage therapy in chronic bacterial prostatitis—Case report. *Folia Microbiol.* **2009**, *54*, 457–461. [CrossRef] [PubMed]
89. Uchiyama, J.; Rashel, M.; Takemura, I.; Wakiguchi, H.; Matsuzaki, S. In silico and in vivo evaluation of bacteriophage ϕEF24C, a candidate for treatment of Enterococcus faecalis infections. *Appl. Environ. Microbiol.* **2008**, *74*, 4149–4163. [CrossRef]
90. Biswas, B.; Adhya, S.; Washart, P.; Paul, B.; Trostel, A.N.; Powell, B.; Carlton, R.; Merril, R.; Merril, C.R. Bacteriophage Therapy Rescues Mice Bacteremic from a Clinical Isolate of Vancomycin-Resistant Enterococcus Bacteriophage Therapy Rescues Mice Bacteremic from a Clinical Isolate of Vancomycin-Resistant Enterococcus faecium. *Infect. Immun.* **2002**, *70*, 204–210. [CrossRef]
91. Cheng, M.; Liang, J.; Zhang, Y.; Hu, L.; Gong, P.; Cai, R.; Zhang, L.; Zhang, H.; Ge, J.; Ji, Y. The bacteriophage EF-P29 efficiently protects against lethal vancomycin-resistant Enterococcus faecalis and alleviates gut microbiota imbalance in a murine bacteremia model. *Front. Microbiol.* **2017**, *8*, 837. [CrossRef]
92. Cheng, M.; Zhang, Y.; Li, X.; Liang, J.; Hu, L.; Gong, P.; Zhang, L.; Cai, R.; Zhang, H.; Ge, J.; et al. Endolysin LysEF-P10 shows potential as an alternative treatment strategy for multidrug-resistant Enterococcus faecalis infections. *Sci. Rep.* **2017**, *7*, 10164. [CrossRef]
93. Weber-Dąbrowska, B.; Mulczyk, M.; Górski, A. Bacteriophage Therapy of Bacterial Infections: An Update of our Institute's Experience. In *Inflammation*; Springer: Dordrecht, The Netherlands, 2001; pp. 201–209.
94. Schooley, R.T.; Biswas, B.; Gill, J.J.; Hernandez-Morales, A.; Lancaster, J.; Lessor, L.; Barr, J.J.; Reed, S.L.; Rohwer, F.; Benler, S.; et al. Development and Use of Personalized Bacteriophage-Based Therapeutic Cocktails to Treat a Patient with a Disseminated Resistant Acinetobacter baumannii Infection. *Antimicrob. Agents Chemother.* **2017**, *61*, e00954-17. [CrossRef] [PubMed]
95. Uchiyama, J.; Matsui, H.; Murakami, H.; Kato, S.; Watanabe, N.; Nasukawa, T.; Mizukami, K.; Ogata, M.; Sakaguchi, M.; Matsuzaki, S.; et al. Potential Application of Bacteriophages in Enrichment Culture for Improved Prenatal Streptococcus agalactiae Screening. *Viruses* **2018**, *10*, 552. [CrossRef] [PubMed]
96. Kavanagh, K.; Fallon, J.P. Galleria mellonella larvae as models for studying fungal virulence. *Fungal Biol. Rev.* **2010**, *24*, 79–83. [CrossRef]
97. Mukherjee, K.; Altincicek, B.; Hain, T.; Domann, E.; Vilcinskas, A.; Chakraborty, T. Galleria mellonella as a model system for studying Listeria pathogenesis. *Appl. Environ. Microbiol.* **2010** *76*, 310–317. [CrossRef]

98. Ramarao, N.; Nielsen-Leroux, C.; Lereclus, D. The insect Galleria mellonella as a powerful infection model to investigate bacterial pathogenesis. *J. Vis. Exp.* **2012**, *70*, e4392. [CrossRef] [PubMed]
99. Kamal, F.; Dennis, J.J. Burkholderia cepacia complex phage-antibiotic synergy (PAS): Antibiotics stimulate lytic phage activity. *Appl. Environ. Microbiol.* **2015**, *81*, 1132–1138. [CrossRef] [PubMed]
100. Manohar, P.; Nachimuthu, R.; Lopes, B.S. The therapeutic potential of bacteriophages targeting gram-negative bacteria using Galleria mellonella infection model. *BMC Microbiol.* **2018**, *18*, 97. [CrossRef] [PubMed]
101. Goh, H.M.S.; Yong, M.H.A.; Chong, K.K.L.; Kline, K.A. Model systems for the study of Enterococcal colonization and infection. *Virulence* **2017**, *8*, 1525–1562. [CrossRef]
102. Eiko Maekawa, L.; Dennis Rossoni, R.; Oliveira Barbosa, J.; Olavo Cardoso Jorge, A.; Campos Junqueira, J.; Carneiro Valera, M.; José Longo, F. Different Extracts of Zingiber Officinale Decrease Enterococcus Faecalis Infection in Galleria Mellonella. *Braz. Dent. J.* **2015**, *26*, 105–109. [CrossRef]
103. Luther, M.K.; Arvanitis, M.; Mylonakis, E.; LaPlante, K.L. Activity of daptomycin or linezolid in combination with rifampin or gentamicin against biofilm-forming Enterococcus faecalis or E. faecium in an in vitro pharmacodynamic model using simulated endocardial vegetations and an in vivo survival assay using Galleria mellonella larvae. *Antimicrob. Agents Chemother.* **2014**, *58*, 4612–4620. [PubMed]
104. Nale, J.Y.; Chutia, M.; Carr, P.; Hickenbotham, P.T.; Clokie, M.R.J. "Get in early"; Biofilm and wax moth (Galleria mellonella) models reveal new insights into the therapeutic potential of Clostridium difficile bacteriophages. *Front. Microbiol.* **2016**, *7*, 1383. [CrossRef]
105. Seed, K.D.; Dennis, J.J. Experimental bacteriophage therapy increases survival of Galleria mellonella larvae infected with clinically relevant strains of the Burkholderia cepacia complex. *Antimicrob. Agents Chemother.* **2009**, *53*, 2205–2208. [CrossRef]
106. Beeton, M.L.; Alves, D.R.; Enright, M.C.; Jenkins, A.T.A. Assessing phage therapy against Pseudomonas aeruginosa using a Galleria mellonella infection model. *Int. J. Antimicrob. Agents* **2015**, *46*, 196–200. [CrossRef]
107. Abbasifar, R.; Kropinski, A.M.; Sabour, P.M.; Chambers, J.R.; MacKinnon, J.; Malig, T.; Griffiths, M.W. Efficiency of bacteriophage therapy against Cronobacter sakazakii in Galleria mellonella (greater wax moth) larvae. *Arch. Virol.* **2014**, *159*, 2253–2261. [CrossRef] [PubMed]
108. Schmelcher, M.; Donovan, D.M.; Loessner, M.J. Bacteriophage endolysins as novel antimicrobials. *Future Microbiol.* **2012**, *7*, 1147–1171. [CrossRef]
109. Fernández-Ruiz, I.; Coutinho, F.H.; Rodriguez-Valera, F. Thousands of Novel Endolysins Discovered in Uncultured Phage Genomes. *Front. Microbiol.* **2018**, *9*, 1033. [CrossRef]
110. Young, R.Y. Bacteriophage holins: Deadly diversity. *J. Mol. Microbiol. Biotechnol.* **2002**, *4*, 21–36.
111. Hill, C.; Mills, S.; Ross, R.P. Phages & antibiotic resistance: Are the most abundant entities on earth ready for a comeback? *Future Microbiol.* **2018**, *13*, 711–726.
112. Finn, R.D.; Clements, J.; Eddy, S.R. HMMER web server: Interactive sequence similarity searching. *Nucleic Acids Res.* **2011**, *39*, W29–W37. [CrossRef] [PubMed]
113. Söding, J.; Biegert, A.; Lupas, A.N. The HHpred interactive server for protein homology detection and structure prediction. *Nucleic Acids Res.* **2005**, *33*, W244–W248. [CrossRef]
114. Oliveira, H.; Melo, L.D.R.; Santos, S.B.; Nóbrega, F.L.; Ferreira, E.C.; Cerca, N.; Azeredo, J.; Kluskens, L.D. Molecular aspects and comparative genomics of bacteriophage endolysins. *J. Virol.* **2013**, *87*, 4558–4570. [CrossRef]
115. Proença, D.; Leandro, C.; Garcia, M.; Pimentel, M.; São-José, C. EC300: A phage-based, bacteriolysin-like protein with enhanced antibacterial activity against Enterococcus faecalis. *Appl. Microbiol. Biotechnol.* **2015**, *99*, 5137–5149. [CrossRef]
116. Uchiyama, J.; Takemura, I.; Hayashi, I.; Matsuzaki, S.; Satoh, M.; Ujihara, T.; Murakami, M.; Imajoh, M.; Sugai, M.; Daibata, M. Characterization of lytic enzyme open reading frame 9 (ORF9) derived from Enterococcus faecalis bacteriophage ϕEF24C. *Appl. Environ. Microbiol.* **2011**, *77*, 580–585. [CrossRef]

Permissions

All chapters in this book were first published by MDPI; hereby published with permission under the Creative Commons Attribution License or equivalent. Every chapter published in this book has been scrutinized by our experts. Their significance has been extensively debated. The topics covered herein carry significant findings which will fuel the growth of the discipline. They may even be implemented as practical applications or may be referred to as a beginning point for another development.

The contributors of this book come from diverse backgrounds, making this book a truly international effort. This book will bring forth new frontiers with its revolutionizing research information and detailed analysis of the nascent developments around the world.

We would like to thank all the contributing authors for lending their expertise to make the book truly unique. They have played a crucial role in the development of this book. Without their invaluable contributions this book wouldn't have been possible. They have made vital efforts to compile up to date information on the varied aspects of this subject to make this book a valuable addition to the collection of many professionals and students.

This book was conceptualized with the vision of imparting up-to-date information and advanced data in this field. To ensure the same, a matchless editorial board was set up. Every individual on the board went through rigorous rounds of assessment to prove their worth. After which they invested a large part of their time researching and compiling the most relevant data for our readers.

The editorial board has been involved in producing this book since its inception. They have spent rigorous hours researching and exploring the diverse topics which have resulted in the successful publishing of this book. They have passed on their knowledge of decades through this book. To expedite this challenging task, the publisher supported the team at every step. A small team of assistant editors was also appointed to further simplify the editing procedure and attain best results for the readers.

Apart from the editorial board, the designing team has also invested a significant amount of their time in understanding the subject and creating the most relevant covers. They scrutinized every image to scout for the most suitable representation of the subject and create an appropriate cover for the book.

The publishing team has been an ardent support to the editorial, designing and production team. Their endless efforts to recruit the best for this project, has resulted in the accomplishment of this book. They are a veteran in the field of academics and their pool of knowledge is as vast as their experience in printing. Their expertise and guidance has proved useful at every step. Their uncompromising quality standards have made this book an exceptional effort. Their encouragement from time to time has been an inspiration for everyone.

The publisher and the editorial board hope that this book will prove to be a valuable piece of knowledge for researchers, students, practitioners and scholars across the globe.

List of Contributors

Bruce R. Levin
Department of Biology, Emory University, Atlanta, GA 30307, USA

Stephen T. Abedon
Department of Microbiology, the Ohio State University, Mansfield, OH 44906, USA

Katarzyna Leskinen and Jenni Horsma-Heikkinen
Department of Bacteriology and Immunology, Medicum, Research Programs Unit, Immunobiology Research Program, University of Helsinki, Helsinki 00290, Finland

Henni Tuomala, Anu Wicklund, Mikael Skurnik and Saija Kiljunen
Department of Bacteriology and Immunology, Medicum, Research Programs Unit, Immunobiology Research Program, University of Helsinki, Helsinki 00290, Finland
Division of Clinical Microbiology, HUSLAB, University of Helsinki and Helsinki University Hospital, Helsinki 00290, Finland

Pentti Kuusela
Division of Clinical Microbiology, HUSLAB, University of Helsinki and Helsinki University Hospital, Helsinki 00290, Finland

Han Lin and Matthew L. Paff
Department of Integrative Biology, University of Texas, Austin, TX 78712, USA

Ian J. Molineux
Institute for Cellular and Molecular Biology, University of Texas, Austin, TX 78712, USA
Department of Molecular Biosciences, University of Texas, Austin, TX 78712, USA
LaMontagne Center for Infectious Disease, University of Texas, Austin, TX 78712, USA

Jacques Goulet
Département des Sciences des Aliments, Faculté des Sciences de L'agriculture et de L'alimentation, Université Laval, Québec, QC G1V OA6, Canada

Shawna McCallin
Department of Musculoskeletal Medicine DAL, Centre Hospitalier Universitaire Vaudois CHUV, Service of Plastic, Reconstructive & Hand Surgery, Regenerative Therapy Unit (UTR), CHUV-EPCR/Croisettes 22, 1066 Epalinges, Switzerland

James J. Bull
Department of Integrative Biology, University of Texas, Austin, TX 78712, USA
Institute for Cellular and Molecular Biology, University of Texas, Austin, TX 78712, USA
Center for Computational Biology and Bioinformatics, University of Texas, Austin, TX 78712, USA
Department of Biological Sciences, University of Idaho, Moscow, ID 83844, USA

Sandra-Maria Wienhold and Jasmin Lienau
Division of Pulmonary Inflammation, Charité–Universitätsmedizin Berlin, Freie Universität Berlin, Humboldt-Universität zu Berlin, and Berlin Institute of Health, 10117 Berlin, Germany

Martin Witzenrath
Division of Pulmonary Inflammation, Charité–Universitätsmedizin Berlin, Freie Universität Berlin, Humboldt-Universität zu Berlin, and Berlin Institute of Health, 10117 Berlin, Germany
Department of Infectious Diseases and Respiratory Medicine, Charité–Universitätsmedizin Berlin, Freie Universität Berlin, Humboldt-Universität zu Berlin, and Berlin Institute of Health, 10117 Berlin, Germany

Brigitte Roy
Département de Biochimie, de Microbiologie et de Bio-Informatique, Faculté des Sciences et de Génie, Université Laval, Québec, QC G1V OA6, Canada
Département des Sciences des Aliments, Faculté des Sciences de L'agriculture et de L'alimentation, Université Laval, Québec, QC G1V OA6, Canada
Félix d'Hérelle Reference Center for Bacterial Viruses and GREB, Faculté de Médecine Dentaire, Université Laval, Québec, QC G1V OA6, Canada

Cécile Philippe and Sylvain Moineau
Département de Biochimie, de Microbiologie et de Bio-Informatique, Faculté des Sciences et de Génie, Université Laval, Québec, QC G1V OA6, Canada
Félix d'Hérelle Reference Center for Bacterial Viruses and GREB, Faculté de Médecine Dentaire, Université Laval, Québec, QC G1V OA6, Canada

Martin J. Loessner
ETH Zurich, Institute of Food, Nutrition and Health, Schmelzbergstrasse, 7CH-8092 Zürich, Switzerland

Dominique Holtappels, Rob Lavigne and Jeroen Wagemans
Laboratory of Gene Technology, KU Leuven, 3001 Heverlee, Belgium

Isabelle Huys
Clinical Pharmacology and Pharmacotherapy, KU Leuven, 3000 Leuven, Belgium
Department of Pharmaceutical and Pharmacological Sciences, KU Leuven, O&N2, Herestraat 49, Box 521, 3000 Leuven, Belgium

David R. Harper
Evolution Biotechnologies, Colworth Science Park, Sharnbrook, Bedfordshire MK44 1LZ, UK

Jean-Paul Pirnay, Gilbert Verbeken and Daniel De Vos, Thomas Rose and Hilde Van Raemdonck
Laboratory for Molecular and Cellular Technology, Queen Astrid Military Hospital, Bruynstraat 1, 1120 Brussel, Belgium

Pieter-Jan Ceyssens
Bacterial Diseases, Unit Antibiotic Resistance, Scientific Institute of Public Health, Rue Engelandstraat 642, 1180 Brussel, Belgium

Alice Maestri
University of Turin, 10124 Turin, Italy

Alan Fauconnier
Federal Agency for Medicines and Health Products, Place Victor Horta 40/40, 1060 Brussels, Belgium
Culture In Vivo ASBL, rue du Progrès, 4, boîte 7, 1400 Nivelles, Belgium

Christine Rohde
Department of Microorganisms, Leibniz Institute DSMZ—German Collection of Microorganisms and Cell Cultures, 38100 Braunschweig, Germany

Grégory Resch
Department of Fundamental Microbiology, University of Lausanne, 1015 Lausanne, Switzerland

Bob G. Blasdel
Laboratory of Gene Technology, Department of Biosystems, 3000 Leuven, Belgium

Laurent Debarbieux
Department of Microbiology, Institut Pasteur, 75015 Paris, France

Daniel Gelman and Ronen Hazan
Faculty of Dental Medicine, The Hebrew University of Jerusalem, Jerusalem 9112001, Israel

Olivier Patey and Alain Dublanchet
Service of Infectious and Tropical Diseases, CHI Lucie et Raymond Aubrac, 94190 Villeneuve Saint Georges, France

Hubert Mazure
HGM Consultants, 63 Rebecca Parade, Winston Hills, NSW 2153, Australia

Andrzej Górski
Bacteriophage Laboratory, Hirszfeld Institute of Immunology and Experimental Therapy, Polish Academy of Sciences, 53-114 Wroclaw, Poland
Department of Clinical Immunology, Transplantation Institute, Medical University of Warsaw, 02-006 Warsaw, Poland

Elene Kakabadze, Khatuna Makalatia and Nina Chanishvili
Eliava Institute of Bacteriophage, Microbiology and Virology, Gotua Street 3, 0160 Tbilisi, Georgia

Małgorzata Łobocka
Institute of Biochemistry and Biophysics, Polish Academy of Sciences, 00-901 Warsaw, Poland
Autonomous Department of Microorganisms' Biology, Faculty of Agriculture and Biology, Warsaw University of Life Sciences—SGGW, 02-787 Warsaw, Poland

Charlotte Ameloot
Federal Agency for Medicines and Health Products, Place Victor Horta 40/40, 1060 Brussels, Belgium

Gabriel Magno de Freitas Almeida
Centre of Excellence in Biological Interactions, Department of Biological and Environmental Science, Nanoscience Center, University of Jyväskylä, Survontie 9C, FI-40014 Jyväskylä, Finland

Danish J. Malik
Chemical Engineering Department, Loughborough University, Leicestershire LE11 3TU, UK

Ivana Mašlaňová and Roman Pantucek
Department of Experimental Biology, Faculty of Science, Masaryk University, 60000 Brno, Czech Republic

Maia Merabishvili
Laboratory for Molecular and Cellular Technology, Queen Astrid Military Hospital, 1120 Brussels, Belgium
Laboratory for Bacteriology Research, Faculty Medicine & Health Sciences, Ghent University, 9000 Ghent, Belgium

Dana Štveráková
Department of Experimental Biology, Faculty of Science, Masaryk University, 60000 Brno, Czech Republic
MB Pharma, 120 00 Prague 2 Vinohrady, Czech Republic

Magali Leroy and Michael S. DuBow
Institute for Integrative Biology of the Cell (I2BC), CEA, CNRS, Université Paris-Sud, Université Paris-Saclay, 91198 Gif-sur-Yvette, France

Frank Oechslin
Department of Fundamental Microbiology (DMF), University of Lausanne, CH-1015 Lausanne, Switzerland

Anthony Smithyman
Cellabs Pty Ltd, and Founder Special Phage Services Pty Ltd, both of 7/27 Dale St, Brookvale, NSW 2100, Australia

Max Liddle
School of Life Sciences, University of Technology, Ultimo, NSW 2007, Australia

Andrei S. Bolocan, Aditya Upadrasta, Pedro H. de Almeida Bettio, Adam G. Clooney, Lorraine A. Draper and Colin Hill
APC Micro biome Ireland, University College Cork, Cork T12 YT20, Ireland
School of Microbiology, University College Cork, Cork T12 YN60, Ireland

Julien Lossouarn, Arnaud Briet, Elisabeth Moncaut, Sylviane Furlan, Astrid Bouteau, Olivier Son, François Lecointe, Pascale Serror and Marie-Agnès Petit
Micalis Institute, INRA, Agro Paris Tech, Université Paris-Saclay, 78350 Jouy-en-Josas, France

R. Paul Ross
APC Micro biome Ireland, University College Cork, Cork T12 YT20, Ireland
School of Microbiology, University College Cork, Cork T12 YN60, Ireland
Teagasc Food Research Centre, Moore park, Fermoy, Cork P61 C996, Ireland

Index

www.ingramcontent.com/pod-product-compliance
Lightning Source LLC
LaVergne TN
LVHW080930210926
848485LV00004B/768
* 9 7 8 1 6 4 6 4 7 5 7 4 2 *

Kaplan Publishing are constantly finding new ways to make a difference to your studies and our exciting online resources really do offer something different to students looking for exam success.

This book comes with free MyKaplan online resources so that you can study anytime, anywhere

Having purchased this book, you have access to the following online study materials:

CONTENT	ACCA (including FFA,FAB,FMA)		AAT		FIA (excluding FFA,FAB,FMA)	
	Text	Kit	Text	Kit	Text	Kit
iPaper version of the book	✓	✓	✓	✓	✓	✓
Interactive electronic version of the book	✓					
Progress tests with instant answers	✓		✓			
Mock assessments online			✓	✓		
Material updates	✓	✓	✓	✓	✓	✓
Latest official ACCA exam questions		✓				
Extra question assistance using the signpost icon*		✓				
Timed questions with an online tutor debrief using the clock icon*		✓				
Interim assessment including questions and answers	✓				✓	
Technical articles	✓	✓			✓	✓

* Excludes F1, F2, F3, FFA, FAB, FMA

How to access your online resources

Kaplan Financial students will already have a MyKaplan account and these extra resources will be available to you online. You do not need to register again, as this process was completed when you enrolled. If you are having problems accessing online materials, please ask your course administrator.

If you are already a registered MyKaplan user go to www.MyKaplan.co.uk and log in. Select the 'add a book' feature and enter the ISBN number of this book and the unique pass key at the bottom of this card. Then click 'finished' or 'add another book'. You may add as many books as you have purchased from this screen.

If you purchased through Kaplan Flexible Learning or via the Kaplan Publishing website you will automatically receive an e-mail invitation to MyKaplan. Please register your details using this email to gain access to your content. If you do not receive the e-mail or book content, please contact Kaplan Flexible Learning.

If you are a new MyKaplan user register at www.MyKaplan.co.uk and click on the link contained in the email we sent you to activate your account. Then select the 'add a book' feature, enter the ISBN number of this book and the unique pass key at the bottom of this card. Then click 'finished' or 'add another book'.

Your Code and Information

This code can only be used once for the registration of one book online. This registration and your online content will expire when the final sittings for the examinations covered by this book have taken place. Please allow one hour from the time you submit your book details for us to process your request.

Please scratch the film to access your MyKaplan code.

Please be aware that this code is case-sensitive and you will need to include the dashes within the passcode, but not when entering the ISBN. For further technical support, please visit www.MyKaplan.co.uk

KAPLAN PUBLISHING